Spiritual Needs in Research and Practice

Arndt Büssing
Editor

Spiritual Needs in Research and Practice

The Spiritual Needs Questionnaire as a Global Resource for Health and Social Care

palgrave
macmillan

Editor
Arndt Büssing
Professorship Quality of Life, Spirituality and Coping, Faculty of Health
Witten/Herdecke University
Herdecke, Germany

IUNCTUS—Competence Center for Christian Spirituality
Philosophical-Theological University of Münster
Münster, Germany

ISBN 978-3-030-70138-3 ISBN 978-3-030-70139-0 (eBook)
https://doi.org/10.1007/978-3-030-70139-0

Cover illustration: Ivan Nesterov / Alamy Stock Photo

This Palgrave Macmillan imprint is published by the registered company Springer Nature Switzerland AG.
The registered company address is: Gewerbestrasse 11, 6330 Cham, Switzerland

Simple things make the difference:
Holding hands
A smile
Some tears
Giving hope
Being there
—Arndt Büssing

Foreword

Systematic research has shown that addressing the spiritual needs of medical and psychiatric patients can improve patient satisfaction and health outcomes. Yet the majority of healthcare professionals still ignores the spiritual needs of their patients, considering them irrelevant to healthcare and not in their area of expertise.

This volume makes a major contribution to clarifying why assessing and addressing spiritual needs are so important and how to do so quickly and efficiently. In addition, this volume addresses a wide range of perspectives on the spiritual needs of patients, from theology to philosophy to medical/psychiatric. Spiritual needs of patients are examined in different settings, countries, religions, and illnesses, and thus will be useful to many different practitioners throughout the world. In addition, the views of physicians, nurses, social workers, volunteers, and chaplains on how to assess and address the spiritual needs of patients are explored, as well as opinions on who should be responsible for doing so. Here are some of my views on how this might work, views that are quite consistent with most of what the authors of this book are presenting.

Every person on the healthcare team has a unique and specific role in identifying and addressing the spiritual needs of patients. Physicians, nurses, and social workers are ideally positioned to early identify patients' spiritual needs through taking a spiritual history, since they will be seeing all patients and will be in charge of taking an initial clinical history (in which the spiritual history should be embedded as part of the social history). The physician should be the person who is responsible for conducting the spiritual history to identify spiritual needs. If the physician fails to do so, then the next person in line is the nurse. However, even if the physician takes a spiritual history, there may be aspects of nursing care that may require that the nurse do one as well, but only after reviewing the information that the physician has collected. Finally, if the physician or nurse both fail to conduct a spiritual history, then the social worker should be next in line. Again, however, there may be specific aspects of the social worker's duties that may require that he or she ask some additional questions to clarify the patient's spiritual needs, particularly when arranging for discharge from the hospital when unmet spiritual needs (that could not be met in the hospital) may need to be addressed in a community setting or at least followed up there. A similar procedure should be followed for medical outpatients, and for patients receiving mental healthcare in various settings.

One might argue why trained pastoral care workers or chaplains shouldn't be those who screen patients for spiritual needs. At least in the United States and also in most European countries, they simply do not have time enough to see everyone. Pastoral care staff is inadequate to meet the great need, so they are often limited only to seeing those who are referred to them.

Except for very simple types of spiritual interventions for addressing immediate spiritual needs (such as praying with a religious patient after being requested by the patient to do so), most spiritual needs should be addressed by the only healthcare professional with the training to do so, i.e., the healthcare chaplain. This is especially true for more complex kinds of spiritual needs, and spiritual needs can become complex very quickly. An example is the patient feeling that their medical or psychiatric illness is a punishment from God or the patient feeling angry at or unloved by God or deserted by their faith community. Such beliefs and feelings require an expert to address them, one who has been extensively trained to do so. The family physician does not do open-heart surgery for someone who needs a coronary artery bypass, but rather refers the person to a surgeon who has been trained to do so. The person in the healthcare system who has the experience and training to address spiritual needs is the healthcare chaplain. That person is equipped to address all but the most simple of spiritual needs. However, in order for the chaplain to address the spiritual needs of patients, other healthcare professionals need to refer the patient to the chaplain. Nurses tend to be the healthcare professional (at least in the United States) who is most likely to refer patients to the chaplain, but it should not only be the nurse or the social worker. Again, the physician is in charge of coordinating the healthcare of the patient, including the addressing of their spiritual needs. The reason is, as I have already noted above, because addressing of spiritual needs affects the mental and physical health of the patient, including the response of the patient's medical condition to treatments that are being prescribed by the physician. In my opinion, if the physician ignores the spiritual needs of patients, then that physician is not practicing the standard of care today, which involves addressing the whole patient and all aspects of their life that can influence their medical condition (psychological, social, and, yes, that includes spiritual influences).

Thus, this volume breaks new ground in providing a comprehensive examination of spiritual needs of patients, whether they are religious or not, needs that are directly related to their medical or mental healthcare. The research that is now showing the powerful effect that religious and spiritual beliefs have on physical and mental health has been ignored for too long. This book is a giant step in mainstreaming the assessment and addressing of spiritual needs into the practice of healthcare across multiple disciplines and multiple religions. Bravo to the many authors who have contributed to this work.

Harold G. Koenig, M.D., M.H.Sc

Professor of Psychiatry &
Behavioral Sciences
Associate Professor of Medicine
Director, Center for Spirituality,
Theology, and Health
Duke University Medical Center,
Durham, NC, USA
Adjunct Professor, Department
of Medicine, King Abdulaziz
University, Jeddah, Saudi Arabia
Adjunct Professor of Public Health,
Ningxia Medical University,
Yinchuan, P.R. China
Visiting Professor, Shiraz University
of Medical Sciences, Shiraz, Iran

Acknowledgment

I am grateful to all contributors, friends, and colleagues from different professions and countries who shared their expertise to make this book possible. This is a wonderful experience of interconnectedness.

I am further grateful to my wife Claudia, my son Oliver, and my daughter Annika for being family and supportive friends. Thanks a lot for being around. May you all be guided and sheltered.

Contents

1 **Introduction** 1
Arndt Büssing

Part I Different Perspectives on Spiritual Needs 7

2 **The Religious Under-Determination of Spiritual Needs from a Theological Perspective and Their Implications for Health and Social Care** 9
Klaus Baumann and Eckhard Frick

3 **Spiritual Care in Health Care: Guideline, Models, Spiritual Assessment and the Use of the ©FICA Spiritual History Tool** 27
Christina Puchalski

4 **Using the Spiritual Needs Questionnaire: A Perspective from the Ethics of Care** 47
Carlo Leget

Part II Assessment of Spiritual Needs 57

5 **Assessing Patients' Spiritual Needs in Healthcare: An Overview of Questionnaires** 59
Ricko Damberg Nissen and Niels Christian Hvidt

6 **Application and Implementation of the Spiritual Needs Questionnaire in Spiritual Care Processes** 79
Arndt Büssing

7 **Structure of the Spiritual Needs Questionnaire in Patients with Chronic Diseases, Elderly and Healthy Persons and Their Association with Quality of Life Indicators** 87
Arndt Büssing

8 **Adapted Spiritual Needs Questionnaire for Adolescents with Chronic Diseases** 103
Arndt Büssing

9 **Structures of Spiritual Needs Questionnaire Versions in Countries with Different Cultural and Religious Backgrounds** 111
Olga Riklikienė, Wilson Correia de Abreu, Tânia Cristina de Oliveira Valente, Maryam Rassouli, Janusz Surzykiewicz, and Arndt Büssing

Part III Findings in Different Populations: Persons with Chronic Diseases 133

10 **Spiritual Needs of Patients with Chronic Pain Diseases** 135
Arndt Büssing and Simon Peng-Keller

11 **Spiritual Needs of Non-terminally Ill Cancer Patients from Lithuania** 147
Olga Riklikienė

12 Spiritual Needs of Cancer Patients in Iran 159
Maryam Rassouli, Azam Shirinabadi Farahani, and Khadijeh Hatamipour

13 Development of Spiritual Needs during Chemotherapy of Breast Cancer Patients 173
Arndt Büssing, Pia Marie Hartmann, Yvonne Beerenbrock, and Daniela Rodrigues Recchia

14 Psychosocial, Existential and Spiritual Needs of Persons with Cystic Fibrosis 183
Jörg Große-Onnebrink and Arndt Büssing

15 Spiritual Needs of HIV-Infected Persons from Brazil 193
Tânia Cristina de Oliveira Valente and Ana Paula Rodrigues Cavalcanti

16 Spiritual Needs in People with Mild to Moderate Dementia 207
Wilson Correia de Abreu, Margarida Abreu, and Arndt Büssing

17 Spiritual Needs in Psychiatry and Psychotherapy 221
Klaus Baumann, Eunmi Lee, and Franz Reiser

18 Spiritual Needs of Tumor Patients During Their Stay at a Palliative Care Unit 239
Arndt Büssing, Klaus Baumann, Jochen Rentschler, and Gerhild Becker

Part IV Findings in Different Populations: Persons with Special Needs in Difficult Situations 249

19 Spiritual Needs of Patients in the Emergency Room 251
Charlotte Wapler, Christoph Dodt, Arndt Büssing, Andreas Beivers, Kristin Härtl, and Eckhard Frick

20 **Spiritual Needs of People with Autism Spectrum Disorder** 265
Jan Christopher Cwik

21 **Spiritual Needs of Persons with Down Syndrome** 281
Arndt Büssing and Janusz Surzykiewicz

22 **Spiritual Needs of Adolescents with Chronic Diseases** 297
Arndt Büssing, Justine Hussong, Jörg Große-Onnebrink, and Alexander von Gontard

23 **Spiritual Needs in Postwar Population Posttrauma Patients in Croatia and Bosnia-Herzegovina** 313
Andrijana Glavas and Klaus Baumann

24 **Spiritual Needs and Life Satisfaction of Refugees in Bavaria** 323
Kathrin Maier and Janusz Surzykiewicz

Part V Findings in Different Populations: Healthy Populations 349

25 **Spiritual Needs of Parents with Health-Affected Children** 351
Arndt Büssing and Olga Riklikienė

26 **Spiritual Needs of Elderly** 369
Arndt Büssing, Renata Spalek, Norbert Gerard Pikuła, Eckhard Frick, and Janusz Surzykiewicz

27 **Spiritual Needs of Patients' Relatives** 397
Arndt Büssing, Charlotte Wapler, Christoph Dodt, Andreas Beivers, Kristin Härtl, and Eckhard Frick

Part VI Relevance of Addressing Spiritual Needs for Clinical Support 407

28 Spiritual Needs, Hopes and Resources: A Chaplain's Mantra 409
Anne Vandenhoeck

29 Relevance of Addressing Spiritual Needs for Clinical Support: Nursing Perspective 419
Linda Ross and Wilfred McSherry

30 Addressing Spiritual Needs in Faith Community Nursing 437
Helen A. Wordsworth

31 Physician's Perspectives on Addressing Patients' Spiritual Needs 447
Lubna Hammoudeh and Tracy Balboni

32 Relevance of Addressing Spiritual Needs for Clinical Support in Palliative Medicine 457
Stephan M. Probst

33 Addressing Spiritual Needs and Spiritual Care from a Volunteers' Perspective 467
Torsten Ernst

34 Concluding Suggestions 473
Arndt Büssing and Harold G. Koenig

Appendix: Questionnaires 477

Index 481

Notes on Contributors

Margarida Abreu is an associate Professor at the Porto School of Nursing and senior researcher at CINTESIS (University of Porto). She teaches community health, elderly care, and occupational health. Her main areas of research include community health interventions, sexual health, and caregivers support at home.

Wilson Correia de Abreu is a full Professor at the Porto School of Nursing and senior researcher at CINTESIS (University of Porto). He teaches mental health of the elderly, anthropology of health, and ethnopsychiatry. His main areas of research include dementia, palliative care, end-of-life care, and spirituality and HIV/AIDS.

Tracy Balboni is a medical doctor and Professor of Radiation Oncology and Clinical Director of the Dana-Farber/Brigham and Women's Cancer Center Supportive and Palliative Radiation Oncology Service. Her primary research interests include advancing quality-of-life outcomes after palliative radiation therapy for symptomatic metastases and the role of psychosocial and spiritual factors in the quality of life and care decision-making of cancer patients.

Klaus Baumann is a Catholic diocesan priest and Professor at the Faculty of Theology at Freiburg University, Germany. His field of research and teaching is Caritas Science and Christian Social Work. He is a trained psychologist and psychotherapist in private clinical practice, in addition to continuous pastoral ministry in parishes and jails, and serving on various scientific and advisory boards. He is Editor-in-Chief of the journal *Religions*.

Gerhild Becker is Professor at the Medical Faculty of University of Freiburg, a physician and theologian, and the Chair and Medical Director of the Clinic for Palliative Care at the University Hospital of Freiburg in Germany. She is board certified in Internal Medicine and Palliative Medicine and, further, is ordained as volunteer Pastor in the Protestant Regional Church, Baden.

Yvonne Beerenbrock is a research assistant at the Witten/Herdecke University, Germany. She is a health educator (2nd state examination in biology and health), health economist (MA, University of Kaiserslautern), molecular biologist (BSc, University of Applied Sciences CUNY—Central University of New York), nurse for intensive medicine and anaesthesia, and yoga teacher.

Andreas Beivers is Professor of Economics and Dean of Studies for Health Economics at the Hochschule Fresenius, Munich. Since 2017, he is associate scientist in the competence area of "Health" at the Leibniz Institute for Economic Research in Essen and since 2015, member of the Academic Board of the University of Salzburg Business School, and lecturer at the Technical University of Munich.

Arndt Büssing is a medical doctor and Professor for Quality of Life, Spirituality, and Coping at the Witten/Herdecke University and has been associated as a research professor at IUNCTUS—Competence Center for Christian Spirituality at the Philosophical-Theological University of Münster since 2016. He is coeditor of the *German Journal for Oncology*, on the editorial board of the journal *Spiritual Care*, and Editor-in-Chief of the journal *Religions*.

Ana Paula Rodrigues Cavalcanti is a nutritionist and social psychologist. She is a full Professor at Religious Sciences Department of Paraíba Federal State University. She teaches spirituality and health, sacred foods, and subjects on religious studies. Her main area of research is spirituality and health and Anthropology of Health.

Jan Christopher Cwik is a psychologist and research associate at the Chair of Clinical Psychology and Psychotherapy at the University of Cologne. He is also a licensed psychotherapist and supervisor with a focus on behavioral therapy. His research focuses primarily on clinical-psychological diagnostics, psycho-oncology, traumatic disorders, and psychophysiology.

Christoph Dodt is head of the Emergency Department of the Munich Clinic Bogenhausen, vice president of the European Society of Emergency Medicine (EUSEM), and past president of the German Federation for Emergency Medicine (DGINA). His research interests focus on Emergency Care and Intensive Care for emergency patients. He is member of the editorial board of the journals *Notfall und Rettungsmedizin* and *Medizinische Klinik—Intensivmedizin und Notfallmedizin*.

Torsten Ernst is a theologian of the Protestant Church of Anhalt and works as head of the Anhaltische Diakonissenanstalt Dessau. In this role he is also in the management of the Anhalt Hospice and Palliative Society and the Deaconess Hospital Dessau. For many years he was chairman of the Thuringian Hospice and Palliative Association and on the board of the German Hospice and Palliative Association.

Eckhard Frick is a medical doctor and Roman Catholic priest, psychiatrist, and Jungian psychoanalyst. As a Professor he teaches anthropology and spiritual care at Munich School of Philosophy and University Hospital, Technical University of Munich. He is coeditor of the journal *Spiritual Care* and the collection *Studies in Spiritual Care*.

Andrijana Glavas is a medical doctor and qualified Caritas scientist. Since 2011, she has been working as a research assistant at the University of Freiburg and is a doctoral candidate at the working group "Caritas Science and Christian Social work." Before she came to Germany, Glavas worked for several years as a general practitioner in Croatia.

Jörg Große-Onnebrink is a medical doctor and pediatrician, and head of the Pediatric Respiratory Unit of the University Children's Hospital in Münster, Germany, whose main areas of research include lung diseases, especially cystic fibrosis and primary ciliary dyskinesia, palliative care, quality of life, and spirituality.

Lubna Hammoudeh is a medical doctor from Mu'tah University, Jordan. After receiving her medical degree she worked in radiation oncology at King Hussein Cancer Centre, and is currently a fellow at the Dana-Farber/Brigham and Women's Hospital (DFCI/BWH). Her research interests are optimizing care in the setting of CNS tumors and palliative oncology care).

Kristin Härtl is Professor of Clinical Psychology at Hochschule Fresenius, University of Applied Sciences, Psychology School. She works in the fields of clinical psychology and psycho-oncology. Her research topics are quality of life, fear of recurrence and distress of women with breast cancer, physical activity during therapy for cancer, and psychosomatic disorders in gynecology and obstetrics.

Pia Marie Hartmann is a family physician and is writing a dissertation on spiritual needs of women diagnosed with breast cancer. Prior to that she spent her residency in obstetrics and gynecology as well as in internal medicine and has worked in different countries on humanitarian projects.

Khadijeh Hatamipour is an assistant Professor in Nursing at the Department of Nursing, Tonekabon Branch, Islamic Azad University, Tonekabon, Iran, Her main research field is health-related issues in spirituality. She has published about 30 peer-reviewed articles in various fields of nursing.

Justine Hussong is a psychologist, and a child and adolescent psychotherapist from the Department of Child and Adolescent Psychiatry, Saarland University Hospital, Homburg, Germany. Besides clinical psychotherapeutic work, she focuses her research on psychiatric disorders in children and adolescents, incontinence, genetic syndromes, and intellectual disability.

Niels Christian Hvidt is a theologian and Professor of Spiritual Care at the University of Southern Denmark. Born in 1969, he defended his doctorate at the Gregorian in Rome in 2001, published with Oxford University Press in 2007 titled *Christian Prophecy.* He was a fellow in Rome and Chicago until 2006 and has been employed at the University of Southern Denmark since 2017 as Professor; he was also a fellow at the Freiburg Institute for Advanced Studies from 2012 to 2014 and Professor at the Ludwig Maximilian University Munich, 2013–2014. He is author of several books on the interplay of spirituality and health.

Harold G. Koenig is a medical doctor and a board-certified general psychiatrist, and formerly boarded-certified in family medicine, geriatric medicine, and geriatric psychiatry. He is Professor of Psychiatry and associate Professor of Medicine at the Duke University Medical Center, Durham, NC. He is an adjunct Professor in the Department of Medicine at King Abdulaziz University, Jeddah, Saudi Arabia, and in the School of Public Health at Ningxia Medical University, Yinchuan, China. He has published more than 50 books.

Eunmi Lee is a theologian and a research co-operator of the Department of Caritas Science and Christian Social Work at the Albert-Ludwigs University in Freiburg. Since 2018, she is also active as a research Professor in the Center for Social Cohesion, Daegu Catholic University of Korea.

Carlo Leget is full Professor of Care Ethics at the University of Humanistic Studies in Utrecht, the Netherlands, where he also holds an endowed Chair in Palliative Care, established by the Netherlands Comprehensive Cancer Organisation (IKNL) and the Association Hospice Care Netherlands (AHZN). He is a member of the Health Council of the Netherlands, was vice president of the European Association for Palliative Care from 2012 to 2019.

Kathrin Maier is a psychologist, pedagogist, and Professor in Educational Psychology in Social Work at the Catholic University of Applied Sciences Munich. Her research and teaching focuses on social-emotional learning of children and youth from disadvantaged backgrounds as well as on the field of healthcare with a special focus on well-being, mental health and spirituality.

Wilfred McSherry is a nursing Professor jointly appointed between Department of Nursing, School of Health and Social Care, Staffordshire University and the University Hospitals of North Midlands NHS Trust United Kingdom. He is also parttime Professor at VID University College, Bergen, Norway. He has published extensively with several books and many articles addressing different aspects of the spiritual dimension. He is a founding and executive member of the British Association for The Study of Spirituality (BASS) and a Principal Fellow of The Higher Education Academy and Fellow of the Royal College of Nursing.

Ricko Damberg Nissen is an anthropologist holding an M.A. in Anthropology and Religious Studies from the University of Aarhus, Denmark, and has defended his PhD in psychiatry and religion. He is currently employed as postdoc at the University of Southern Denmark with research on spiritual care.

Simon Peng-Keller is a theologian and Professor of Spiritual Care at the University of Zürich. His primary research focus is on healthcare chaplaincy and interprofessional spiritual care at the end of life and in the context of severe chronic disease. With Springer Nature he has published a volume entitled *Charting Spiritual Care—The Emerging Role of Chaplaincy Records in Global Healthcare.*

Norbert Gerard Pikuła is Professor of Pedagogy and Social Work at the Pedagogical University of Krakow, Department of Social Sciences, Krakow, Poland, and doctor honoris causa at the Tiraspol State University of Moldova. As Director of the Institute of Social Affairs, a scholarship holder of the Canadian Government, he did research internships at the Universities of Toronto and Ottawa. His main research interests are in pedagogy, gerontology, and social policy, particularly the perception of the meaning of life among older adults, their quality of life, the labor market, and the state policy toward seniors.

Stephan M. Probst is a medical doctor and Senior Physician in Charge in the Department of Hematology, Oncology, and Palliative Medicine of the Clinicum Bielefeld, Germany, head of the Palliative Care Unit and chairman of the clinical ethics committee, and member of the central ethics committee of the German Medical Association. He is a specialist in internal medicine, hematology, oncology, emergency medicine, and palliative medicine, and an expert in Jewish medical ethics and author of several books on dying, death, and mourning from the Jewish perspective.

Christina Puchalski is Professor of Medicine and Health Sciences and Founder and Executive Director of The George Washington University's Institute for Spirituality and Health (GWish). She is board certified in Palliative Care and Internal Medicine, directs an interdisciplinary outpatient supportive and palliative clinic and is a medical hospice director in Washington, DC. She is widely published in academic journals and has authored numerous book chapters and published the book *Time for Listening and Caring: Spirituality and the Care of the Seriously Ill and Dying*.

Maryam Rassouli is a professor of nursing at Cancer Research Center, Shahid Beheshti University of Medical Sciences, Tehran, Iran. Her main research fields are scale development, palliative care, and spirituality in the context of cancer. She has published more than 150 peer-reviewed articles in these fields. She is associate editor of the *International Journal of Cancer Management*.

Franz Reiser is a Catholic priest and psychotherapist, and also a postdoc researcher in cooperation with the department of Caritas Science and Christian Social Work at the Theological Faculty of the Albert-Ludwigs University, Freiburg. He has written his doctoral thesis on spiritual needs of patients with psychiatric diagnoses.

Jochen Rentschler is a medical doctor working as Leading Senior Physician in the Department of Hematology, Oncology, and Palliative Medicine at Ortenau-Klinikum Offenburg, Germany. He is board certified in Internal Medicine, Hematology/Medical Oncology and Palliative Medicine and responsible for the Palliative Care Unit in Offenburg as well as for the Specialized Outpatient Palliative Care Team.

Olga Riklikienė is a nurse and Professor from the Faculty of Nursing, Lithuanian University of Health Sciences, Lithuania. Her main duties are teaching research methodology, quality of nursing care, nursing management and clinical mentorship. In the field of scientific investigations she focuses on spiritual well-being and spiritual care of different groups of patients, women's mental health and birth-related trauma, missed nursing care, and clinical training of student nurses.

Daniela Rodrigues Recchia is a researcher at the Chair of Research Methods and Statistics in Psychology at the Witten/Herdecke University and a statistician at the German Center for Neurodegenerative Diseases (DZNE) in Witten, Germany. She has academic background in statistics with PhD in theoretical medicine. Her interests lie in the fields of psychometrics, structural equation modeling, moderation and mediation modeling.

Linda Ross is a Professor of Nursing at the School of Care Sciences, Faculty of Life Sciences and Education, University of South Wales, Pontypridd, UK. She has been researching and publishing on spirituality and nursing for 30 years, focusing particularly on nursing practice and education. She is a founding member and Membership Secretary for the British Association for the Study of Spirituality and an executive editor for its affiliated journal. She co-led an Erasmus-funded 3 year project to establish best practice in spiritual care nurse education across Europe (www.epicc-project.eu).

Azam Shirinabadi Farahani is an assistant Professor in Nursing at School of Nursing and Midwifery, Shahid Beheshti University of Medical Sciences, Tehran, Iran. She is working on spirituality as well as palliative care as her research fields. She has published many books and articles about the above-mentioned subjects.

Renata Spalek is the director and Professor for the BSc Occupational Therapy program at the University Cattolica del Sacro Cuore, Rome, and the clinical and administrative lead of the Occupational Therapy department in the rehabilitation centre "Mons L. Novarese", in Moncrivello, Italy. She has worked and promoted the role of the occupational therapist in geriatric rehabilitation setting underlying the interconnection and reciprocal influence between spirituality and elder people.

Janusz Surzykiewicz is a social scientist and theologian and a Professor at the Catholic University of Eichstätt-Ingolstadt, and the Cardinal Stefan Wyszynski University, Warsaw, Poland. His main research areas focus on resource-oriented health and social behavior issues. He combines educational and psychological aspects to analyze current questions regarding the role of spirituality and well-being as well as social inequality and social change. As a specialist and coach of the international coaching associations ICI and EASC he is engaged in counseling and pastoral care.

Tânia Cristina de Oliveira Valente is a psychiatrist. She is full associate Professor at the Medical and Surgical School, and Chief of Laboratory of Medical Anthropologic Interdisciplinary Studies and Research of the Public Health Department of Rio de Janeiro Federal State University. She teaches Medical Psychology, Anthropology of Health, and Science Studies. Her main areas of research include science studies, ethnopsychiatry, quality of health, and anthropology of health.

Anne Vandenhoeck is a Professor of Pastoral Care and Diaconia at the Faculty of Theology and Religious Studies, KU Leuven, Belgium, and has worked as a chaplain in several hospitals. She teaches spiritual care to students in medical faculties. She is the Chair of the Academic Centre for Practical Theology and the director of the European Research Institute for Chaplains in HealthCare.

Alexander von Gontard is a pediatrician, as well as a child and adolescent psychiatrist and psychotherapist. He was Chair and Director at Saarland University Hospital, Germany, and continues to be affiliated with Saarland University and works now in his own practice. He has published widely on various topics of child and adolescent mental health, including spirituality.

Charlotte Wapler is a medical student at the Ludwig Maximilian University, Munich, and is writing her doctoral thesis at the Chair for Psychosomatic Medicine and Psychotherapy at the Technical University of Munich on spiritual needs of patients in the emergency room.

Helen A. Wordsworth is a Baptist minister who has combined her nursing career with her interest in Christian spiritual care to found the charitable organization Parish Nursing Ministries UK. It encourages churches and Christian organizations to take an active role in whole-person health promotion and support by appointing a specially trained nurse to their ministry team. She is the International Parish Nurse Specialist for the Westberg Institute for Faith Community Nursing.

List of Figures

Fig. 6.1	Schematic representation of spiritual needs categories and related topics	81
Fig. 6.2	Schematic representation of implementation processes and their different phases	83
Fig. 7.1	Mean values of spiritual needs in the sample	93
Fig. 10.1	Principles of the concept of total pain according to Cicely Saunders (1993) with its four basic, interacting components. Here, pain is understood multidimensionally and not restricted as a bodily experience only	136
Fig. 10.2	Spiritual needs of patients with chronic pain conditions who reported on their age	140
Fig. 16.1	Spiritual needs in people with mild (level 1) or moderate (level 2) dementia	212
Fig. 18.1	Spiritual needs of patients at the start and end of their PCU stay	242
Fig. 21.1	Comparison of relational needs in persons with DS from Poland and Germany	287
Fig. 22.1	Expression of spiritual needs in adolescents depending on treatement condition and gender	302
Fig. 24.1	Visualization of the conditional effects in the moderator model. The black vertical lines indicate the low (two standard deviations below the mean) and high levels of spiritual needs (two standard deviations above the mean), which were used to calculate the conditional effects of home countries on life satisfaction.	334

Fig. 25.1 Comparison of spiritual needs among the three samples of mothers from Germany (GER) and Lithuania (LITH) 354
Fig. 26.1 Spiritual needs in the elderly (n=345) from different regions in Germany 375
Fig. 26.2 Spiritual needs in the elderly from Germany (n = 345), Poland (n = 292) and Italy (n = 164) 380
Fig. 26.3 Spiritual needs in the elderly from Germany, Poland and Italy (n = 766) differentiated for their self-care abilities 384

List of Tables

Table 3.1	Spiritual distress or concerns	31
Table 3.2	FICA spiritual history tool©	36
Table 5.1	List of questionnaires that aim to address spiritual needs, spiritual well-being, spiritual distress, and so on (alphabetically listed)	63
Table 5.2	Implementation of instruments in different countries	71
Table 7.1	Factor loading and mean values of items	89
Table 8.1	Exploratory factor and reliability analyses	106
Table 9.1	The structure of SpNQ when adapting it for different cultural and religious backgrounds and in various samples	114
Table 11.1	Spiritual needs of non-terminally ill cancer patients in relation to their importance (very strong or strong need) and gender and religiosity	150
Table 12.1	A comparison of the SpNQ with the "Spiritual Needs Assessment Scale of Patients with Cancer" (SNAS)	165
Table 13.1	Quality-of- life indicators and spiritual needs within the course of treatment	176
Table 14.1	Spiritual needs scores in the sample	187
Table 15.1	SpNQ domains and items responses among PLWHA from Rio de Janeiro and João Pessoa samples of PLWHA	198
Table 15.2	SpNQ Scores among Brazillian Rio de Janeiro and João Pessoa samples of PLWHA	200
Table 16.1	Correlations (*r*) between the subscales of the Portuguese version of the SpNQ	213
Table 17.1	Spiritual needs of 248 patients from clinical survey at University Hospital, Department of Psychiatry and Psychotherapy, Freiburg, Germany	224

Table 19.1	Expression of spiritual needs in patients in the emergency room	255
Table 20.1	Range, means, and standard deviations of measures in adult people with ASD	271
Table 20.2	Correlations between spiritual needs, frequency of spiritual practices, and indicators of quality of life	273
Table 22.1	Correlations analyses in female and male adolescents	305
Table 23.1	Frequency and Strength of spiritual needs	316
Table 23.2	Strength of spiritual needs in subgroups	317
Table 24.1	Means, standard deviations, standard errors, and correlations between life satisfaction and spiritual needs	331
Table 24.2	Hierarchical linear regression analysis of the proposed mediator model for spiritual needs	333
Table 27.1	Expression of spiritual needs in relatives and patients	401
Table 30.1	Nursing action plan based on the Spiritual Needs Questionnaire	443
Table 31.1	National Consensus Project for Quality Palliative Care spiritual, religious, and existential aspects of care components and the corresponding role of physicians	449
Table 31.2	Top ten spiritual care barriers perceived by physicians and adjusted odds ratios estimating barriers' associations with actual spiritual care provision	451

CHAPTER 1

Introduction

Arndt Büssing

Background

During the last decades there has been a significant increase in the number of studies that underline the relevance of a person's spirituality as a strategy to cope with difficult life situations, as a general resource of hope, hold and orientation in life, and, depending on the religious background and worldview, as a source to connect with that which is Sacred, with others and with creation (nature/environment).

However, spirituality is a complex and multilayered construct. And because of its complexity, its definitions and also the measures involved are heterogeneous and diverse (ranging from inclusive to exclusive definitions and approaches, and from unidimensional to multidimensional constructs) (Büssing 2019). The different layers of spirituality could be exemplified as *Faith/Experience* as the core, related *Attitudes* and subsequent *Behaviors.* With respect to the core aspect, a person may have specific own

A. Büssing (✉)
Professorship Quality of Life, Spirituality and Coping, Faculty of Health, Witten/Herdecke University, Herdecke, Germany

IUNCTUS—Competence Center for Christian Spirituality, Philosophical-Theological University of Münster, Münster, Germany
e-mail: Arndt.buessing@uni-wh.de

A. Büssing (ed.), *Spiritual Needs in Research and Practice*,
https://doi.org/10.1007/978-3-030-70139-0_1

experiences with that which is Sacred or might have to follow the belief concepts of a religious tradition. Both the own experience which has to be integrated into a person's life concept and the adopted belief concepts of specific religions may shape peoples' *Faith*, which in turn could influence their *Attitudes*, "their (cognitive) beliefs, their (emotional) hopes and also their trust in a transcendent source" (Büssing 2019). The aforementioned layers will further influence their *Behaviors*, "the related ethics, social and health behaviors, and the use of distinct rituals (i.e., prayer, meditation)" (Büssing 2019). The experiential core aspect of spirituality is difficult to access (best in narratives), while the secondary indicators (i.e., religious trust, belief in a helping God, feelings of awe, compassion, altruism and charity, prayer and meditation) can be more easily assessed and measured with standardized instruments. Several of these indicators are not exclusive for religious persons but can be found also in nonreligious persons. These indicators *are* not 'spirituality' but they may be related to its distinct aspects and layers.

To assess a person's spirituality, one has to thus assume a complex set of 'indicators' which may all have differential meanings in one's life. These are shaped by a person's religious socialization, cultural influences, certain life experiences, personality factors and so on. In-depth biographic interviews may elucidate that a person's spirituality is not a fixed state, but a continuous development process (with phases of standstill, growth and decline). During the different phases of one's life (the biography), certain aspects may change their relevance—and the centrality of specific beliefs and practices may also change. Some may have lost their faith, others may experience phases of religious struggles and spiritual dryness, and some may reach states of 'enlightenment' or closeness with the Sacred.

While it is true that certain aspects of spirituality are related to positive health behaviors and lower risk factors, and more effective coping strategies and higher well-being, it is nevertheless problematic to recommend becoming 'more' spiritual in order to improve health and revert illness, or to assume that 'being' spiritual protects against the unpredictability of life. Generally, spirituality cannot be prescribed and used as a remedy, while for some spirituality-based treatments it can nevertheless be appropriate and beneficial. As most of us live in rather pluralistic societies with different worldviews, religious beliefs, social standards and ethical values, it is difficult to establish concepts that are ubiquitously valid. Spiritual issues and concerns might be important for several persons, but not for all. Some would see themselves as neither religious nor spiritual, while others are either religious or spiritual, or both. However, even the putatively nonreligious/non-spiritual individuals may be interested in distinct 'spiritual' issues, but these are mostly not related to specific religious doctrines and faith traditions. They might be too rapidly labeled as 'nonreligious' and thus disregarded.

Therefore, it might be more appropriate to ask people what they need instead of providing what they might not want. The latter attitude refers to a paternalistic approach (which is often found in health-care professionals and religious leaders), while the former refers to a person-centered attitude of respect and humbleness. One attitude means "You should follow my recommendations!", and the other, "How may I help you?". In 1970, Zen master Shunryu Suzuki recommended a "beginner's mind" instead of an expert mind (Suzuki 2006). One mind is open to face the world as it is and listens, while the other already knows and gives answers because of the acquired expertise. "In the beginner's mind there are many possibilities, but in the expert's there are few" (Suzuki 2006). This means, when we listen to what people need and then ask how we may help and support them, we show interest in their specific concerns and value them as individuals with their own biography, hopes and expectations, as well as fears and worries, and try to find ways to care compassionately. This rather open and contemplative view "allows us to discover in each thing a teaching which God wishes to hand on to us, since 'for the believer, to contemplate creation is to hear a message, to listen to a paradoxical and silent voice'", said Pope Francis citing Pope John Paul II (Francis 2015, Chapter 85). Mindfully listening to the "silent voices" of others thus approves their dignity and respects their value and purpose (even if they cannot see these by themselves), and is also a spiritual act of humility and compassion that may enrich and transform the life of both the caregiver who receives and the receiver who gives, too. This underlines the interconnectedness within the field of spiritual care.

This book focuses on the assessment of a person's spiritual needs using the *Spiritual Needs Questionnaire* (SpNQ), an established and internationally used standardized questionnaire. Experts from different professions and cultures discuss the theoretical background of spiritual needs (from philosophical, anthropological, theological, ethical and health care perspectives), describe the tool's application in different groups of persons from varying cultural and religious backgrounds and with different health conditions (those with chronic diseases or special needs, and healthy persons, whether they are adolescents, adults or elderly) and subsequent consequences of treatment and support. This book thereby differs from other important approaches like George Fitchett's 2002 book *Assessing Spiritual Needs*, which is intended primarily for pastoral caregivers, or Rachel Stanworth's 2003 book *Recognizing Spiritual Needs in People Who Are Dying*, which focuses on interviews with dying people in palliative care, or Judith Allen Shelly's 1984 book *Spiritual Needs of Children*, which deals only with children.

Using a standardized tool to assess a person's spiritual needs does not replace communication; it provides a reason to start talking about what is stated as important and unmet. Further, it can be a useful tool for documentation as the intensity of unmet needs is recorded and can be used for better planning of specific support and treatment. It also encourages research to compare the spiritual needs of persons from different cultural, religious and health groups, and thus to find specific interventions and culture-sensitive support. It facilitates learning processes to be more aware of the uniqueness of the person in question. This would further underline the relevance of this topic for a more comprehensive health-care system, which too often ignores addressing a person's spirituality because of 'professional neutrality' and lack of time, expertise or even interest (Curlin et al. 2006; Lee & Baumann 2013), thereby ignoring patients' fundamental concerns and dignity (Koslander et al. 2009). Assessing patients' spiritual needs thereby encourages health-care professionals, psychologists, social workers, pastoral workers, volunteers and relatives to start communication about an oft-neglected and avoided topic, namely persons' spiritual needs, and how these can be best supported.

References

Büssing A (2019) Measuring spirituality and religiosity in health research. In: Lucchetti G, Prieto P, Mario F, Damiano RF (eds) Spirituality, religiousness and health. From research to clinical practice. Springer, Cham, Chapter 2, pp 11–31

Curlin FA, Chin MH, Sellergren SA, Roach CJ, Lantos JD (2006) The association of physicians' religious characteristics with their attitudes and self-reported behaviors regarding religion and spirituality in the clinical encounter. Med Care 44(5):446–453

Fitchett G (2002) Assessing spiritual needs. A guide for caregivers. Academic Renewal Press, Lima, OH

Koslander T, da Silva AB, Roxberg A (2009) Existential and spiritual needs in mental health care: an ethical and holistic perspective. J Holist Nurs 27:34–42. https://doi.org/10.1177/0898010108323302

Lee E, Baumann K (2013) German psychiatrists' observation and interpretation of religiosity/spirituality. Evidence-based complementary and alternative medicine, Article ID 280168. https://doi.org/10.1155/2013/280168

Pope Francis (2015) Encyclical letter *Laudato si'* of the Holy Father Francis on care for our common home. Libreria Editrice Vaticana, Vatican City. http://www.vatican.va/content/francesco/en/encyclicals/documents/papa-francesco_20150524_enciclica-laudato-si.html. Accesses 21 Aug 2020

Shelly JA (1984) Spiritual needs of children. Scripture Union Publishing, Milton Keynes

Stanworth R (2003) Recognizing spiritual needs in people who are dying. Oxford University Press, Oxford

Suzuki S (2006) Zen Mind, Beginner's Mind. Shambhala, Boulder

PART I

Different Perspectives on Spiritual Needs

CHAPTER 2

The Religious Under-Determination of Spiritual Needs from a Theological Perspective and Their Implications for Health and Social Care

Klaus Baumann and Eckhard Frick

Introduction

Spiritual needs are included in the 2002 WHO definition of palliative care. Palliative care, according to this definition, should also take care of the spiritual needs and issues of patients facing terminal illness and death, of their relatives, and of staff. Before this acknowledgment by the WHO,

K. Baumann (✉)
Caritas Science and Christian Social Work, Faculty of Theology, Alberts Ludwig-University, Freiburg, Germany
e-mail: klaus.baumann@theol.uni-freiburg.de

E. Frick
Research Unit Spiritual Care, Clinic and Policlinic for Psychosomatic Medicine and Psychotherapy, Klinikum rechts der Isar, Technical University of Munich, Munich, Germany
e-mail: eckhard.frick@tum.de

A. Büssing (ed.), *Spiritual Needs in Research and Practice*,
https://doi.org/10.1007/978-3-030-70139-0_2

Cicely Saunders had successfully introduced heeding the spiritual dimension in the concept of 'total pain', embracing all pain dimensions including physical, psychic, social, and spiritual aspects. The World Health Organization's questionnaire on Quality of Life (WHOQOL) was extended to include issues on spiritual, religious, and personal beliefs as relevant aspects which impact the quality of any human life (WHOQOL-SRPB), especially as far as they give meaning and a sense of coherence (Antonovsky 1987) to individuals' lives. In the meantime, there is plenty of research on correlations and causalities between religious and spiritual practices on the one hand, and health and disease, mortality and quality of life, prevention and healing, or coping with disease and with critical life events on the other hand, many of which will also be reported and reflected on in this volume.

This chapter intends to offer a few concepts and reflections on spiritual needs from a theological perspective by two authors who are themselves Catholic theologians and priests as well as researchers and practicing depth-psychological psychotherapists; the second author is also a physician and psychiatrist. This predominantly interdisciplinary theological perspective will reflect on the reality and implications of spiritual needs in the context of health and disease and of social care.

The Anthropological Concept of (Spiritual) Needs

The concept of 'spiritual needs' can be considered a part of the underlying anthropological assumptions which are frequently presupposed more than reflected or openly displayed in the context of secular health care and social care. The WHO remains at a descriptive (empirical) level with regard to spiritual needs as well as spiritual, religious, and personal beliefs.

Obviously, there is a vast range of needs of the human body and mind which we may coin "spiritual needs" of the human person. A need indicates that something whatsoever is missing. A felt need indicates an awareness of the individual that something is missing even if it cannot be exactly defined. A felt need in this sense can also be called a wish, a want, or a lack of something. This implies that there are innumerous wishes and needs. Without pretending an exhaustive taxonomy, such needs can be physical, emotional, cognitive, psychosocial, behavioral—and spiritual. In a less differentiated manner, they could also be summarized as bodily and mental needs of the human person. Physical, emotional, cognitive, psychosocial, and behavioral needs can always resonate as 'spiritual' in the human mind, and vice versa: spiritual needs can resonate or express themselves physically, emotionally, cognitively, psychosocially, and behaviorally. This interdependence might best be captured in the concepts of symbols and of the human being as a symbolizer of the inseparable union of body and soul, matter and spirit, who connects and interweaves all of these dimensions with personal and intersubjective 'meaning', importance, or 'value'. Spiritual needs, then, are and remain ubiquitous in human realities, as well as in secularized cultures.

Spiritual needs therefore imply that there is a lack which may be felt (more or less strongly) and which makes the individual search for cognitive, emotional, psychosocial, and behavioral meaning and its realization in his or her life, relationships, and vicissitudes. Becoming aware of an undefined, vague need or of a palpable lack is feeling a wish and can become the starting point of a new thinking process, of a new search and exploration, cognition, reflection, and self-awareness. In other words, felt needs motivate further behavior: Psychoanalysis even hypothesizes that the felt lack of milk, which disrupts the blissful feeling of complete satisfaction and safety of the baby, is the stimulus for the first thought of the human being awaking to conscious life (Loch 1984):

> *I shall limit the term 'thought' to the mating of a pre-conception with a frustration. The model I propose is that of an infant whose expectation of a breast is mated with a realization of no breast available for satisfaction. This mating is experienced as a no-breast, or 'absent' breast inside. The next step depends on the infant's capacity for frustration: in particular it depends on whether the decision is to evade frustration or to modify it. If the capacity for toleration of frustration is sufficient the 'no-breast' inside becomes a thought, and an apparatus for 'thinking it' develops.* (Bion 1962/2003: 306)

This hypothesis, in consequence, already indicates and implies the role of biography which is more or less happily formed by the personal history of the fate of one's multiple and multifaceted bodily and mental needs, including spiritual needs, especially as experienced and marked in relationship with significant others. It also indicates the biographical starting point of the continuous experience expressed by the author and poet Ingeborg Bachmann (1926–1973): "In everything there is too little" (Bachmann 1978, 68)—In everything and all, something is missing.

This leads to an important distinction of terms following two French authors, the psychoanalyst Jacques Lacan and the philosopher Emmanuel

Levinas (Frick and Baumann 2017): needs and wishes in general versus spiritual needs and desires in particular ("besoin vs désir"). For Lacan, a need and a wish (as "besoin") are directed to a "real" (biological) object, while "desire" (as "désir") is connected to phantasy and directed to the imagined other (as object) by which the subject desires to be regarded unconditionally. For Levinas, a need and wish (as "besoin") can be stilled by their satisfaction, while desire ("désir") is directed to the other; its satisfaction creates new hunger and can never be stilled; it always goes beyond and implies the "idea of infinity" as the relationship between self and other (Levinas 1963/1986; cf. 1983).

Ingeborg Bachmann likewise indicates a ubiquitous felt (spiritual) need and a kind of ubiquitous longing (desire) which cannot be satisfied by "anything". And with her, Abraham Maslow's idea (1954) to confine spirituality to peak experiences, considered possible only after the satisfaction of the other needs of his needs pyramid, would be contradicted in principle. Three philosophically anthropological approaches of the twentieth century can exemplify spiritual needs as "anthropological givens" (Pleger 2018). They focus the realities of human deficits and compensation (Arnold Gehlen), of the specifically human eccentric position (Helmuth Plessner), and of feeling values by the human spirit in its openness for the world (Max Scheler).

The German anthropologist Arnold Gehlen (1904–1976), in a philosophical tradition dating back to Platon and to German romanticists (e.g. Herder, eighteenth and nineteenth centuries), defined the human being as a being that continuously feels lacks as it is not fixed by instincts. By the experience of these lackings, the human being actively experiences, explores, and transforms the world from a "natural" to a "cultural" one which compensates for the experienced shortcomings and which better fits with the manifold human needs. Culture, hence, is a product of the compensation for the needs and deficits, experienced by the open human mind in a world which is not instinctually determined. Rather, living in this world calls for decisions and actions by human beings in order to satisfy the felt needs and wants. This indicates the basic reality of needs for orientation in the world in combination with freedom and values, especially in connection with the psychosocial needs and vital challenges in contact with fellow humans and the environment.

Helmuth Plessner (1892–1985) phenomenologically defined a double aspectivity of being a lived body (Leib) and having a physical body (Körper). Humans are not only centered in their body (like animals). They can also become aware of the double aspectivity of their bodily life. This "eccentric positionality" or "human brokenness" entails a "constitutive homelessness of the human being" who must make himself into what he already is: "The human lives only insofar as he leads a life" (Plessner 1928/2019: 287).

The eccentric form of this existence drives the human to cultivation and creates needs that can only be satisfied by a system of artificial objects, which it stamps with the mark of transience. Human beings attain what they want all the time. And as they attain it, the invisible human within them has already gone beyond them. The reality of world history testifies to his constitutive rootlessness (Plessner 1928/2019: 316).

Max Scheler (1874–1928), building on Aristotelian ontology, defined a special position of human beings among and beyond anorganic, vegetative, and animal beings due to the human spirit which unties the human being from drives and the environment. The human spirit opens human beings to the world, enables them to distance themselves from the world (and from themselves), and to 'have' the world and themselves. Human beings are able to transcend the world and themselves, in feeling values and acting according to values—like "love and hatred", "happiness and despair", "peace and conflict"—which motivate human behavior and direct human needs and drives, wishes, and desires to goals considered meaningful, important, or worthwhile.

Experience of Spiritual Needs and Religions

Seizing on the observation of anthropological phenomena and on reflections on the human being, on the human mind and spirit, which arrive at assertions such as the human mind or spirit is able to transcend the here and now, to mentally or cognitively go beyond any limitation, and that the horizon of the human mind or spirit is unlimited and open to the infinite and to the transcendent, for example transcendent truth, goodness, beauty, and oneness, philosophy questions whether there *is* God and whether God can be proven, for example, as the ultimate being "greater than which cannot be conceived" (Anselm of Canterbury (2008), Proslogion, ch. II, "Ontological Argument"; twelfth century). Phenomenological observations have been extended to philosophical attempts like this 'ontological argument' to prove God's existence or at least to prove the plausibility of an infinite reality beyond the human spirit. There is nothing 'unreasonable' about asking such questions and following their logics while being aware of their ultimate limitations. Existentialist philosophers such as Jaspers (1932) remind theologians that we can never attain the goal of our longing for transcendence. In front of boundary situations there is no human mastery but failure.

Attempts of philosophical 'theology' differ from what can be called religious and spiritual experiences in their many varieties (James 1997) and which constitute a necessary dimension in any religion. The other dimensions of religions—their narratives and doctrines, their rituals and community celebrations, as well as their ethos and rules for living (Glock and Stark 1971)—are nourished by, and in their turn stimulate, new experiences which modify, strengthen, or loosen the personal adherence to a religion or religious group. The French mathematician Blaise Pascal (1623–1662) can epitomize the cogent or convincing power of religious experiences for the individual. Due to an extraordinary personal joyful experience (dated 23-11-1654, 10.30 pm) marked as "Memorial" in a personal note which he secretly sewed into his coat, he characterized an existential difference between the "God of the philosophers and scholars" and the "God of Abraham, Isaac and Jacob", noting the following: "Certitude, heartfelt joy, peace. God of Jesus Christ. God of Jesus Christ. 'My God and your God.' ... Joy, Joy, Joy, tears of joy ... Jesus Christ. Jesus Christ. May I never be separated from him" (Pascal 1937, 247–248). Much depends on the interpretation of such an experience. Pascal interpreted what he went through (without giving us a more detailed report) in terms of his previous personal history in a Christian context; for him, this Christian interpretation was immediately and intrinsically evident. He wanted to make sure he would never forget it. Although Pascal's "Memorial" may be called a report of an extraordinary religious ("mystical") experience, Christian faith expresses the conviction that "homo capax Dei" ("the human person is capable of God") in every religion, time, and culture, including for agnostics and atheists.

What does this conviction mean? It interprets the aforementioned anthropological phenomena as indications that the human person is searching for the sacred (Pargament 2005), and that there is not only a cognitive openness for the infinite, but also an insatiable spiritual (need and) desire for God in the human heart which becomes a desire once it is felt. Ultimately there is the divine reality—God—who wants to meet the human person in her or his spiritual needs and desires. For the Catechism of the Catholic Church (CCC), this theological perspective is its very starting point, right from the beginning of everything that follows: "The desire for God is written in the human heart, because man is created by God and for God; and God never ceases to draw man to himself. Only in God will he find the truth and happiness he never stops searching for" (CCC n. 27). The Old Testament psalm 42,2 turns the praying person's spiritual needs toward God into their ultimate fulfillment: "My soul thirsts for God, for the living God. When shall I come and appear before God?" (Transl. English Standard Version). Spiritual needs in all their multiple forms and expressions are ultimately considered as expressions and veiled synonyms of this specific human "need" and "desire for God" (Wolff 1973; Schroer and Staubli 1998; Frevel 2006; Benedict XVI 2012).

Kearney (1999) resumes Levinas' thinking about desire differentiating between two ways of desiring God: onto-theological and eschatological. The onto-theological paradigm construes desire as lack and striving for fulfillment: This is what we call 'need' and 'wish' in the present contribution. Conversely, eschatological desire does not fulfill or adhere to the lack of human needs. St. Augustine of Hippo impressively gave prayerful voice to this eschatological desire with its unrest in his autobiographical *Confessions* (I,1): "You have made us for yourself, O Lord, and our hearts are restless until they rest in You." (Augustinus 1987) Augustine understands the duplicity of the genitive "desire of God": His desire of God (genitivus obiectivus) has its origin in God's desire (genitivus subiectivus) of (genitivus obiectivus) Augustine.

Kearney (1999) calls eschatological desire "desire beyond desire" (114):

> *"God, it seems, is the other who seeks me out before I seek him, a desire beyond my desire, bordering at times, in the excess of its fervor, on political incorrectness! 'You have searched me and you know me Lord … You search out my path and are acquainted with all my ways' [Ps 139]. This desire beyond desire I call eschatological to the extent that it alludes to an alterity that already summons me yet is not yet, that is already present yet always absent (Philippians 2:12), a deus adventurus who seeks me yet is still to come, unpredictably and unexpectedly, "in the twinkling of an eye" (I Corinthians 15:52). "Like a thief in the night" (I Thessalonians 5:2).*

Philosophically spoken, human desire is following "trace(s) of the Other" (Levinas 1963/1986), "chiffres of transcendence" (Jaspers 1970), bringing transcendence into daily experience, without the need for it becoming an object of perception or fulfillment. According to Augustine, human desire presupposes the divine desire, which may be conceptualized as God's "tracing" the human being. Karl Rahner (1949/1997), talking about the need and the blessing of prayer, insinuates that we become more sensitive to God's desire with increasing age "as if we had the impression that we could no longer elude the love of God, that the divine Hunter had already surrounded his game that always wants to escape from him, so that it can only wait in blissful trembling for the moment when it finally becomes his catch" (67).

The equivalence (but also the gap!) between the divine and the human desires is expressed by the relationship between the Creator and his creature or, as a rabbinic metaphor says, *God and the human being are twins.*

The fundamental affirmation of the bible that God created human beings "in the image of God" (Gen 1,26–27) first of all claims a divine dignity of the human person to be universally protected, both as man and woman (Schmidt 2011). In the same instant, however, as summarized by the 2nd Vatican Council, the notion of "being created in the image of God" implies the social (and psychosexual) nature of men and women and that the human person is "capable of knowing and loving his Creator" (Vatican II (1965b), Gaudium et spes, 12, italics added). Hence, an innate capacity of (to be developed) and an infinite desire for mutual love—being loved and loving—are theologically considered intrinsic elements of every human being by her or his very being called into existence. This implies love of God for God's own sake as well as love between human persons for their own sake, too, also in sexual relationships. And for spirituality, in this sense, it implies that spiritual needs do not seek fulfillment for themselves, but imply a continuous openness and thrust toward God for God's sake.

The Religious Under-Determination of Spiritual Needs Is Theologically Needed for the Sake of Freedom

Pascal's Memorial, the CCC, and the affirmations of St. Augustine are explicitly Christian. Religious experiences are open to many interpretations, depending on many individual dispositions and biographical, cultural, and historical circumstances. Religions therefore seek to stimulate spiritual experiences which favor the conversion, adherence, and consent, as well as the believing, bonding, behaving, and belonging of their members (cf. Saroglou 2011; Saroglou et al. 2020), building on their spiritual needs in general, and providing a context of interpretation in the light of the respective religious faiths and their holy texts (Theissen 2000). Obviously, then, the anthropological realities called 'spiritual needs' and desires have found manifold reactions, answers, hues, and expressions in the history and cultures of humanity, in the many religions, within and beyond all of these religions, but also in plenty of secular varieties. This means that spiritual needs are religiously under-determined. By themselves, spiritual needs and even a conscious desire for God as ultimate, eschatological fulfilment ("greater than which cannot be conceived") cannot prove the truth of any religion.

This is no contradiction to the Christian stance and perspective of the authors. Our theological intention is not to make an apology for Christian faith, but rather to offer and indicate a theological perspective which deals with both spiritual needs and desires and their 'religious under-determination". The religious under-determination of spiritual needs, their openness to the sacred, and their earthly incompleteness allows for a maximum of personal freedom regarding religious commitments, and it does so for theological reasons from a Christian perspective and interpretation.

In biblical perspectives of both the Old and New Testaments, God offers a covenant to Israel, first, and to all human beings in the New Covenant established by and in Jesus Christ. Such a covenant, by its very nature and definition of mutual obligation, is only possible as a free commitment on both sides. Neither God's People nor individuals can be forced to enter and to persevere in this covenant with God by other means but only with the free inner consent of their hearts and minds. They can also do otherwise. This becomes even more evident in the Christian perspective with its central tenet that God is love and calls the human partners to accept God's love and to answer it with their own love which cannot be done but in freedom—in loving God with all their capacities and their neighbor as themselves.

This aspect of freedom deserves further explanation, seizing on the teaching of philosopher and theologian Thomas Aquinas and from the perspective of the 2nd Vatican Council. Although biblical and Christian anthropology state a fundamental responsiveness of human hearts and minds to God's love and human interpersonal love in their 'desire for God', God's call to respond in freedom corresponds to an 'ontological indifference' of human will. This means human will—in its openness for the ultimate good—is indifferent and undetermined as to whether it really wants some specific object or not, whether it decides and undertakes the steps to gain it, and this is most fundamentally (ontologically) true for the ultimate good or goal, too, at least in earthly times.

Furthermore, there is a 'responsive' difference between God's desire and human beings' spiritual quest, that is, the incapacity to adequately respond to God's initiative. This responsive difference can be considered an anthropological given (Waldenfels 1994). For God is always beyond and different from what human beings imagine God to be (with the exception of Jesus Christ) and always transcends human capacities and realities of love, "Deus semper maior".

In addition, there are many appearances of the good; every being has a resemblance of the good and therefore can become an object of will (Siewerth 1954, 28–30). In consequence, both in specific decisions and in questions of ultimate bearing, of meaning and religious faith, every human person is not only called to ask for what is good and evil, but also what is truly good and what is less than truly good but 'only' apparently good. Theologically, this means not only an obligation to search for what is truly good, but also the human right and duty "to seek the truth in matters religious" (Vatican II (1965a), Dignitatis humanae 3), and hence, the human right of religious freedom as "the right of the person and of communities to social and civil freedom in matters religious" (Vatican II (1965a), Dignitatis humanae, subtitle; Schockenhoff 2012).

In consequence, in the under-determination of spiritual needs we can find an empirical anthropological correlate and precondition of the human right to religious freedom. They can find some fulfillment in many ways which appear desirable. Spiritual needs and desires, in other words, can find some fulfillment in receiving God's attention, love, and mercy, in dwelling in this reality of being loved, in meditation and reflecting on the Gospel, in worshipping God in joy and grief, in cherishing the beauty of creation and in struggling for more social justice, in taking care of the needs of neighbors and drawing close to them in their needs and sorrows, in enjoying the community of faith, in listening and in being listened to. This list of spiritual activities could be continued, for example, with items operationalized in the SpNQ (Büssing et al. 2010, 2018), or found in qualitative research (Milner et al. 2020), or taken from the history of Christian or other religious practices, not only of contemplative 'specialists' or 'mystics', but also and especially in the social care of charitable actions, biographies, and organizations where contemplation is translated into (pro-)social, altruistic action which finds joy in the well-being of others.

The religious under-determination of spiritual needs and desires implies that there can be manifold spiritual practices as attempts to meet these needs and desires. These practices can be more or less fulfilling, more or less sustainable, more or less ‘authentic’. Many of these practices can be independent and separated from religions, inspired by various religious and spiritual traditions and new inventions which seem to fit better than former practices of tradition. Spiritual needs can also be numbed, narcotized, and suffocated. In their ‘neediness’, they can be filled with surrogates and apparent fulfillments which can even do harm to the individual, to others, to the group. As an expression of freedom, individuals can do away with less than authentic satisfactions of their spiritual needs and desires, with instant narcotization, or painful consequences rather than long-lasting and sustainable joy. In the majority of cases, however, there will be a manifold individual mix of what are felt as spiritual needs and what is sought for and experienced as authentic, fitting to self, helpful, or fulfilling.

Spiritual needs, in accordance to what Gehlen said about human nature in general, are not determined by what satisfies them; they indicate the need for self-transcendence implied by the eccentric position according to Plessner, and the search for what is truly worthwhile and meaningful as put into relief by Scheler. By themselves, again, they cannot, however, tell which kind and which object of self-transcendence and which values and meanings are ‘truly’ fulfilling. In addition, they are ‘insatiable’: after moments or experiences of fulfillment, new neediness and new desires ensue, and call for further and maybe other fulfillment. They continue to call for self-transcendent going beyond and for verification that these values and meanings are really worthwhile and meaningful for the person.

Spiritual Needs and Health/Disease

What about the relationship between spiritual needs and health or disease, then, theologically? Empirical research is not unanimous on a ‘health effect’ of spirituality and religiosity. In the majority of cases, there are significant moderate positive correlations between intrinsic religiosity and indicators of health. There are also specific conditions of religiosity which correlate weakly negatively with health, especially if this religiosity is predominantly anxiety-driven. Intrinsic religiosity and spiritual practices (statistically) tend to go along with healthy lifestyles and positive, hopeful coping with disease as well as responsible compliance with treatment

(Matthews and Clark 1999). However, neither intrinsic religiosity nor spiritual practices which increase quality-of-life outcomes can be shown to result in better health apart from the preventive healthy behavioral aspects. Both religious and spiritual practices in response to spiritual needs can increase the mental balance of individuals and decrease the impact of stressors. These are important side effects with empirical evidence that should be acknowledged wholeheartedly as they can be preventive and therapeutic factors of resilience. Nevertheless, there is no theological promise that an authentic Christian or other religiously and spiritually engaged individual may not fall prey to some incurable disease. Such a misleading promise would postulate a psychosomatic causality that spiritual needs and their orthodox fulfillment lead to and ensure somatic health. Such causality, then, would contradict the theological meaning of the under-determination of spiritual needs and the freedom of the spiritual search for the meaning of the human person and her/his encounter with realities interpreted as transcendent and divine. 'Healing' in a theological sense does not focus on elimination of illness symptoms. It concerns another 'sickness', coined "unto death" by Søren Kierkegaard (1849/2013) alluding to John 11:4: This sickness is despair, consciously or unconsciously not to will to be oneself or in despair to will to be oneself, that is, avoiding the response to God's desire.

Disease catalyzes spiritual needs. Some theories of religion (Luhmann 1977) consider religions' main function in dealing and coping with experiences of 'contingency', of the limits of life, especially in failure, disease, and any kind of suffering, and finally of death of beloved others and self, with the help of faith in transcendence. Though there is more about religions and spiritualities, the diagnosis and experience of life-threatening illness shake the personal existence and its everyday securities; they throw ajar the door to existential questions, needs, and doubts about one's life and its meaning. Exploring the spiritual needs of patients dying of lung cancer or heart failure, Murray et al. (2004, 39) stated: "Spiritual concerns were important for many patients in both groups, both early and later in the illness progression. Whether or not patients and carers held religious beliefs, they expressed needs for love, meaning, purpose and sometimes transcendence."

It is a part of appropriate patient care, then, to uncover and address these needs and to discuss them with patients, if they like and with whom they like in the multidisciplinary team. In this sense, with Murray et al. (2004, 40 Fig. 1), we can succinctly state that "[s]piritual care is about helping people whose sense of meaning, purpose, and worth is challenged by illness." It is done for the patients' own sake for their spiritual needs, not expecting miraculous healing, yet possibly an increase in their quality of life and in coping with their illness. In our Christian-theological perspective, spiritual care is mandatory as part of the impulse and divine mandate to assist the sick and the suffering, the needy and the poor, in their afflictions.

Spiritual Needs and Social Care

There are strong needs in many people to reach out to and help others in need. This can be interpreted as transcending oneself for the others in need, and such self-transcending is considered as most valuable and meaningful. Indeed, there is no point in claiming love of one's neighbor as specifically or exclusively Jewish and Christian, notwithstanding its contrast with Ancient Greek–Roman philosophy and ethos (Baumann 2008). Lists of so-called works of mercy (Mt 25:31–46) can be found in extra-biblical oriental writings, especially in Ancient Egypt (about 600 BC), about the obligations first of sovereigns, then of all members to help each other within the religious or cultic community, not yet transcending toward the social environment of all Egyptians (Brunner-Traut 1990). Such transcending toward the social environment without regarding kin or cultic community is then accomplished in the Old Testament commandment of love of neighbor and even of stranger (Leviticus 19:18.34)—and universalized in the ethos of the Christian Gospel, for example in the parable of the Good Samaritan (Luke 10:25–37; and again Mt. 25:31–46). This democratization and universalization make evident that helping others in need is intrinsically "a sovereign expression of humanity" by the human person as such (Theissen 1990) and at the same time contains a transcendent meaning. In some form and with some relevance, social care is part of the ethos of most religions (König and Waldenfels 1987). This is so perhaps because it is the face of the other—for the other's own sake way beyond oneself—which inevitably calls for my responsibility (Casper 2020, with Levinas) or which concerns me ultimately and unconditionally (Tillich 1958).

Social care, at any rate, seizes on the spiritual needs to give and to foster the well-being of others, in other words, on the need not only and not primarily to be loved oneself but to love, to take care of others, to give oneself for others' sake (cf. De Lubac 1983). This is strongly present even in the personal prayer of patients dealing with chronic illness including cancer (Jors et al. 2015). These needs, captured in the SpNQ basically in the scale of *Giving/Generativity* needs, are under-determined, too, and prone to be mixed with many other motivations and needs (Baumann 2003), to the extent of distorting originally intended self-giving love to compulsory self-exploitation, for example due to missing self-esteem, or of perverting it into economic self-interests which alienate and reduce empathy and care for others in need and make social care a business.

Thanks to the connection of spiritual giving and generativity needs with other needs and resources of spirituality—in other words, because of the longing of the human heart to love and be loved, and the meeting with what it experiences as truly human and truly transcendent love—there remains the continuous potential and opportunity for healing such distortions systemically (Baumann 2015) and for growth in the love of neighbor and the love of who we may call God. This God is whom Christians, even in a secular age and due to their interpretations of their manifold experiences, their needs, and their desire (as "désir"), believe in and trust as life-giving (threefold) Love that is most caring—more than which cannot be conceived—for the spiritual and other needs of God's images and that calls them to meet their spiritual needs by becoming instruments of this divine Love (cf. Baumann 2017).

References

Anselm of Canterbury (2008) Proslogion. In: Davies B, Evans GR (eds) Anselm of Canterbury. The major works. Oxford University Press, Oxford, pp 82–104

Antonovsky A (1987) Unraveling the mystery of health. How people manage stress and stay well. Jossey-Bass, San Francisco

Augustinus A (1987) Bekenntnisse (Confessiones). Insel, Frankfurt

Bachmann I (1978) Sämtliche Erzählungen. Piper, München

Baumann K (2003) Persönliche Erfüllung im Dienen? Zeitschrift für medizinische Ethik 49:29–42

Baumann K (2008) Hilfekultur als Kulturhilfe. Die organisierte Nächstenliebe (Caritas/ Diakonie) der Kirche als Kulturfaktor. In: Eurich J, Oelschlägel C (eds) Diakonie und Bildung. Kohlhammer, Stuttgart, pp 109–126

Baumann K (2015) Wie kann „caritas" systemisch werden? Zu einer zentralen Herausforderung an kirchliche Einrichtungen im Gesundheitssystem und im Dienst der Kirche. In Büssing A, Surzykiewicz J, Zimowski Z (eds) Dem Gutes tun, der leidet. Springer, Heidelberg, pp 181–189

Baumann K (2017) Focusing on the basic elements of Christian faith in the Service of Renewal. The scope and effects of the encyclical Deus caritas Est more than ten years after its publication. Rozniki Teologiczne 64(6):5–25. https://doi.org/10.18290/rt.2017.64.6-1

Benedict XVI (2012) The year of faith. The desire for GOD. General audience of 7 November 2012. http://www.vatican.va/content/benedict-xvi/en/audiences/2012/documents/hf_ben-xvi_aud_20121107.html. Accessed 13 Sept 202

Bion WR (1962/2003) A theory of thinking. In: Raphael-Leff J (ed) Parent-infant psychodynamics: wild things, mirrors and ghosts. Whurr Publishers, Philadelphia, pp 74–82

Brunner-Traut E (1990) Wohltätigkeit und Armenfürsorge im Alten Ägypten. In: Schäfer GK, Strohm T (eds) Diakonie. Biblische Grundlagen und Orientierungen. HVA, Heidelberg, pp 23–43

Büssing A, Balzat HJ, Heusser P (2010) Spiritual needs of patients with chronic pain diseases and Cancer—validation of the spiritual needs questionnaire. Eur J Med Res 15:266–273

Büssing A, Recchia DR, Koenig H, Baumann K, Frick E (2018) Factor structure of the spiritual needs questionnaire (SpNQ) in persons with chronic diseases, elderly and healthy individuals. Religions 9:13. https://doi.org/10.3390/rel9010013

Casper B (2020) „Geisel für den Anderen—vielleicht nur ein harter Name für Liebe“. Emmanuel Levinas und seine Hermeneutik diachronen *da*-seins. Alber, Freiburg

De Lubac H (1983) Le drame de l'humanisme athée, 7ème ed. du Cerf, Paris

Frevel C (2006) Anthropologie. In: Berlejung A, Frevel C (eds) Handbuch theologischer Grundbegriffe zum Alten und Neuen Testament (HGANT). Wissenschaftliche Buchgesellschaft, Darmstadt, pp 1–7

Frick E, Baumann K (2017) Spiritualität—Bedürfnis und Begehren. Empirische Forschung und theologisch-philosophische Reflexion können voneinander lernen. In: Nauerth M, Hahn K, Tüllmann M, Kösterke S (eds) Religionssensibilität in der Sozialen Arbeit: Positionen, Theorien, Praxisfelder. Kohlhammer, Stuttgart, pp 227–245

Glock CY, Stark R (1971) Religion and Society in Tension, 5th edn. Rand McNally, Chicago

Jaspers K (1970) Chiffren der Transzendenz. Hrsg. von Hans Saner. Piper, München.

James W (1997) The varieties of religious experience. Introduction by Reinhold Niebuhr. Simon & Schuster, New York

Jaspers K (1932) Philosophie II (Existenzerhellung). Springer, Berlin

Jors K, Büssing A, Hvidt NC, Baumann K (2015) Personal prayer in patients dealing with chronic illness: a review of the research literature. Evid Based Complement Alternat Med:927973. https://doi.org/10.1155/2015/927973
Kearney R (1999) Desire of god. In: Caputo JD, Scanlon MJ (eds) God, the gift, and postmodernism. Indiana University Press, Bloomington, pp 112–163
Kierkegaard S (1849/2013) Sickness unto death: a Christian psychological exposition for upbuilding and awakening. De Gruyter, Berlin
König F, Waldenfels H (eds) (1987) Lexikon der Religionen. Herder, Freiburg
Levinas E (1963/1986) The trace of the other. In: Taylor MC (ed) Deconstruction in context. Literature and philosophy. University of Chicago Press, Chicago, pp 345–359
Levinas E (1983) Die Spur des Anderen. In: Krewani WN (ed) Die Spur des Anderen. Untersuchungen zur Phänomenologie und Sozialphilosophie. Alber, Freiburg, pp 209–235
Loch W (1984) Psychoanalytische Perspektiven. Hirzel, Stuttgart
Luhmann N (1977) Fuktion der Religion. Suhrkamp, Frankfurt
Maslow AH (1954) Motivation and personality. Harper & Row, New York
Matthews DA, Clark C (1999) The faith factor. Proof of the healing power of prayer. Penguin Books, London
Milner K, Crawford P, Edgley A, Hare-Duke L, ML S (2020) The experiences of spirituality among adults with mental health difficulties: a qualitative systematic review. Epidemiol Psychiatr Sci 29:e34. https://doi.org/10.1017/S2045796019000234
Murray SA, Kendall M, Boyd K, Worth A, Benton TF (2004) Exploring the spiritual needs of people dying of lung cancer or heart failure: a prospective qualitative interview study of patients and their carers. Palliat Med 18:39–45. https://doi.org/10.1191/0269216304pm837oa
Pargament KI (2005) The sacred and the search for significance: religion as a unique process. J Soc Issues 61:665–687
Pascal B (1937) Über die Religion und über einige andere Gegenstände (Pensées). Lambert Schneider, Berlin
Pleger W (2018) Handbuch der Anthropologie, 3rd edn. WBG Academic, Darmstadt
Plessner H (1928/2019) Levels of organic life and the human: an introduction to philosophical anthropology. Fordham University Press, New York
Rahner K (1949/1997) The need and the blessing of prayer. Liturgical Press, Collegeville
Saroglou V (2011) Believing, bonding, behaving, and belonging: the big four religious dimensions and cultural variation. J Cross-Cult Psychol 42(8):1320–1340. https://doi.org/10.1177/2F0022022111412267
Saroglou V, Clobert M, Cohen AB, Johnson KA, Ladd KL, Van Pachterbeke M, Adamovova L, Blogowska J, Brandt PY, Çukur CS, Hwang KK, Miglietta A,

Motti-Stefanidi F, Muñoz-García A, Murken S, Roussiau N, Valladares JT (2020) Believing, bonding, behaving, and belonging: the cognitive, emotional, moral, and social dimensions of religiousness across cultures. J Cross-Cult Psychol 51(7–8):551–575. https://doi.org/10.1177/0022022120946488

Schmidt WH (2011) Alttestamentlicher Glaube, 11th edn. Neukirchener Verlag, Neukirchen-Vluyn

Schockenhoff E (2012) Das Recht, ungehindert die Wahrheit zu suchen. Die Erklärung über die Religionsfreiheit *Dignitatis humanae*. In: Tück JH (ed) Erinnerung an die Zukunft. Das Zweite Vatikanische Konzil. Herder, Freiburg, pp 601–642

Schroer S, Staubli T (1998) Die Körpersymbolik der Bibel. Wissenschaftliche Buchgesellschaft, Darmstadt

Siewerth G (ed) (1954) Thomas von Aquin. Die menschliche Willensfreiheit. Verlag L. Schwann, Düsseldorf

Theissen G (1990) Die Legitimitätskrise des Helfens und der barmherzige Samariter. In: Röckle G (ed) Diakonische Kirche. Neukirchener Verlag, Neukirchen-Vluyn, pp 46–76

Theissen G (2000) Die Religion der ersten Christen. Eine Theorie des Urchristentums. Gütersloher Verlagshaus, Gütersloh

Tillich P (1958) The dynamics of faith. Harper, New York

Vatican II (1965a) Dignitatis humanae. Declaration on religious freedom. On the right of the person and of communities to social and civil freedom in matters religious. http://www.vatican.va/archive/hist_councils/ii_vatican_council/documents/vat-ii_decl_19651207_dignitatis-humanae_en.html. Accessed 20 Sept 2020

Vatican II (1965b) Gaudium et spes. Pastoral Constitution on the Church in the Modern World. http://www.vatican.va/archive/hist_councils/ii_vatican_council/documents/vat-ii_const_19651207_gaudium-et-spes_en.html. Accessed 20 Sept 2020

Waldenfels B (1994) Antwortregister. Suhrkamp, Frankfurt

Wolff HW (1973) Anthropologie des Alten Testaments. Kaiser, München

CHAPTER 3

Spiritual Care in Health Care: Guideline, Models, Spiritual Assessment and the Use of the ©FICA Spiritual History Tool

Christina Puchalski

Background

Tom is a 58-year-old male who presents for a new patient visit with a physician. His wife had died of COVID-19 two months prior to the visit. Three weeks prior to the visit, Tom had severe chest pain and shortness of breath. He is worried he might have COVID-19 or that it might be a heart attack since he had a history of hypertension and several of his family members had had heart attacks. At the emergency department when he describes his symptoms to the triage nurse, his voice trembles as he tells her about his wife's illness and death. "Do you think I have COVID-19?" he says to the nurse. "I can hardly breathe; everything hurts so much." All his tests, including a stress test, are normal. Tom has a history of mild anxiety, mostly exacerbated by stress but says he has never felt as bad as he does

C. Puchalski (✉)
The George Washington University Institute for Spirituality and Health (GWish), Washington, DC, USA
e-mail: cpuchals@email.gwu.edu

A. Büssing (ed.), *Spiritual Needs in Research and Practice*,
https://doi.org/10.1007/978-3-030-70139-0_3

now. Tearfully he notes that he feels like he cannot go on anymore and that the "pain inside is too great." He denies suicidal ideation, affirms insomnia, and has had decreased appetite since his wife died. He has lost 10 pounds within three weeks of his wife's death. "Doctor, I know the tests are normal but can you help me. I am really suffering. Why is this happening to me?"

How can we help Tom and patients like him who experience deep spiritual and existential suffering? Tom was discharged and went home with a referral to a therapist felt but still alone, still in distress. Addressing spiritual distress and providing compassionate presence is one way to begin to help Tom in the midst of his loss, anguish, and aloneness. This article will review the role of spirituality in health care and provide a model for how to begin to help patients like Tom.

Spirituality, religion, and health were interconnected for centuries, as evidenced by the healing role of priests and shamans, and by the history of hospitals often founded by religious organizations that emphasized health, healing, and the whole person. In 1910 in the United States, the Flexner Report emphasized the important role of grounding clinical practice in science. As a result, the spiritual and humanistic areas were disassociated from medical practice (Flexner, 1910). In the late twentieth century, several important events began to reintegrate spirituality into the care of patients. In the 1970s the hospice movement was created in England by Dame Cicely Saunders, who coined the concept of "total pain"—physical, psychological, social, and spiritual pain that make up the "total pain" experience and distress (Clark 2014). In the United States the growth of the alternative medicine movement and the preference of a large part of the society for alternative medicine over established allopathic medicine highlighted the need for a whole-person approach to care and not a strictly biomedical one. In 2020 the whole world faced the COVID-19 pandemic, which shed greater light on the importance of spiritual care as patients experienced deep spiritual and existential suffering, particularly in the face of death of and isolation from loved ones (Puchalski et al. 2020a). In the early 1990s The John Templeton Foundation funded award programs for medical schools in the United States in Spirituality and Health, which I directed. This program laid the groundwork for the formation of the first charted university institute in spirituality and health: The George Washington University's Institute for Spirituality and Health (GWish). A key work of this institute was to develop the education, clinical tools, and guidelines for clinicians to address patients' spiritual pain as part of total care but also to understand patients' spiritual beliefs, values, and practices as part of whole-person well-being.

Why Spiritual Care in Health Care?

As noted earlier, Dame Saunders recognized that the suffering of patients with serious illness or the end-of-life experience is not only physical pain but also deep psychosocial and spiritual pain. The treatment for suffering is found in a concept known as accompaniment—clinicians accompany patients in the midst of their suffering. We may not be able to fix another's suffering, but by offering our compassionate service, our patients may feel more supported, and in that space of compassionate support they may find answers to their suffering and may even discover healing. As the Dalai Lama wrote, "[w]hen people are overwhelmed by illness, we must give them physical relief, but it is equally important to encourage the spirit through a constant show of love and compassion. It is shameful how often we fail to see that what people desperately require is human affection. Deprived of human warmth and a sense of value, other forms of treatment prove less effective. Real care of the sick does not begin with costly procedures, but with the simple gifts of affection, love, and concern" (HH Dalai Lama 2006). The Dalai Lama speaks to the core of what spirituality means in the care of all patients, particularly those who are suffering from chronic illness and facing dying. Illness can, in and of itself, trigger profound spiritual questions and issues. The diagnosis of a lifelong condition stirs within people the awareness that they will no longer be the same and that their lives will change. Illness can provoke the deepest of spiritual pain—aloneness, abandonment, self-doubt, loss of a sense of wholeness and dignity, and hopelessness. It can throw someone into a deep existential crisis of meaninglessness and despair. In the midst of this suffering, an attentive and compassionate health-care professional can be an important anchor in whom the patient can find solace and the strength to move through distress to peace and acceptance.

Theoretical, ethical, and philosophical literature as well as empirical research demonstrate the impact of religious and spiritual beliefs on people's decision-making, way of life, ability to transcend suffering, deal with life's challenges, interactions with others, and life choices (Koenig et al. 2010; Powell et al. 2003). Spirituality has been demonstrated to impact health outcomes including pain, pain interference, pain catastrophizing, and quality of life and has been associated with decreased mortality and morbidity (McCabe et al. 2018; Siddall et al. 2015). Spiritual distress is associated with worse quality of life, physical pain, depression, and anxiety (Hadi et al. 2018). Addressing spiritual needs improves physical, functional, and emotional outcomes (Garschagen et al. 2015).

Patients would like their spiritual beliefs addressed by physicians and other health-care professionals in a variety of health-care circumstances (Best et al. 2015). Patients feel increased trust in their clinicians if a spiritual history is obtained, as is noted in many US surveys. Patients also note that they experience an increased sense of being listened to (McCord et al. 2004). Interestingly, a study by Balboni et al. showed that 75% of dying cancer patients did not have their spiritual needs met even when 95% of them said spirituality was important to them (Balboni et al. 2007). These data indicated the importance of developing guidelines and resources for patients and clinicians.

National and International Guidelines for Addressing Spirituality in Health Care

Many national and international guidelines have been developed for addressing spiritual care as part of whole-person care, especially in the field of palliative care (Puchalski et al. 2014; World Health Organization Executive Board 2014; National Consensus Project for Quality Palliative Care 2020 [Domain 5]; Meaningful Ageing Australia 2016; Selman et al. 2010). The clinical models described in these guidelines are based on addressing spiritual health as a part of whole-person care, and identifying spiritual distress as a part of symptom management (Puchalski et al. 2009). In these guidelines, spirituality is defined broadly as a “dynamic and intrinsic aspect of humanity through which persons seek ultimate meaning, purpose, and transcendence, and experience relationship to self, family, others, community, society, nature, and the significant or sacred. Spirituality is expressed through beliefs, values, traditions, and practices” (Puchalski et al. 2014b). Religion is one type of expression of spirituality and it relates to the participation in beliefs and practices of a community of faith, but there are many other expressions of spirituality, including secular humanism, nature, cultural beliefs and practices, meditation, mindfulness, and so on. This broad definition and the aforementioned guidelines support an inclusive model of interprofessional spiritual care.

These guidelines focused on the clinical aspect of spirituality, identifying spiritual distress as a clinical symptom to be assessed and treated. The experience of chronic pain, including physiological and existential suffering, is multidimensional, such as questioning why I have to go through this painful existence (Shukla 2020). The need for intervention in the spiritual or existential dimension of pain appears to be common across nationalities, belief systems, and cultures (Ferreira-Valente et al. 2020). There is significant evidence documenting spiritual pain and its relationship to other forms of pain, as well as the influence of spiritual distress and spiritual coping on the pain experience (Delgado-Guay et al. 2013). Spiritual pain can be defined as pain deep in the soul. It is one dimension of what is now understood as the multidimensionality of pain. The clinical aspect of spirituality that is critical, especially in patients with serious and chronic illness, is spiritual distress, which is seen as a symptom that must be managed with the same intensity as physical pain. The National Comprehensive Cancer Network (NCCN) defined spiritual distress symptoms, and in the 2009 consensus conference a list of these diagnoses along with others were defined as spiritual distress diagnoses (NCCN Guidelines for Patients 2020; Puchalski et al. 2009).

These Spiritual Distress Diagnoses include the concerns listed out in Table 3.1.

The focus on spiritual distress as a symptom has been critically important is establishing the need for clinicians such as physicians, nurses, physician assistants, and social workers to address spiritual needs and issues of

Table 3.1 Spiritual distress or concerns

Diagnoses (Primary)
Existential
Abandonment God or others
Anger at God or others
Concerns about relationship with deity
Conflicted or challenged belief systems
Despair/Hopelessness
Grief/loss
Guilt/shame
Reconciliation
Isolation
Religious-specific
Religious/Spiritual Struggle

patients in clinical care. The medical model of most health-care systems primarily focuses on assessment and treatment of presenting symptoms and secondarily on inclusion of resources that are supportive to the patients. This medical and perhaps reductionist approach is becoming increasingly dominant given the time pressures of physicians in most clinical settings. Efficiently diagnosing presenting symptoms of patients and then treating the patient appropriately is of paramount importance.

Increasingly, the concept of spiritual health is gaining recognition as a part of 'Whole-Person Care' (Hutchison 2012; Puchalski and Ferrell 2010). Hubner and colleagues developed an international consensus-based definition of health as "the ability to adapt and to self-manage." They further recognized health as being able to cope with chronic illness and being healthy even in the presence of ongoing chronic illness or conditions; having the ability to perform relative to the condition; being able to achieve individual fulfillment, meaning, purpose; and being able to negotiate demands of social environments. Achieving individual fulfillment, meaning, and purpose is to be in the "spiritual health" domain (Hubner et al. 2011). Thus, spiritual beliefs, values, and practices that support the overall health of patients can be understood as being a part of "spiritual health." Examples of spiritual health might include the ability to seek forgiveness or the willingness to forgive; experiencing a connection to or relationship with the sacred or significant; living a life that is consistent with one's values and beliefs; participating in spiritual practices that contribute to positive coping or well-being; or having a spiritual community that is supportive to the person. Spiritual communities might include the church, temple, or mosque, or could be like-minded friends, family, or other spiritual support groups (e.g., a Parkinson or cancer support group could be thought of by some as a spiritual support group). Spiritual practices, including meditation, connection with nature, music, or arts, may also help people find a sense of wholeness and experience transcendence or healing. All these aspects of spirituality help patients cope, find hope in the midst of suffering, find joy in life, and/or find the ability to be grateful.

Interprofessional Model of Spiritual Care: A Consensus-Based Model of Care

In 2009, the National Consensus Conference for Spiritual Care in Palliative Care (NCC) developed recommendations for improving spiritual care in palliative care settings, with palliative care broadly defined as care for patients with chronic or life-threatening illness. The NCC also described the concept of spiritual distress as a diagnosis, which should be treated with the same intensity as physical pain. An algorithm was developed whereby clinicians could evaluate patient distress in the biopsychosocial–spiritual framework.

The model of interprofessional spiritual care developed from these guidelines is based on a generalist-specialist model of care called the Interprofessional Spiritual Care Model (Puchalski et al. 2020b). Spiritual care involves the assessment and treatment of spiritual distress, identifying and supporting spiritual resources of strength, and in-depth spiritual counselling when appropriate (Puchalski et al. 2019b). Spiritual screening identifies whether a patient is in spiritual distress and might therefore need an urgent chaplain referral. Spiritual history, a more complete assessment made by clinicians conducting a treatment or care plan, further identifies types of spiritual issues that cause the distress, as well as spiritual resources of strength. Clinicians can diagnose spiritual distress, begin to treat that distress, as well as enhance spiritual well-being as appropriate. Clinicians can also consider referral to chaplains for a more complete spiritual assessment and treatment for spiritual distress. Ideally, the treatment or care plan is developed by the interdisciplinary team, which should include a chaplain along with other members of the team involved in the care of the patient.

Spiritual care refers to many different aspects of care ranging from the intrinsic (presence in patients' suffering, honoring dignity of patients, recognition of the concept of healing, and the role of spirituality in the healing process) to the extrinsic (doing a spiritual history, integration of spirituality into the treatment plan, and follow-up on spiritual issues as appropriate). Practicing the extrinsic part of spiritual care requires training in assessment; practicing the intrinsic part of spiritual care requires an awareness of the clinician's or chaplain's own spirituality and vocation to serve others, and training in reflective listening and presence.

Spiritual Assessment

When people face serious or chronic illness or the prospect of dying, such as is currently experienced by so many people all over the world, questions such as the ones Tom voiced often arise:

- Why did this happen to me?
- Will I die?
- What will happen to me after I die?
- Why would God allow me to suffer this way?
- Will I be remembered?
- Will I be missed?

This questioning can result in fears, anxieties, and unresolved feelings, which in turn can result in despair and suffering as people face themselves and their eventual mortality. How do we invite people to ask these questions in a busy clinical setting? How do we help people in the midst of the resultant suffering they may be experiencing.

The NCC guidelines for taking a spiritual history and for the formulation of spiritual treatment or care plans, include the following:

- All health-care professionals should be trained in doing a spiritual screening or history as part of their routine history and evaluation.
- Spiritual screenings, histories, and assessments should be communicated and documented in patient records (e.g., charts and computerized databases shared with the interprofessional health-care team).
- Follow-up spiritual histories or assessments should be conducted for all patients whose medical, psychosocial, or spiritual condition changes and as part of routine follow-up in a medical history.
- A spiritual issue becomes a diagnosis if the following criteria are met: (1) the spiritual issue leads to distress or suffering (e.g., lack of meaning, conflicted religious beliefs, and inability to forgive); (2) the spiritual issue is the cause of a psychological or physical diagnosis, such as depression, anxiety, or acute or chronic pain (e.g., severe meaninglessness that leads to depression or suicidality, and guilt that leads to chronic physical pain); and (3) the spiritual issue is a secondary cause or affects the presenting psychological or physical diagnosis (e.g., hypertension is difficult to control because the patient refuses to take medications because of his or her religious beliefs).

- Treatment or care plans should include but not be limited to referral to chaplains, spiritual directors, pastoral counselors, and other spiritual care providers, including clergy or faith-community healers for spiritual counseling; development of spiritual goals; meaning-oriented therapy; mind–body interventions; rituals, spiritual practices; and contemplative interventions.
- Spiritual diagnosis, resources of strength, as well as the spiritual treatment plan should be documented in the chart.

Obtaining a spiritual history is one way of listening to what is deeply important to the patient. The spiritual history affords the patient the space and opportunity to share the questions of "why me?' and feelings of despair or hopeless, and helps the clinician address the patient's suffering and hopes. It also enables the clinician to connect with the patient on a deep, caring level. Finally, it helps the clinician to identify spiritual distress and begin to treat it through compassionate presence and reflective listening, and through referral to spiritual care professionals for more in-depth assessment and treatment. It also helps the clinician to address the spiritual health of the patient and discuss spiritual wellness as part of total health with spiritual resources of strength.

There are several spiritual history tools that have been developed. These include SPIRIT (Maugans 1996), FICA (Puchalski and Romer 2000), and HOPE (Anandarajah and Hight 2001). FICA, described in Table 3.2, is more a communication tool than a checklist. This acronym helps clinicians to structure questions that help elicit patients' spiritual beliefs and values. The tool is primarily used as a way to invite the patient to share their spiritual beliefs and values with their clinician, if they would like to do so. The questions in each section of the tool are designed to offer clinicians options of how to ask a question that can be contextualized to the clinical situation of the patient they are treating. In general, the spiritual history is imbedded in the personal or social history of the clinical interview. This section also includes relationships, occupational history, sexual history, nutrition, exercise, smoking, drug and alcohol use, and goals of care.

There are several other spiritual assessment tools that can be used by clinicians or chaplains including the Spiritual Needs Questionnaire (SpNQ) (Büssing et al. 2018), which differentiates four factors: religious needs, need for inner peace, existential needs, and need for generativity, and the

Table 3.2 FICA spiritual history tool©

FICA Spiritual History Tool©
The acronym FICA can help structure questions in taking a spiritual history by health-care professionals
F—Faith and Belief and Meaning
"Do you consider yourself spiritual or religious?" or "Is spirituality something important to you" or "Do you have spiritual beliefs that help you cope with stress/difficult times?" (Contextualize to reason for visit if it is not the routine history)
If the patient responds "No," the health-care provider might ask, "What gives your life meaning?" Sometimes patients respond with answers such as family, career, or nature (The question of meaning should also be asked even if people answer yes to spirituality)
I—Importance
"What importance does your spirituality have in your life? Has your spirituality influenced how you take care of yourself, your health? Does your spirituality influence you in your health-care decision-making? (advance directives, treatment, etc.)
C—Community
"Are you part of a spiritual community? Communities such as churches, temples, and mosques, or a group of like-minded friends, family, or yoga can serve as strong support systems for some patients. Can explore further: Is this of support to you and how? Is there a group of people you really love or who are important to you?"
A—Address in Care
"How would you like me, your healthcare provider, to address these issues in your healthcare?" (With the newer models including diagnosis of spiritual distress A also refers to the "Assessment and Plan" of patients' spiritual distress or issues within a treatment or care plan)
© C. Puchalski, 1996

Spiritual Distress Assessment Tool (SDAT) (Monod et al. 2010), which addresses meaning, transcendence, values, and psychosocial identity.

The FICA© Spiritual History Tool

The FICA Spiritual History Tool was developed by Dr. Puchalski and a group of primary care physicians to help physicians and other health-care professionals address spiritual issues with patients (Puchalski and Romer 2000). Spiritual histories are taken as part of the regular history during an annual exam or new patient visit but can also be taken as part of follow-up visits, as appropriate. The FICA tool serves as a guide for conversations in the clinical setting.

Whole-Person Assessment and Treatment Plan

Once a clinician does a spiritual history, they can use communication strategies such as deep listening, presence, and reflective listening to invite the patient to share more about their spirituality. If the clinician identifies the spiritual distress, as well as spiritual resources of strength or resources for coping, the clinician should then integrate that into the patient treatment or care plan and document this in the chart. The clinician must attend to spiritual distress with the same urgency as for any other distress. Thus, patients with moderate or severe spiritual distress or with religious-specific needs should be referred to the trained chaplain. Some types of spiritual distress, which one might classify as minimal or mild, might be able to be attended to by other clinicians on the team, such as art therapists. The patient might also share spiritual practices that are important to the patient. The clinician can then incorporate these practices into the treatment plan as appropriate. All issues, whether simple or complex, should be documented in the patient's chart appropriately and shared with the patient's health-care team. The clinician can summarize the findings or their inquiry without necessarily revealing more detailed confidential aspects of the spiritual history.

Spiritual care may include such practices as reflective listening and being present for patients. Treatment options might include referral to spiritual care professionals, art therapists, meaning-oriented therapy, and meditation. If the patient identifies specific spiritual or religious practices that are important to them, then encouraging those practices might be appropriate, such as reconnecting with nature, prayer, meditation, community support, or rituals. Part of wellness coping strategies might include spiritual coping strategies such as mindfulness practices, or reestablishing priorities (Kruizinga et al. 2018).

This refers to the extrinsic spiritual care that assesses for spiritual distress, identifies spiritual health or resources of strength, and develops an appropriate assessment and treatment plan for spiritual health as part of the whole-person plan. Intrinsic spiritual care refers to the intentional practice of presence. The clinician has an intention to openness and to connection with the patients. An intention to openness refers to the willingness to listen to the patient with a sense of curiosity, without a preconceived agenda, with full respect for the patient as an individual with a unique story, and a commitment to be fully present in the encounter with the patient. An intention to connection refers to the willingness and ability to actively and appropriately form a connection with the patient on a spiritual and emotional level, thereby affording the patient the opportunity to experience a sense of belonging, care, and love. By relating on a humanitarian level, we can help form deeper and more meaningful connections with our patients.

The outcomes of spiritual care may simply be helping the person feel less lonely and despair less in their suffering. Perhaps spiritual care may facilitate the individual's eventual ability to come to an understanding with their suffering at a deeper level, connecting with a source or sources of meaning and purpose, and perhaps reconnecting with a sense of transcendence or that which is sacred or significant in their lives. Often my patients have talked about their illness, loss, and stress from the COVID pandemic as transformative. These events in people's lives may trigger a period of self-reflection about what matters most in their life. But this process requires accompaniment by their clinicians and others so that people can move from a sense of aloneness and darkness to one of possibility and hope. This is why we as clinicians or spiritual care professionals need to engage with our patients and with ourselves on that spiritual level. Spirituality is concerned with a transcendental or existential way of living one's life at a deeper level. All people seek meaning and purpose in life; this search may be intensified when someone is facing serious illness, the possibility of death, or dying, as is so evident during the current pandemic.

Case Examples of FICA© History in the Clinical Setting

Case 1: Tom

Tom had scheduled a visit with his doctor's office a few days after the emergency department visit via a telehealth call due to the COVID-19 pandemic. Because his doctor was away, he was scheduled to see another physician in the practice, Dr. Smith. Dr. Smith listened intently to Tom's story about his wife, her dying, and his sense of deep suffering. Tom shared his profound sense of loss, abandonment, and fear. After giving Tom the time and space to share, and affirming the loss and offering condolences, Dr. Smith asked more about Tom's living situation (social or person-centered history). Tom lives alone now, has a son in the area, and two daughters who live in other states. Due to COVID, however, he has not seen anyone. He works as a teacher in a high school and is conducts classes virtually. He does not exercise as much as he use to and his appetite is poor. Dr. Smith then asks him if spirituality is something important in his life to which the patient answers "Yes." The following is his complete FICA© spiritual history:

- F: Raised Episcopalian, was very involved in his faith community, but since the COVID-19 pandemic he has not been able to attend services. His meaning is in his family and his work.
- I: His personal faith is more important than organized religion so he is not particularly missing the faith community except that he is lonely now. He likes to meditate but since his wife's death he has not been able to do that. He talks about the intense emptiness he feels since his wife died. "Is there really a God? Why did this happen to me?" He talks of wanting to deepen his spiritual journey but feels "stuck in sadness."
- C: He feels very lonely and would like to connect with his children but due to the COVID 19 pandemic, they can only connect by digital media and that is "not the same."
- A: Would be interested in speaking with a pastoral counselor or spiritual director.

The Assessment and Treatment Plan is as follows:

Biopsychosocial–Spiritual Model Assessment and Plan	
Tom is a 58-year-old male with h/o hypertension and anxiety, recent loss of his wife from COVID, for a follow-up from an Emergency department visit for chest pain and shortness of breath. COVID, stress and other tests all normal; he was diagnosed with a panic attack. He has lost some weight, insomnia likely from spiritual distress, grief and anxiety	
Physical	Exercise, healthy eating, regular hours of sleep, developed diet plan
Emotional	Referral to a therapist, begin mirtazapine for situational depression, insomnia and to stimulate appetite
Social	Encouraged to build a support community via digital media, continue to connect with family

(*continued*)

(continued)

Spiritual	Bereavement spiritual distress (Why me?), spiritual longing, referral to pastoral counselor and also gave names of spiritual directors. Discussed resuming meditation practices

Tom was open to taking medication and trying to do exercises regularly, he agreed with the referrals to both pastoral counseling and spiritual direction, and welcomed further discussion with Dr. Smith. He felt listened to, had a sense that maybe he could manage this huge loss, and requested a 2-week follow-up visit with Dr. Smith.

Case 2: Jessica

Jessica is a 27-year-old who comes for a new patient visit. She recently moved to DC to work with the government as a computer analyst. She is single and currently not in a relationship. Her chief concern is her anxiety, which she rates as 6–10/10. It is beginning to affect her sleep and work. She denies depression but does not deny that she has a history of anxiety and feels that it is active now. She is beginning to make friends but has not yet established a good support system.

Her family history is significant as many members had anxiety disorders: father was an alcoholic, brother has schizophrenia and was autistic since birth.

In her first visit her FICA© assessment was as follows:

- F: Not religious does not relate to the word spiritual. Meaning: has no meaning in life, no sense of purpose
- I: no values or beliefs that impact her health
- C: no spiritual community, very little support from family
- A: not interested in talking with anyone

Jessica was interested in starting medication for her anxiety, which her doctor prescribed. In a follow-up visit one month later, she noted that she was thinking about the question of meaning from her previous visit and wondered whether there was some connection of lack of meaning with her lifelong anxiety. Her physician posed the FICA questions again and asked her to share more thoughts about meaning and spirituality. The following is the result of that conversation.

- F: I was raised Catholic but not interested in going back to Catholicism or any faith. My parents also left the church shortly after my brother was born. I have not had any meaning in life, no sense of purpose but since my last visit I have been exploring that and would like to find some meaning in my life, and something that would guide me in my life.
- I: I see a connection between lack of meaning and my anxiety
- C: I would love to find some spiritual ("in a broad sense") community
- A: I would like some resources from you but I am not interested in therapy or chaplain visit. I would like to continue working with you on this.

The Assessment and Treatment plan is as follows:

Biopsychosocial–Spiritual Model Assessment and Plan

Jessica is a 28-year-old here for a follow-up visit for anxiety. She is interested in mind-body resources; searching for a community. She is also dealing with complicated family issues

Physical	Exercise, healthy eating, regular hours of sleep
Emotional	Suggested a therapist and she declined
Social	Encouraged building a support community of friends
Spiritual	Offered list of resources including mindfulness sessions, ACOA meetings given family history of alcoholism, Unitarian Community that is very diverse, inclusive of religious and nonreligious people, referral to meaning-oriented therapy

Jessica was open to the physician's suggestions, and on subsequent visits told her doctor she found them helpful. She joined a mindfulness meditation community and attended Adult Children of Alcoholics (ACOA) meetings, which she found helpful. She appreciated the secular ACOA group she joined and felt comfortable sharing with that group. She continued to follow up with her physician on these spiritual and existential issues, along with her other health issues.

Training

While data, guidelines, and patient preferences support the practice of interprofessional spiritual care, clinicians often meet obstacles in addressing spirituality in patient care. These obstacles include lack of time and lack of training. Through a partnership with the John Templeton Foundation, we at GWish have developed medical school curricula in spirituality and health, and developed competencies in this area (Puchalski et al. 2014b). We also developed and piloted a professional development program called GWish Templeton Reflection Rounds (GTRR) which is based on contemplative facilitation to help students and clinicians explore their own spirituality as part of their professional development and learn the inner and practical skills for compassionate presence. These initiatives have culminated in a global education program called Interprofessional Spiritual Care Education Curriculum (ISPEC) (Puchalski et al. 2020b). This curriculum includes an online course composed of six modules, available on the Relias Academy website https://reliasacademy.ocm/rls/ispec. It also consists of a train-the-trainer course in which clinician–chaplain pairs from different clinical settings learn knowledge, teaching, and leadership skills in interprofessional spiritual care. They continue to work with GWish for one year implementing their goals in spiritual care in their clinical settings. To date we have taught this course to participants from many countries. Program evaluation has demonstrated that ISPEC is a much-needed and effective resource to improve spiritual care for patients.

Conclusion

Spiritual care is an essential aspect of whole-person care, particularly for patients dealing with serious and chronic illness, end-of-life, or serious life stresses. Spiritual health is an important domain of whole health and should be addressed at clinical visits. Clinicians should assess for spiritual distress as part of a whole-person assessment and treatment plan and identify spiritual resources of strength. The importance of spiritual care has been evident especially during the COVID-19 pandemic when patients, families, and clinicians are exposed to issues that can raise deep spiritual and existential crises. Spiritual distress is associated with worse health outcomes and is often expressed as deep suffering. All health-care professionals have an obligation to attend to the spiritual distress and the spiritual health of their patients. Global Guidelines have supported a clinical integrated model of care whereby all members of the patient's health-care team address spiritual issues, identify spiritual resources of strength, and diagnose and treat spiritual distress if present. Spiritual care is an interprofessional model of spiritual care whereby clinicians of different disciplines and spiritual care professionals work together to provide holistic spiritual care to patients.

It is very important to ground the work of interprofessional spiritual care in guidelines and models. What underlies spiritual care is the compassionate presence that each of us brings to our patients. As one of my patients, who recovered from a difficult course of COVID-19, said to me, "Thank you for walking with me all these months." The simple act of love and concern underlies all we do in our care for patients and their families.

References

Anandarajah G, Hight E (2001) Spirituality and medical practice: using HOPE questions as a practical tool for spiritual assessment. Am Fam Physician 63(1):81–89

Balboni TA, Vanderwerker LC, Block SD, Paulk ME, Lathan CS, Peteet JR, Prigerson HG (2007) Religiousness and spiritual support among advanced cancer patients and associations with end-of-life treatment preferences and quality of life. J Clin Oncol 25(5):555–560

Best M, Butow P, Olver I (2015) Do patients want doctors to talk about spirituality? A systematic literature review. Patient Education and Counseling 98(11):1320–1328

Büssing A, Recchia DR, Koenig HG, Baumann K, Frick E (2018) Factor structure of the spiritual needs questionnaire (SpNQ) in persons with chronic diseases, elderly and healthy individuals. Religions 9:13. https://doi.org/10.3390/rel9010013

Clark D (2014) 'Total pain': the work of Cicely Saunders and the maturing of a concept. http://endoflifestudies.academicblogs.co.uk/total-pain-the-work-of-cicely-saunders-and-the-maturing-of-a-concept/. Accessed 28 Aug 2020

Delgado-Guay MO, Parsons HA, Hui D, De la Cruz MG, Thorney S, Bruera E (2013) Spirituality, religiosity, and spiritual pain among caregivers of patients with advanced cancer. Am J Hosp Palliat Care 30(5):455–461

Ferreira-Valente A, Damião C, Pais-Ribeiro J, Jensen MP (2020) The role of spirituality in pain, function, and coping in individuals with chronic pain. Pain Med 21(3):448–457

Flexner A (1910) Medical education in the United States and Canada: a report to the Carnegie Foundation for the advancement of teaching. Bulletin No. 4. Carnegie Foundation for the Advancement of Teaching, New York

Garschagen A, Steegers MAH, van Bergen AHMM, Jochijms JAM, Skrabanja TLM, Vrijhoef HJM, Smeets RJEM, Vissers KCP (2015) Is there a need for including spiritual Care in Interdisciplinary Rehabilitation of chronic pain patients? Investigating an innovative strategy. Pain Practice: The Official Journal Of World Institute Of Pain 15(7):671–687

Hadi MA, McHugh GA, Closs SJ (2018) Impact of chronic pain on patients' quality of life: a comparative mixed-methods study. J Patient Exp 6(2):133–141. https://doi.org/10.1177/2374373518786013

HH Dalai Lama (2006) Forward in time for listening and caring. Puchalski C (ed) Oxford University Press, New York

Huber M, Knottnerus JA, Green L, van der Horst H, Jadad AR, Kromhout D, Schnabel P (2011) How should we define health? BMJ 343:d4163

Hutchinson TA (2012) Whole person care. In: Hutchinson TA (ed) Whole person care, vol 1. Springer, Chapter, pp 1–8

Koenig HG, McCullough ME, Larson DB (2010) Handbook of religion and health. Oxford University Press, New York, NY

Kruizinga R, Scherer-Rath M, Schilderman HJBAM, Puchalski CM, van Laarhoven HHWM (2018) Toward a fully fledged integration of spiritual care and medical care. J Pain Symptom Manag 55(3):1035–1040

Maugans TA (1996) The SPIRITual history. Arch Fam Med 5(1):11–16

McCabe R, Murray R, Austin P, Siddall P (2018) Spiritual and existential factors predict pain relief in a pain management program with a meaning-based component. Journal of Pain Management 11(2):163–170

McCord G, Gilchrist V, Grossman S, King BD, McCormick KE, Oprandi AM, Schrop SL, Selius BA, Smucker WD, Weldy DL, Amorn M, Carter MA, Deak AJ, Hefzy H, Srivastava M (2004) Discussing spirituality with patients: a rational and ethical approach. Ann Fam Med 2(4):356–361

Meaningful Ageing Australia (2016) National guidelines for spiritual care in aged care. Ageing Australia, Parkville. https://meaningfulageing.org.au/national-guidelines-for-spiritual-care-in-aged-care/ Accesses 28 Aug 2020

Monod S, Rochat E, Büla CJ, Jobin G, Martin E, Spencer B (2010) The spiritual distress assessment tool: an instrument to assess spiritual distress in hospitalised elderly persons. BMC Geriatr 10(88). https://doi.org/10.1186/1471-2318-10-88

National Consensus Project for Quality Palliative Care (2020) Domain 5: spiritual, religious, and existential aspects of care. In: National Consensus Project for Quality Palliative Care (eds) Clinical practice guidelines for quality palliative care, 4th edn. http://nchpc.conferencespot.org/67968-nchpc-1.4266595/t009-1.4266773/f009-1.4266774/a054-1.4266785. Accesses 28 Aug 2020

NCCN Guidelines for Patients: Distress. https://www.nccn.org/patients/guidelines/content/PDF/distress-patient.pdf. Accessed 4 June 2020

Powell LH, Shabbi L, Thoreson CE (2003) Religion and spirituality linkages to physical health. Am Psychol 58:36–52

Puchalski CM, Ferrell B (2010) Making healthcare whole. Templeton Press, West Conshohoken, PA

Puchalski CM, Romer AL (2000) Taking a spiritual history allows clinicians to understand patients more fully. J Palliat Med 3(1):129–137

Puchalski C, Ferrell B, Virani R, Otis-Green S, Baird P, Bull J, Chochinov H, Handzo G, Nelson-Becker H, Prince-Paul M, Pugliese K, Sulmasy D (2009) Improving the quality of spiritual care as a dimension of palliative care: the report of the consensus conference. J Palliat Med 12:885–904

Puchalski C, Blatt B, Kogan M, Butler A (2014a) Spirituality and health: the development of a field. Acad Med 89(1):10–16

Puchalski CM, Vitillo R, Hull SK, Reller N (2014b) Improving the spiritual dimension of whole person care: reaching national and international consensus. J Palliat Med 17(6):642–656

Puchalski CM, Sbrana A, Ferrell B, Jafari N, King S, Balboni T, Miccinesi G, Vandenhoeck A, Silbermann M, Balducci L, Yong J, Antonuzzo A, Falcone A, Ripamonti CI (2019) Interprofessional spiritual care in oncology: a literature review. ESMO Open 4(1):e000465–e000465

Puchalski C, Bauer R, Ferrell B et al (2020a) Interprofessional spiritual care in the time of COVID-19. http://globalpalliativecare.org/covid-19/uploads/briefing-notes/briefing-note-interprofessional-spiritual-care-in-the-time-of-covid-19.pdf. Accesses 28 Aug 2020

Puchalski C, Jafari N, Buller H, Haythorn T, Jacobs C, Ferrell B (2020b) Interprofessional spiritual care education curriculum: a milestone toward the provision of spiritual care. J Palliat Med 23(6):777–784

Selman LE, Harding-Swale R, Agupio G, Fox P, Galimaka D, Mmoledi K, Higginson I, and the Spiritual Care in sub-Saharan Africa Advisory Group (2010) Spiritual care recommendations for people receiving palliative care in sub-Saharan Africa: with special reference to South Africa and Uganda. Cicely Saunders International, London. https://www.kcl.ac.uk/cicelysaunders/attachments/Spiritual-care-Africa-Full-report.pdf. Accesses 28 Aug 2020

Shukla S (2020) Spirituality in Ayurveda. Spirituality in Clinical Practice 7(2):103–113

Siddall PJ, Lovell M, MacLeod R (2015) Spirituality: what is its role in pain medicine? Pain Med 16(1):51–60

World Health Organization Executive Board (2014) Strengthening of palliative care as a component of comprehensive care throughout the life course. Paper presented at: WHO sixty-seventh world health assembly 2014. J Pain Palliative Care Pharmacothe 28(2):130–134

CHAPTER 4

Using the Spiritual Needs Questionnaire: A Perspective from the Ethics of Care

Carlo Leget

Introduction

There is no question that any assessment of personal views, perspectives and behavior of patients and clients, including the use of a spiritual care questionnaire, has a moral dimension. Like any human action that is deliberately and freely chosen it is related to moral values like respect and justice. In the context of health and social care, there are also issues of vulnerability, autonomy and confidentiality. And when we speak about spirituality, all this is intensified, since we are dealing with the ultimate concern of what a human life is about: existential meaning, transcendence and what is sacred to people (Puchalski et al. 2014).

An ethical perspective on spiritual care in health care is often limited to the four famous principles of respect for autonomy, beneficence, non-maleficence and justice (Beauchamp and Childress 2012). This approach is helpful for making a quick analysis. Based on these four moral principles that are generally agreed upon, the most important questions regarding

C. Leget (✉)
University of Humanistic Studies, Utrecht, The Netherlands
e-mail: C.Leget@UvH.nl

A. Büssing (ed.), *Spiritual Needs in Research and Practice*,
https://doi.org/10.1007/978-3-030-70139-0_4

the spiritual needs questionnaire seem to be the following: (1) Does the questionnaire respect the autonomy of the patient or client? (2) Is it likely that the questionnaire adds to the well-being of the patient or client? (3) Is there any risk that the questionnaire does any harm to the patient or client? (4) Do all patients or clients have an equal opportunity to benefit from the questionnaire?

Questions like these are important to ask. It is a good thing that as a reaction to the involuntary medical experiments on human beings in the twentieth century, medical research worldwide is nowadays subjected to approval by ethical committees (Ten Have 2016). In this way, an attempt is made to protect patients and clients in vulnerable positions. So far so good. From a philosophical perspective, however, such an ethical approach remains a rather formal one. It is similar to a legal perspective that focuses on the question of whether moral boundaries are transgressed rather than the moral dimension of what happens inside those boundaries.

In this contribution, I will develop a perspective on the spiritual needs questionnaire that focuses on the moral dimension of what happens inside the boundaries of the four principles that have been listed earlier. I will assume that the reader has sufficient moral awareness to identify examples of using the questionnaire in a way that does not respect the autonomy of the patient or is in contradiction with the principles of beneficence, non-maleficence or justice. Even if all these principles apply, more can be said about the moral dimension of a spiritual needs questionnaire. For this I will focus on different kind of questions: What is care? What are (spiritual) needs? What ethical awareness is needed to use the spiritual needs questionnaire in a good way? My intention is not so much to formulate definitive and universal answers, but to promote moral sensitivity and ethical questioning.

For this task I will use an interdisciplinary field of studies that is known as 'care ethics' or 'ethics of care' (Held 2006). Care ethics is not to be confused with ethics in health or social care. Ethics in health or social care is any kind of ethics focusing on a specific domain in society. Many different traditions and approaches in ethics can do this job, like we have just seen in the case of the four principles of Beauchamp and Childress that are often used in the domain of health and social care. Care ethics, on the other hand, is an ethical perspective itself; a lens—so to speak—that can be used to look at any domain in society, including the domain of health and social care (Leget et al. 2019).

In the field of care ethics the view on care is far from romantic. Care is not seen as a soft ideal exemplified in, for example, the loving relationship between mother and child. Neither is care seen as intrinsically good in itself. Care is seen as an essential and universal human practice full of complexity and potential conflicts. In care relationships there are always issues of vulnerability, power, responsibility and inequality. Care relationships are always embedded in cultural and political contexts and they mirror the morally good and bad features of these conditions. This makes care a helpful lens for moral reflection and evaluation.

Setting the Stage: What Is Care?

Because ethics focuses on the moral dimension of human action, any moral evaluation of using the spiritual needs questionnaire will come across the question of how to delineate the use of the questionnaire and define this action? Where does it start and where does it end? How important is the context in which it is used? How important are the intentions of the user? And should any unforeseen and unintended consequences of using the questionnaire also be included in a moral evaluation? There are many questions and they ask for a coherent view on what is actually done when using a spiritual needs questionnaire. How can care ethics be helpful in developing such a coherent view?

In care ethics, care is often defined in a broad way as "a species activity that includes everything that we do to maintain, continue, and repair our 'world' so that we can live in it as well as possible. That world includes our bodies, ourselves, and our environment … all of which we seek to interweave in a complex, life-sustaining web" (Tronto and Fisher 1990). Following this definition care is a phenomenon that can be seen in many different forms in many different contexts. From this perspective it is clear that the use of a spiritual needs questionnaire can be seen as a form of care. Using the questionnaire is an activity and this complex, life-sustaining web is composed of formal and informal caring relations, crossing the boundaries of the private and public sphere that hold together our societies. From a care ethical perspective, the activity of caring connects the personal with the professional dimension of our lives, and the private with the political. Caring comprises both my personal motivation and intentions (the things I care about) and my actions (the things I take care of).

One of the defining insights in care ethics is that caring is both a disposition and a practice (Tronto 1993). By seeing caring as a disposition, the relation with intention, motivation, character and virtue is secured. Considering the use of the spiritual needs questionnaire as a form of care implies that the instrument is used in a caring or careful way. Instruments can do harm if they are used in a wrong way, as anyone who has ever struggled with a hammer would know. Care without this caring attitude is experienced as cold and painful. People may suddenly feel like a piece of flesh instead of a patient. In medical education this dimension is often addressed in terms of empathy or compassion.

By defining care as a practice, care ethics views caring as a coherent set of actions aimed at a goal that holds these actions together (Rouse 2006). Considering the use of the spiritual needs questionnaire as a practice means that the use of this questionnaire is embedded in a larger context of caring for a patient. Using the spiritual needs questionnaire without such a context raises questions. The use of the questionnaire should make sense and be connected to a larger goal in which the well-being of the patient is intended (in the case of care) or safeguarded (in the case of research). So by considering the use of the instrument as a practice, one becomes sensitive to the nature of caring as a process and the elements that can be discerned in that process. Let us take a closer look at the different steps in this process and see what questions they can generate about the use of the spiritual needs questionnaire.

Phases of Caring

Few insights from care ethics have been quoted more often than the four phases of caring that were defined by Joan Tronto and Berenice Fisher (Tronto and Fisher 1990). In her book *Moral Boundaries* Joan Tronto connected these four phases with four moral qualities or ethical elements (Tronto 1993), and in her book *Caring Democracy* she added a fifth phase of a somewhat different nature, connecting them all with democratic commitments to justice, equality and freedom for all (Tronto 2013). In this contribution we will focus on the four phases of caring that can be distinguished, but need all to be there in order to consider a practice as a form of care and not a fragment of care.

Caring About

Caring starts with identifying unmet caring needs. This first phase is connected with the moral quality of attentiveness. In the case of health care, it is noteworthy that responding to spiritual needs has been under the radar for many decades. In the 1990s many considered it a step forward when the focus of health care was expanded from attention to physical problems and needs to attention to the psychosocial dimension of needs. Since then, partly fueled by developments in palliative care, an attempt has been made to broaden the focus to include the spiritual dimension as well (Sulmasy 2006). From these developments one might learn that identifying needs presupposes awareness of the existence of these needs and a language to express them.

From the perspective of care ethics this raises the question of whether this attentiveness to spiritual needs (or rather the spiritual dimension of needs) can be seen as a professional competency that might be expected from every professional working in health and social care. This is a political-ethical question, referring to the way we organize society and allocate money to and within health and social care (education). Professional caring practices are always embedded in institutional structures and the question of attentiveness starts from this institutional dimension.

But professional caring practices are also always full of relations of power and inequalities. Attentiveness to spiritual needs may have a risk of projecting and proselytizing. Is there really a spiritual need of a patient or client, or rather a preoccupation, 'mission' or wishful thinking of a caregiver? Care professionals have authority and power connected to their professional status, and being aware of this is part of their professional responsibility.

This said, one of the benefits of the spiritual needs questionnaire can be that it helps professionals to develop a sense of what spiritual needs may be about. It can be helpful in education as it presents concrete questions that have been validated as being helpful for a large group of patients in different situations and cultures. In that sense the instrument may help to promote its own use in practice by preparing the first phase of caring, and the moral quality of attentiveness.

Caring For

The next step in the caring process is to take responsibility and make sure that the right steps are taken so that care needs are met. But what are the right steps? And when is the use of the questionnaire the right step in taking care of spiritual needs? From a care ethical perspective, a central question is who defines what a need is. People might disagree about the importance of the spiritual dimension: some people consider care for the soul as the core of whole-person care, others see it as an add-on that has no place inside medicine because it lacks a solid scientific basis. Is a need whatever the patient says it is, or is a need something that has to be distinguished from wishes or desires? The resources in health and social care are scarce and a hospital is not a wellness hotel.

Once one agrees with the idea that spiritual needs belong to health and social care, what is the right way of organizing taking care of them? Is the spiritual needs questionnaire the right way to address needs because it is based on solid research, or does the questionnaire itself prematurely frame unarticulated patient feelings of uneasiness in predefined categories? Is the questionnaire open enough to secure the spiritual process of the patient finding his or her own words? If the free text fields in the questionnaire are rarely used, what does this tell us? Is the questionnaire open enough for this specific and individual patient who is not easily allocated to one of the versions of the instrument?

Here we touch upon another interesting set of questions regarding the use of the spiritual needs questionnaire as a practice. Should the use of this instrument be a standard procedure with all patients (with the risk of burdening patients unnecessarily)? Or should it be dependent on the attentiveness and sensitivity of particular caregivers (with the risk of not giving all patients equal access to care in this dimension)? There is no universal answer to this question: it depends on the context of the practice of caring about what a good decision is. But part of the answer will be connected with the overarching view of the institutional context on what is considered to be good health and social care. And different cultural contexts bring different sensitivities: tools from a country where the majority of the population belongs to a religious community may meet resistance in more secularized countries.

Reflecting on the phase of 'caring for' and the moral quality of responsibility, an important feature of care ethics comes to the fore: the right thing to do is always dependent on a great number of contextual elements, and the moral quality of responsibility cannot be replaced by a textbook or a code (Walker 2007). Responsibility, just like attentiveness, is a quality of a person by which he or she is able to respond to particular situations in a morally good way. In classical terms, they are virtues that need practice in order to be learned and perfected. The same is applicable for the next phase of the caring process and its ethical element.

Caregiving

The phase of caregiving is when the caring activity is actually done. It is connected with the moral quality of competence. Incompetent caregiving can be harmful or dangerous. Competent caregiving requires certain skills. When we consider the spiritual needs questionnaire, we can raise the question of whether the use of the questionnaire itself is a caring practice, or rather the preparation for a caring practice. Since the instrument can be used either as a diagnostic tool or a research instrument, it is obvious that it can be used as a preparation for a caring practice. From a care ethical perspective, however, the use of the instrument is also a caring practice itself, used either as a diagnostic tool or a research instrument. The reason for this is that the goal of the questionnaire is the identification of needs that are related to what is sacred to people.

Competent use of the questionnaire involves responsibility on the side of the professional in a number of ways. It should be used respectfully, voluntarily, in the right version, at the right time, in an atmosphere of patience and confidentiality, with attention to what it might evoke, and taking care of possible aftercare. This responsibility has a moral dimension (being related to respect), but also an impact on the quality of the results. It makes a difference both to the process and the outcome of the use of the questionnaire if a patient or client is asked to fill in the questionnaire knowing that there is no further time to discuss or explore spiritual needs, or if the same thing is done with a caregiver who is present and signals that there is time to explore possible questions or issues that might come up.

Competence has both professional and personal elements. Apart from their personal qualities, professionals from different professions have different positions, responsibilities and competencies. For this reason distinction can be made between three ways of providing spiritual care (IKNL 2018).

The first way is spiritual caregiving as a dimension of other caring activities or practices; it is a shared responsibility of all caregivers. When a patient is washed, for example, a spontaneous conversation may come up in which the spiritual dimension of becoming a grandmother is touched upon. For some patients or clients just listening and sharing a moment of attentiveness may be enough to fulfill their spiritual needs. Central to spiritual care as a dimension are the virtues of attentiveness and nonjudgmental openness. In this embedded and often implicit way of providing spiritual care, using the spiritual needs questionnaire is not appropriate.

The second way of spiritual caregiving is related to the practice of accompaniment. In this case the conversation on the spiritual dimension is more explicit. There are many ways of accompaniment, depending on the profession, education and possibilities of the caregivers: from the more spontaneous series of conversations with a nurse who happens to be from the same religious background to the spiritual assessment by a chaplain. In spiritual accompaniment the use of the questionnaire may be a good way of exploring spiritual needs, but there may also be situations in which this is not fitting.

The third way of spiritual caregiving pertains to situation of a spiritual crisis. When a patient or client shows signs of great restlessness, feelings of guilt, fear or forms of spiritual distress, a caregiver who is specialized in spiritual caregiving should be contacted. In this situation the spiritual needs questionnaire may be a useful instrument and a great help. But also, then, its use should be embedded in a practice of attentiveness and competence.

Care-Receiving

The fourth phase of caring makes it very clear that caring is a relational practice and is connected with the moral quality of responsiveness. Even if a spiritual need has been identified, the question remains as to what the appropriate way of responding to this need might be. A patient or client may confirm that they are wrestling with spiritual issues, just as the questionnaire has demonstrated, but still decide not to talk about it. Or once a need has been identified, and there are many more needs in different dimensions of health, one might consider the right order to address these needs. The fourth phase of caring is inherently ethical in putting the patient or client in the lead again. Caring is not a one-sided or one-way activity. It is a relational practice between two or more parties that attune to each other.

The fourth phase of caring is connected to another phenomenon of importance. Caregiving may not only have impact on the care receiver, but also on the caregiver. While in conversation about what is sacred to people one may be confronted with one's own philosophy of life or religious background. Good conversations open up new horizons in both partners of a dialogue (Gadamer 1975). Being involved in a spiritual conversation is a process of giving and receiving. In that sense, using the spiritual needs questionnaire may also lead to becoming aware of one's own spiritual needs.

Conclusion

In this contribution we reflected on the spiritual needs questionnaire from a care ethical perspective. We explored the ethical dimension of using the questionnaire by understanding this use as a caring practice that comprises four phases. Each phase is connected with the moral quality of the one who provides care. Working with the spiritual needs questionnaire (either in care or in research) asks for attentiveness to its ethical dimension, the characteristics of the context and the particularities of each unique patient or client. Using the spiritual needs questionnaire in an ethically good way entails more than having one's care practice or research plans checked by an ethical committee. It requires a caring attitude that is characterized by attentiveness, responsibility, competency and responsiveness. The practice of caring is an open encounter of two or more unique people who are moral actors capable of free decisions and initiatives (van Heijst 2011). Using the spiritual needs questionnaire is a practice with an intrinsically moral dimension that requires a professional who takes responsibility for what this practice might do to the patient or client.

References

Beauchamp T, Childress J (2012) Principles of biomedical ethics, 7th edn. Oxford University Press, Oxford

Gadamer HG (1975) Truth and method. Seabury Press, New York, NY

Held V (2006) The ethics of care. In: Copp D (ed) Oxford handbook of ethical theory. Oxford University Press, Oxford, pp 537–566

Integraal Kancercentrum Nederland (IKNL) (2018) Existential and spiritual aspects of palliative care. National guideline. https://www.pallialine.nl/. Accessed 31 Aug 2020

Leget C, van Nistelrooij I, Visse M (2019) Beyond demarcation: care ethics as an interdisciplinary field of inquiry. Nurs Ethics 26:17–25

Puchalski CM, Vitillo R, Hull SK, Reller N (2014) Improving the spiritual dimension of whole person care: reaching national and international consensus. J Palliat Med 17:642–656

Rouse J (2006) Practice theory. In: Turner S, Risjord M (eds) Philosophy of anthropology and sociology. Elsevier, Dordrecht, pp 639–681

Sulmasy DP (2006) The rebirth of the clinic: an introduction to spirituality in health care. Georgetown University Press, Washington, DC
Ten Have H (2016) Global bioethics: an introduction. Routledge, New York
Tronto J (1993) Moral boundaries: an ethic of care. Routledge, New York
Tronto J (2013) Caring democracy. Markets, equality, justice. New York University Press, New York and London
Tronto J, Fisher B (1990) Toward a feminist theory of caring. In: Abel EK, Nelson MK (eds) Circles of care: work and identity in women's lives. State University of New York Press, Albany, pp 36–54
Van Heijst A (2011) Professional loving care: an ethical view of the healthcare sector. Peeters, Leuven
Walker MU (2007) Moral understandings. A feminist study in ethics. Oxford University Press, Oxford

PART II

Assessment of Spiritual Needs

CHAPTER 5

Assessing Patients' Spiritual Needs in Healthcare: An Overview of Questionnaires

Ricko Damberg Nissen and Niels Christian Hvidt

Introduction

Assessing the spiritual needs of patients is, and has, over the last decades been a growing area of attention in both healthcare research and clinical practice. Research has shown that spiritual and/or religious existential considerations and needs increase with life-threatening illness, and that these needs intensify with the severity of disease and the prospect of (immanent) death (Cadge and Bandini 2015; Gijsberts et al. 2019; Harrad et al. 2019). Research has also argued, however, that spirituality is an important coping resource, and that quality of life increases when spiritual needs are addressed and when spiritual care is provided in appropriate ways (Balboni et al. 2010; Büssing and Koenig 2010; Jafari et al. 2013). This kind of care is now widely known internationally as *spiritual care*. Success has many fathers though, and there are many different

R. D. Nissen (✉) • N. C. Hvidt
Research Unit of General Practice, Department of Public Health, University of Southern Denmark, Odense, Denmark
e-mail: rnissen@health.sdu.dk; nchvidt@health.sdu.dk

A. Büssing (ed.), *Spiritual Needs in Research and Practice*,
https://doi.org/10.1007/978-3-030-70139-0_5

understandings of what spiritual care is, what it can be, and what it ought to be (El Nawawi et al. 2012; Greasley et al. 2001; Hummel et al. 2008; Nolan et al. 2011; Ramezani et al. 2014; Østergaard Steenfeldt 2018). This resides partly in the fact that defining spirituality in an international context has proven continuously elusive (Hall et al. 2004; Hill et al. 2000; la Cour et al. 2012; la Cour and Hvidt 2010), and partly in the fact that spiritual care is not a 'quick fix', but rather a continuous process (Nissen et al. 2020; Burkhart et al. 2011).

Furthermore, but just as importantly, spiritual care is a relationship between patient and healthcare professional (HCP) and is realized in trust and empathy, demanding a level of knowledge from the HCP of both the secular/spiritual/religious existential domains (la Cour and Hvidt 2010) and of how the individual patient relates to these domains. As this is (often) a private area and intrinsic to the individual, it is not easily approachable, and ethical considerations and professional boundaries also need to be taken into account (Nissen et al. 2018). Following this, it might not come as a surprise that research also shows that patients often find their spiritual needs unmet (Gibson et al. 2004; Sharma et al. 2012), and that patients and HCPs alike find it difficult to express and address spiritual needs (Assing Hvidt et al. 2018; Balboni et al. 2014; Pedersen and Post 2012; Rushton 2014; Slort et al. 2011), illustrating a 'gap' between the spiritual and religious domains and the secular grounding of healthcare. Finally, an understanding of and an approach to spiritual care need not only be able to include the various religious and spiritual orientations, but also to consider that people who are grounded in a secular worldview may still have needs of an existential character that does not include spiritual beliefs or practices, but interpret their needs as existential or in humanistic terms (Büssing and Koenig 2010). Therefore, it is necessary to ascertain an understanding of patients' secular/spiritual/religious beliefs and practices before the individual-specific approach to spiritual care can be developed.

Even though we see spirituality[1] as an elusive concept defying exact definition, it is an approach we entertain to keep in sight that spirituality is a constructed concept that does not automatically 'fit' the individual

[1] In this study we focus exclusively on the concept of spirituality, and even though the concepts of existential and religious are intertwined with spirituality they fall outside the aim of this paper and are thus not included in this discussion. For differentiation and discussion of the concepts in relation to health, see la Cour and Hvidt (2010).

patient who is in need of spiritual care. We will counterbalance this understanding with the European Association for Palliative Cares (EAPC) definition of spirituality, which is based on and adjusted from the North American Consensus Project for Quality Palliative Care definition of spirituality (Puchalski et al. 2009): "Spirituality is the dynamic dimension of human life that relates to the way persons (individual and community) experience, express and/or seek meaning, purpose and transcendence, and the way they connect to the moment, to self, to others, to nature, to the significant and/or the sacred" (Nolan et al. 2011).

This definition suggests spiritual care should not be taken lightly or addressed without serious reflection, which is also likely to be part of the explanation as to why so many approaches to and understandings of spiritual care have been developed (Nissen et al. 2020). It also illustrates that spiritual care is a process.

The aim of this paper is to present an overview of questionnaires developed to assess the spiritual needs of patients and to place them in relation to a discussion of international relevance. The understanding of spiritual care as a process is one of the criteria for inclusion of the instruments as outlined here. The instruments are drawn from the Catalogue of Spiritual Care (Nissen et al. 2020), which will also be presented in this chapter.

Approach

The Catalogue of Spiritual Care Instruments (CSCI) (Nissen et al. 2020) is employed in the initial search for literature. The CSCI is a scoping review (Daudt 2013) aimed at locating instruments used in the healthcare context in the process of providing spiritual care. The CSCI, which is available online (https://faith-health.org/catalogue), has 182 entries, located in a wide range of healthcare areas and international contexts, employing a variety of approaches.

As mentioned, an understanding of spiritual care as a process is entertained in this study. This understanding sees spiritual care spanning (at least) four phases that potentially involve (1) the identification/assessment of spiritual needs, hereunder understanding the individual patient's specific needs; (2) developing the individual spiritual care treatment plan, hereunder involving the relevant HCPs; (3) the provision of spiritual care in terms of concrete support or interventions; and (4) evaluating the spiritual care provided (Nissen et al. 2020). This is not to be seen as a definition of spiritual care, rather, it is a way to bring into view what may seem evident, namely, that providing spiritual care takes time, and that various approaches and instruments are necessary in order to provide adequate and appropriate spiritual care. Burkhart and colleagues, for instance, who also identified spiritual care as a process, developed the Spiritual Care Inventory as an instrument to evaluate the process of spiritual care from the nurses' perspective (Burkhart et al. 2011). Through this understanding it becomes clear that the assessment of spiritual needs is likely to be located in phase 1, but also that a later assessment is relevant in order to evaluate whether the provided spiritual care has had the desired effect.

Spiritual Needs Assessment Questionnaires

In this overview we have included questionnaires assessing spiritual needs selected from the CSCI, based on the criteria for inclusion that they were located in phase 1 (identifying spiritual needs) employed or applicable in clinical practice, and the articles and questionnaires had to be available in English. Table 5.1 presents the 22 questionnaires in this overview. The questionnaires are listed alphabetically and further include the article reference, year, national context, and healthcare area. The Comment column provides a short description of the questionnaires.

Discussion of Questionnaires

As was argued in the introduction, spirituality is an elusive concept, continuously defying international consensus on its definition. When seen from the macro level this understanding can be regarded as an expression of the immense cultural variation of the human world(s), and the general difficulties of defining concepts internationally and cross-culturally. When seen from the micro level the elusiveness of the concept can be seen as an expression of the existential (ontological) grounding of the individual worldview of both patient and HCP. The following discussion will look at what the questionnaires assess, which healthcare areas the questionnaires are located in, who is doing the assessment and when the assessment is taking place, and a broader discussion of spirituality in relation to spiritual care in an international and cross-cultural context.

Most of the included questionnaires employ a Likert scale response, ranging from a 4-point Likert scale to a 7-point Likert scale. Two questionnaires (PSNAS and SpNQ) employ a varied type of Likert scale, combining a yes/no answer with a Likert scale response. One questionnaire,

Table 5.1 List of questionnaires that aim to address spiritual needs, spiritual well-being, spiritual distress, and so on (alphabetically listed)

Questionnaire name/ abbreviation	*Author/year/ origin*	*Healthcare area*	*Comment*
Existential Distress Scale (EDS)	Lo et al. (2017) CAN	Oncology	10-item, 5-point Likert scale. Measures existential distress in patients with advanced cancer. Not validated but showing promising psychometric properties
Functional Assessment of Chronic Illness Therapy-Spiritual Well-Being (FACIT-Sp-12)	Peterman et al. (2002) USA	Oncology, Chronic illness	12-item, 5-point Likert scale. Brief measure of spiritual well-being. Two subscales, one measuring sense of meaning and the other, peace. Psychometrically sound measure of spiritual well-being
Holistic Health Status Questionnaire (HHSQ)	Chan et al. (2016) HKG	Chronic illness	45-item, 4-point Likert scale. 8-factor holistic health status measurement including religion/ spirituality. Demonstrated content validity and acceptable internal consistency. Culturally sensitive to Chinese-speaking populations
JAREL Spiritual Well-Being Scale (JAREL SWBS)	Hungelmann et al. (1996) USA	General health; Elderly	21-item, 6-point Likert scale. 3-factor assessment of spiritual well-being or spiritual distress. Developed to assist in formulating nursing diagnoses and interventions
Meaning in Life Scale (MILS)	Jim et al. (2006) USA	Oncology	21-item, 6-point Likert scale. Psychometrically sound measure of meaning in life, including spiritual concerns and resources
Psychosocial and Spiritual Needs Evaluation Scale (ENP-E)	Mateo-Ortega et al. (2018) ESP	End-of-life, Palliative care, Oncology	12-item, 6-point Likert scale. Holistic assessment of the psychosocial and spiritual needs of end-of-life patients to enable psychosocial and spiritual/ religious-specific individualized interventions
Quality-of-Life Questionnaire Spiritual Well-Being-32 (QLQ-SWB-32)	Vivat et al. (2017) EU/EORTC[a]	Oncology, Palliative care	32-item, 4-point Likert scale. An internationally validated cross-cultural stand-alone measure of spiritual well-being. Suitable for various religions and none-religious

(*continued*)

Table 5.1 (continued)

Questionnaire name/ abbreviation	*Author/year/ origin*	*Healthcare area*	*Comment*
Religious Spiritual Screening Protocol (RSSP)	Fitchett and Risk (2009) USA	General health	Brief screening protocol to enable non-chaplain HCP to identify patients experiencing religious/ spiritual struggle, who may need spiritual care services and/or a visit from a chaplain
Spirit 8	Selman et al. (2012) RSA	Palliative care	8-item, 5-point Likert scale. A brief, psychometrically robust measure of spiritual well-being for use in South African and Ugandan palliative care and palliative care research
Spiritual Assessment Scale (SAS)	O'Brien (1993) USA	Chronic illness	21-item, 5-point Likert scale. Enables the nurse to get a broad overview of the patient's personal beliefs, the type of spiritual support the patient receives from religious practice, and the type and degree of spiritual contentment/distress the patient is currently experiencing
Spiritual Care Needs Inventory (SCNI)	Wu et al. (2016) TWN	Acute care	21-item, 5-point Likert scale. Assessing spiritual care needs of acute care patients in a multi-faith context. Internal consistency for measuring the spiritual care needs in acute care hospital patients
Spiritual Care Needs Scale (SCNS)	Otuzoglu and Talas (2019) TUR	Oncology, Chronic illness	24-item, 5-point Likert scale. A valid and reliable measurement tool to determine the spiritual care needs of patients with cancer and chronic illness. Clinical practice and research
Spiritual Distress Scale (SDS)	Ku et al. (2010) TWN	Oncology	30-item, 4-point Likert scale. 4-factor subscales. Established content and construct validity. Developed in oncology for nurses to assess spiritual distress of cancer patients

(*continued*)

Table 5.1 (continued)

Questionnaire name/ abbreviation	*Author/year/ origin*	*Healthcare area*	*Comment*
Spiritual Interests Related to Illness Tool (SpIRIT)	Taylor (2006) USA	Oncology, Palliative care	42 items, 5-point Likert scale. Self-report, spiritual needs assessment of whether religious/ spiritual needs are being met in care
Spiritual Needs Assessment for Patients (SNAP)	Sharma et al. (2012) USA	Oncology, General health	23-item, 4-point Likert scale. 3 domains. A valid and reliable instrument for assessing spiritual needs of patients in a culturally diverse population
Spiritual Needs Inventory (SNI)	Hermann (2006) USA	End-of-life, Oncology, Palliative care	17-item, 5-point Likert scale. A valid and reliable assessment of spiritual needs of patients near the end of life and whether those needs are met in care. Useful in the clinical setting and in studies of spiritual needs
Spiritual Needs Questionnaire for Palliative Care (SNQPC)	Vilalta et al. (2014) ESP	Oncology, Palliative care	28-item, 5-point Likert scale. Assessing spiritual needs of terminal cancer patients
Spiritual Needs Questionnaire (SpNQ)	Büssing et al. (2010, 2018) GER	Chronic illness, Elderly, Palliative care Pediatrics	20- to 27-item varied Likert scale. 4-factor structure. Measures psychosocial, existential and spiritual needs. Validated in persons with chronic illness, elderly and healthy stressed persons. Various healthcare settings
Spiritual Needs Survey (SNS)	Galek et al. (2005) USA	Palliative care, General health	29-item, yes/no and 4-point Likert scale. 7 constructs assessing spiritual needs. Designed for religiously heterogeneous populations, inclusive of traditional religion and non-institutionally based spirituality

(*continued*)

Table 5.1 (continued)

Questionnaire name/ abbreviation	*Author/year/ origin*	*Healthcare area*	*Comment*
Spiritual Needs Scale (Korea) (SNS (K))	Yong et al. (2008) KOR	Oncology	26-item, 5-point Likert scale. 5 subconstructs. Spiritual needs measurement. Provides nurses and other HCPs with an appropriate way to identify spiritual needs of patients in practice and research settings
Spiritual Transformation Scale (STS)	Cole et al. (2008) USA	Oncology	40-item, 7-point Likert scale. Across 4 domains. A reliable and valid method to measure spiritual growth and spiritual decline following a cancer diagnosis
Thai Spiritual Well-being Assessment Tool for Elders with Chronic Illnesses (TSWBATECI)	Unsanit et al. (2012) THA	Elderly, Chronic illness	41-item, 5-point Likert scale. A valid and reliable instrument for assessing spiritual well-being of elderly Thais with chronic illnesses. Developed using chronically ill elders who were Buddhist, Islamic or Christian

[a]The European Organisation for Research and Treatment of Cancer

the RSSP, is a yes/no screening protocol to be used by the HCP to determine whether a patient has spiritual distress and whether the patient wants to see a chaplain. In relation to the validity of the included questionnaires, the referral to validity in the comment box in Table 5.1 is taken from the articles and thus represents the authors' referral to the validity of the questionnaires. This means that there is no congruence in Table 5.1 in relation to validity and the individual articles will have to be visited to research the individual criteria for validation as there are, of course, large discrepancies between the various questionnaires. As an example, the QLQ-SWB-32 was validated by an international project group over several phases in a large and varied population ($N = 451$) from 14 countries in four continents (Vivat et al. 2017). The EDS on the contrary was pilot-tested on 21 patients, showing some promising psychometric properties, and the authors call for future validation studies to be made (Lo et al. 2017).

The questionnaires in this overview was, of course, included on the basis that they are aimed at assessing spiritual needs. However, the way this aim is formulated varies, with respect to and considering local understandings of the concept of *spirituality*. Two overriding categories emerge:

- Instruments assessing/measuring spiritual needs: ENP-E, RSSP, SCNI, SCNS, SDS, SNAP, SNI, SNQPC, SNS, SNS (K), SpIRIT, SpNQ
- Instruments assessing/measuring spiritual well-being: Facit-Sp-12, JAREL SWBS, QLQ-SWB-32, Spirit 8, TSWBATECI

This is not meant to imply that these two categories are in opposition; assessing for spiritual needs might show spiritual well-being, just as assessing spiritual well-being might show spiritual needs. Two questionnaires are aimed at spiritual contentment/distress/growth/decline (SAS, STS), one is focused on existential distress (EDS) and two are aimed at spiritual needs as part of a larger assessment instrument (HHSQ, MILS). Except for the RSSP, the questionnaires are applicable as self-/patient-reported outcome measures or can be answered with the assistance of an HCP. The included questionnaires are located in phase 1 in the process of spiritual care, as a spiritual needs assessment tool after being diagnosed or after hospitalization.

The questionnaires have been developed and employed in a variety of healthcare areas. The healthcare areas are Oncology (N = 13), Palliative care (N = 8), Chronic illness (N = 6), General health (N = 5), Elderly (N = 3), End-of-life (N = 2), Acute care (N = 1). Some questionnaires are employed in more than one healthcare area, which is why the total number of areas (N = 38) exceeds the number of questionnaires (N = 22) (see Table 5.1). It is expected that spiritual needs arise in healthcare areas which involve life-threatening conditions and the prospect of immanent death such as in oncology and palliative care, where existential questions are almost forced to the surface, be they secular, spiritual or religious. The category End-of-life includes the two instruments SNI and ENP-E. The SNI was developed in hospice settings and with patients dying of cancer. Even though End-of-life is not technically a health area, the authors mention End-of-life, thereby implying that the questionnaire is not exclusively for patients dying of cancer, and there are no questions in the questionnaire specifically aimed at cancer, hence the questionnaire is applicable in other healthcare settings as well. The ENP-E was also developed with an End-of-life focus primarily in oncology and palliative care settings. Again, there are no questions in the questionnaire relating to cancer specifically and the ENP-E is therefore also applicable in other healthcare settings. One questionnaire, the TSWBATECI, is aimed specifically at the elderly (60+ years), who suffer from a chronic illness. The combination of chronic illness and the elderly is also found in the SpNQ, which has been applied to patients and relatives in emergency room settings. None of the included questionnaires addresses geriatrics specifically, even though it is expected that people dying of old age also experience spiritual needs. One instrument, the SCNI, was developed specifically within acute care, particularly to assess spiritual care needs in an acute care setting in Taiwan. As Wu et al. point out, acute care patients also experience spiritual needs and distress, even though little is known about this area. Wu et al. invoke transition theory to argue that people in any kind of health crisis are likely to undergo a transition and face increased vulnerability, hopelessness, and, potentially, spiritual crisis (Wu et al. 2016). The PSNAS was developed in general health and was specifically designed to be applicable in hospital settings, and the JAREL SWBS was developed specifically for nursing and is not focused on a specific health area. The RSSP was developed in chaplaincy, as a questionnaire enabling the HCP to screen patients for spiritual struggles and determine whether there is need for a visit from the chaplain.

This raises a general question of who is the appropriate person to assist in the assessment of spiritual needs. Several of the instruments have been developed with the nurse as the primary HCP (EDS, JAREL SWBS, SAS, SCNI, SDS, SNI, SNS (K), SpIRIT). As Hungelmann et al. (1996), among others, argue, assessment of spiritual well-being is within the domain of nursing and is an integral component of a thorough nursing assessment, and they suggest JAREL SWBS assessment data may assist in both formulating nursing diagnoses and interventions (Hungelmann et al. 1996). In both hospitalized and palliative care settings the nurse is the HCP most often in contact with the patients and is in position to assess spiritual needs. Knowing the patient is an important aspect of making a successful assessment as spirituality is often a private area (Nissen 2019). However, as Lo et al. (2017) point out, the spiritual distress and needs that patients may be experiencing are not necessarily communicated to HCPs during daily routine interactions, and therefore an explicit spiritual assessment can be argued as necessary. As illustrated by Fitchett and Risk (2009), the chaplain may not be in a position to screen all patients for spiritual struggles, and may not always be the appropriate one to do so either, considering the secular and pluralistic setting of many hospitals. Therefore a 'neutral' HCP in terms of religious/spiritual orientation may be preferable, and, as Fitchett and Risk argue, a religious specialist of a specific religious orientation can be called upon when necessary (Fitchett and Risk 2009). The question is not so much who should make an assessment of spiritual needs, as any HCP, in theory, can be in a position to assess for spiritual needs, just as long as they come appropriately prepared. The question is rather whether an assessment for spiritual needs should be a compulsory part of a general assessment once an individual has been diagnosed with a serious illness or life-threatening or chronic condition? And, following that, when is the appropriate time to make this assessment? As Mateo-Ortega et al. (2018) argue, spiritual care is (should be) a holistic assessment to determine spiritual needs and enable psychosocial and spiritual/religious-specific individualized interventions and this process should be monitored over time. In relation to spiritual care as a process, it is clear that this process is not argued in relation to the point in time when a person is diagnosed with a life-threatening condition, but rather when spiritual needs arise. From this perspective, spiritual care can start at any time, also implying that spiritual needs are something HCPs should be continuously aware of, especially considering the multiplicity character of the human inner life, where needs may change rapidly (Johannessen-Henry 2012; Johannesen-Henry and Iversen 2019). This may not be an easy task in the busy daily life and routines of hospital settings. Then again, the secular setting of the hospital/hospice in a pluralistic world (Berger 2015) may be open for the variety of spirituality at the individual level, and as Wu et al. point out, people may still have spiritual needs whether they are religious or not (Wu et al. 2016).

In their study, Vilalta et al. locate two spiritual needs which emerged as the most relevant for patients participating in the study: the need to be recognized as a person until the end of their life and the need to know the truth about their illness (Vilalta et al. 2014). This brings forth the question of 'spirituality', as it can certainly be argued to what extent these two needs are spiritual. As Seddigh et al. (2016) point out, spirituality is not the same in China as it is in Germany. For some playing or listening to music is a spiritual activity, for others spirituality may be the act of giving, finding inner peace, doing yoga, or something else, and one approach (here questionnaire) may be more appropriate than another, depending on the cultural context and the existential grounding of the patient. The point here is that spirituality is 'merely' a word needed to conceptualize and approach the inner lives of human beings, and that these inner lives do not easily render themselves to such constructs (Descola 2011), and just as spirituality is not the same in China and in Germany, neither is it the same for patient A and patient B. The multiplicity of the human inner life (Iversen 2019; Johannesen-Henry and Iversen 2019) and the ability of the individual to psychologically move between spheres of relevance, to be simultaneously spiritual and secular (Berger 2015), complicates formulating and delivering spiritual care. It illustrates the difficulty and necessity of developing approaches applicable in, and sensitive to, different cultural contexts and healthcare areas (Chan et al. 2016), and in the end to the individual patients. It seems imperative that one must be aware of the effect words have and that two persons are not automatically or necessarily on par in their understandings of concepts such as spirituality and religiosity, not the least in a pluralistic world. Things are likely to be missed or misunderstood if the HCP is not very cautious in the approach to assessing spiritual needs. The study on the Existential Distress Scale showed this difficulty of communicating existential distress between patient and HCP as nurses were unable to comment on patient distress frequency in 24–38% of participants (Lo et al. 2017). Of the 22 included questionnaires, 3 consist of secular questions (EDS, ENP-E, Spirit 8). The remaining 19 questionnaires include explicit questions in relation to spirituality or religiosity, such as the sacred, the divine, karma, religious activities (praying being the prominent activity), and higher beings (God, Allah, Dharma, Angels, Adonai). In this sense, they aim at being pluralistic and inclusive, while also reflecting a grounding in spiritual/religious concepts and contexts and at being inclusive of the world's major religions. These spiritual and/or religious-oriented questions are then often intertwined with secular existential and nonexistential questions, again illustrating the difficulty of assessing religion and spirituality in a pluralistic setting, and the need for the HCPs to be aware of the existential grounding of the individual patient.

The translation and adaptation of the questionnaires in other cultural settings than the original (Table 5.2) show that international exchange of experiences and best practices between cultures and languages is going on. This is not easily done, however, especially because of the earlier argument on the elusiveness and situatedness of the concept of *spiritual* and because this needs to be adjusted to both the local cultural and individual contexts. Table 5.2 shows where the instruments have been developed, followed by the other contexts in which the instruments have been implemented (to our current knowledge).

Table 5.2 Implementation of instruments in different countries

Instrument	*Implemented*
Existential Distress Scale (EDS)	CAN
Functional Assessment of Chronic Illness Therapy-Spiritual Well-Being (Facit-Sp-12)	USA, AUS, BRA, CAN, IND, JOR, KOR, POR
Holistic Health Status Questionnaire (HHSQ)	HKG, CHN
JAREL Spiritual Well-Being Scale JAREL SWBS)	USA, TUR
Meaning in Life Scale (MILS)	USA
Psychosocial and Spiritual Needs Evaluation Scale (ENP-E)	ESP
Quality of Life Questionnaire Spiritual Well-Being-32 (QLQ-SWB-32)	EU, BRA, CHI, CRO, DEN, ESP, NED, ENG, FRE, GER, GRE, ICE, ITL, JAP, MEX, NOR, PER, POR, RUS
Religious Spiritual Screening Protocol (RSSP)	USA
Spirit 8	RSA, UGA
Spiritual Assessment Scale (SAS)	USA
Spiritual Care Needs Inventory (SCNI)	TWN
Spiritual Care Needs Scale (SCNS)	TUR
Spiritual Distress Scale (SDS)	TWN, BRA
Spiritual Interests Related to Illness Tool (SpIRIT)	USA, CHN
Spiritual Needs Assessment for Patients (SNAP)	USA, BRA, CHN
Spiritual Needs Inventory (SNI)	USA
Spiritual Needs Questionnaire for Palliative Care (SNQPC)	ESP
Spiritual Needs Questionnaire (SpNQ)	GER, BRA, CHN, CRO, DEN, ESP, FAR, FRA, GRE, IND, IRN, ITL, LTH, MYS, NGA, POL, PRT, PAK
Spiritual Needs Scale (Korea) (SNS (K))	KOR, IRN
Spiritual Needs Survey (SNS)	USA, TUR
Spiritual Transformation Scale (STS)	USA
Thai Spiritual Well-being Assessment Tool for Elders with Chronic Illnesses (TSWBATECI)	THA

An inclusion criterion for this study was that the questionnaire and the article should be written in English. This is a limitation and a bias as it excludes questionnaires developed in other languages. Some questionnaires originate from contexts outside the language criteria, with articles written in English, thereby giving an insight into these contexts. An example of a questionnaire that was excluded on the basis of the language criterion is the Hope Scale for Korean Cancer Patients (HS_KCP) (Tae et al. 2017). This article was written in Korean but the abstract and the included factor analysis was written in English, reflecting a questionnaire that may very well be applicable as a spiritual assessment questionnaire outside Korea. It is mentioned here to illustrate the language bias and barrier/difficulties between different languages in sharing knowledge and experiences.

Since 2001, the Joint Commission on Accreditation of Healthcare Organizations (JCAHO), the largest and most influential healthcare accrediting body in the USA, requires that a minimum of spiritual assessment be done in healthcare settings (Hodge 2006). An effect of this is that today more than 90% of medical schools in the USA include courses or content on spirituality and health, and 70% with spirituality content in required courses, which has presumably led to an increasing focus in clinical practice. This could be part of the explanation why 10 out of the 22 questionnaires are from the USA, the other part being the language bias.

The SpNQ and QLQ-SWB-32 are by far the two questionnaires most translated and employed in other cultural contexts. QLQ-SWB-32 was developed by the European Organization for Research and Treatment of Cancer, which was supplemented by an international research group with participants from all over the world, who validated the questionnaire as a stand-alone measure of spiritual well-being for palliative cancer patients, cross-culturally applicable in 14 countries and in 10 languages (Vivat et al. 2017). The SpNQ was developed in Germany in 2010 (Büssing et al. 2010) for measuring spiritual, existential, and psychosocial needs of patients with chronic illness, and has been translated into a number of languages, where the different language versions are sensitive to cultural and religious variations (Büssing et al. 2018). The SpNQ was highlighted by Seddigh and colleagues in their review of questionnaires measuring patients' spiritual needs as one of the most important questionnaires in the field, which can be seen reflected in the many and very diverse cultural settings of translation and implementation, such as Iran, China, and Nigeria (Seddigh et al. 2016). The HHSQ is also focused on the importance of local cultural variations and the need for a questionnaire to be both culturally sensitive and context-relevant (Chan et al. 2016).

It is clear from these observations that spiritual needs assessment is an important part of health care, and that spiritual care promotes better coping with the secular/spiritual/religious existential considerations and needs that may follow when diagnosed with a life-threatening or chronic illness. A spiritual needs assessment is only as good as the involved parties, however, and the interpersonal follow-up on an assessment is, of course, essential. Few patients would have any positive effects from answering a questionnaire where they express that they have spiritual needs, if nobody follows up on these expressed needs. This becomes evident when considering spiritual care as a process. A spiritual needs assessment is the first step in the process of delivering spiritual care, to be followed by the development of a spiritual care treatment plan. This plan needs to be relevant for the individual patient and adjusted to and inclusive of the patient's understanding of spirituality, be it secular, spiritual, or religiously grounded. The questionnaires included in this overview have all been developed and implemented in the assessment of spiritual needs and they are important not only from the perspective of delivering spiritual care to the individual patient, but also from the perspective of exchanging knowledge and best practices internationally and cross-culturally.

Conclusion

From the understanding of spiritual care as a process, this study has shown that assessing spiritual needs through the use of a questionnaire is both an approach often used internationally and an appropriate way to address the difficult topic of spiritual needs assessment. The 22 questionnaires included in this overview represent a variety of cultural and healthcare contexts assessing spiritual needs or spiritual well-being, through which spiritual needs may also be expressed. The cultural variety and origins of the 22 questionnaires show that spiritual needs assessment is regarded as an important part of health care across cultural and geographical settings, and that they are prominent in critical areas such as oncology and palliative care. A language bias was located and argued as hindering the cross-cultural exchange of questionnaires and best practice. The study argued that a spiritual needs assessment is ultimately a matter between the individual patient and the HCP. It is an area of intimacy and privacy, not easily approachable, demanding great empathy on behalf of the involved HCP as well as knowledge of the secular, spiritual, and/or religious grounding of the individual patient. Spiritual needs assessment questionnaires play an important part in locating patients' spiritual needs, in delivering spiritual care to the individual patient, and in the continuing development of spiritual care internationally and cross-culturally.

References

Assing Hvidt E, Søndergaard J, Gulbrandsen P, Ammentorp J, Timmermann C, Hvidt NC (2018) We are the barriers': Danish general practitioners' interpretations of why the existential and spiritual dimensions are neglected in patient care. Commun Med 14(2):108–120. https://doi.org/10.1558/cam.32147

Balboni TA, Paulk ME, Balboni MJ, Phelps AC, Loggers ET, Wright AA, Block SD, Lewis EF, Pette JR, Prigerson HG (2010) Provision of spiritual care to patients with advanced cancer: associations with medical care and quality of life near death. J Clin Oncol 28(3):445–452. https://doi.org/10.1200/JCO.2009.24.8005

Balboni MJ, Sullivan A, Enzinger AC, Epstein-Peterson ZD, Tseng YD, Mitchell C, Niska J, Zollfrank A, VanderWeele TJ, Balboni TA (2014) Nurse and physician barriers to spiritual care provision at the end of life. J Pain Symptom Manag 48(3):400–410. https://doi.org/10.1016/j.jpainsymman.2013.09.020

Berger PL (2015) The hospital: on the Interface between secularity and religion. Society 52(5):410–412. https://doi.org/10.1007/s12115-015-9941-z

Burkhart L, Schmidt L, Hogan N (2011) Development and psychometric testing of the spiritual care inventory instrument. J Adv Nurs 67(11):2463–2472. https://doi.org/10.1111/j.1365-2648.2011.05654.x

Büssing A, Koenig HK (2010) Spiritual needs of patients with chronic diseases. Religions 1(1):18–27. https://doi.org/10.3390/rel1010018

Büssing A, Balzat HJ, Heuser P (2010) Spiritual needs of patients with chronic pain diseases and Cancer—validation of the spiritual needs questionnaire. Eur J Med Res 15(6):266–273. https://doi.org/10.1186/2047-783x-15-6-266

Büssing A, Recchia D, Koenig H, Baumann K, Frick E (2018) Factor structure of the spiritual needs questionnaire (SpNQ) in persons with chronic diseases, elderly and healthy individuals. Religions 9(1):13. https://doi.org/10.3390/rel9010013

Cadge W, Bandini J (2015) The evolution of spiritual assessment tools in healthcare. Society 52(5):430–437. https://doi.org/10.1007/s12115-015-9926-y

Chan CW, Wong FK, Yeung SM, Sum F (2016) Holistic health status questionnaire: developing a measure from a Hong Kong Chinese population. Health Qual Life Outcomes 14:28. https://doi.org/10.1186/s12955-016-0416-8

Cole BS, Hopkins CM, Tisak J, Steel JL, Carr BI (2008) Assessing spiritual growth and spiritual decline following a diagnosis of cancer: reliability and validity of the spiritual transformation scale. Psycho-Oncology 17:112–121. https://doi.org/10.1002/pon.1207

la Cour P, Hvidt NC (2010) Research on meaning-making and health in secular society: secular, spiritual and religious existential orientations. Soc Sci Med 71(7):1292–1299. https://doi.org/10.1016/j.socscimed.2010.06.024

la Cour P, Ausker NHR, Hvidt NC (2012) Six understandings of the word "spirituality" in a secular country. Arch Psychol Relig 34(1):63–81. https://doi.org/10.1163/157361212X649634

Daudt VM (2013) Enhancing the scoping study methodology. BMC Med Res 13:48. https://link.springer.com/article/10.1186/1471-2288-13-48

Descola P (2011) Beyond nature and culture. University of Chicago Press, Chicago

El Nawawi NM, Balboni MJ, Balboni TA (2012) Palliative care and spiritual care: the crucial role of spiritual care in the care of patients with advanced illness. Curr Opin Support Palliat Care 6(2):269–274. https://doi.org/10.1097/SPC.0b013e3283530d13

Fitchett G, Risk JL (2009) Screening for spiritual struggle. J Pastoral Care Counsel 63(1–2):4-1-12

Galek K, Flannelly KJ, Vane A, Galek RM (2005) Assessing a Patient's spiritual needs. A comprehensive instrument. Holist Nurs Pract 19(2):62–69

Gibson CA, Pessin H, McLain CS, Shah AD, Breitbart W (2004) The unmet need: addressing spirituality and meaning through culturally sensitive communication and intervention. In: Moore RJ, Spiegel D (eds) Cancer, culture, and communication. Kluwer Academic/Plenum Publishers, New York, pp 281–298

Gijsberts MHE, Liefbroer AI, Otten R, Olsman E (2019) Spiritual Care in Palliative Care: a systematic review of the recent European literature. Med Sci (Basel) 7(2):25. https://doi.org/10.3390/medsci7020025

Greasley P, Chiu LF, Gartland M (2001) The concept of spiritual care in mental health nursing. J Adv Nurs 33(5):629–637

Hall DE, Koenig HG, Meador KG (2004) Conceptualizing "Religion". Perspect Biol Med 47(3):386–401

Harrad R, Cosentino C, Keasley R, Sulla F (2019) Spiritual care in nursing: an overview of the measures used to assess spiritual care provision and related factors amongst nurses. Acta Biomed 90(4-S):44–55. https://doi.org/10.23750/abm.v90i4-S.8300

Hermann CP (2006) Development and testing of the spiritual needs inventory for patients near the end of life. Oncol Nurs Forum 33(4):737–744. https://doi.org/10.1188/06.ONF.737-744

Hill PC, Pargament K II, Hood RW, McCullough JME, Swyers JP, Larson DB, Zinnbauer BJ (2000) Conceptualizing religion and spirituality: points of commonality, points of departure. J Theory Soc Behav 30(1):51–77. https://doi.org/10.1111/1468-5914.00119

Hodge DR (2006) A template for spiritual assessment: a review of the JCAHO requirements and guidelines for implementation. Soc Work 51(4):317–326. https://doi.org/10.1093/sw/51.4.317

Hummel L, Galek K, Murphy KM, Tannenbaum HP, Flannelly LT (2008) Defining spiritual care: an exploratory study. J Health Care Chaplain 15(1):40–51. https://doi.org/10.1080/08854720802698509

Hungelmann J, Kenkel-Rossi E, Klassen L, Stollenwerk R (1996) Focus on spiritual well-being: harmonious interconnectedness of mind-body-Spirit use of the JAREL spiritual well-being scale assessment of spiritual well-being is essential to the health of individuals. Geriatr Nurs 17:262–266

Iversen HR (2019) Kirkelige handlinger for mennesker med forskellige religioner og livstydninger. In: Johannesen-Henry CT, Iversen HR (eds) Mangefoldet tro. Eksistensen Akademisk, Copenhagen. Multiplicitet Som Vilkår for Mennesker, Møder Og Samtaler. Eksistensen Akademisk, Copenhagen, pp 111–136

Jafari N, Zamani A, Farajzadegan Z, Bahrami F, Emami H, Loghmani A (2013) The effect of spiritual therapy for improving the quality of life of women with breast cancer: a randomized controlled trial. Psychol Health Med 18(1):56–69. https://doi.org/10.1080/13548506.2012.679738

Jim HS, Purnell JQ, Richardson SA, Golden-Kreutz D, Andersen BL (2006) Measuring meaning in life following cancer. Qual Life Res 15(8):1355–1371

Johannesen-Henry CT, Iversen HR (2019) Mangefoldet tro. Eksistensen Akademisk, Copenhagen

Johannessen-Henry CT (2012) Polydox eschatology: relating systematic and everyday theology in a cancer context. Studia Theologica-Nordic Journal of Theology 66(2):107–129

Ku YL, Kuo SM, Yao CY (2010) Establishing the validity of a spiritual distress scale for cancer patients hospitalized in southern Taiwan. Int J Palliat Nurs 16(3):133–137

Lo C, Panday T, Zeppieri J, Rydall A, Murphy-Kane P, Zimmermann C, Rodin G (2017) Preliminary psychometrics of the existential distress scale in patients with advanced cancer. Eur J Cancer Care 26:e12597. https://doi.org/10.1111/ecc.12597

Mateo-Ortega D, Limonero JT, Mate-Mendez J, Beas E, Gonzalez-Barboteo J, Barbero E, Ela S, Gomez-Batiste X (2018) Development of a tool to identify and assess psychosocial and spiritual needs in end-of-life patients: the ENP-E scale. Palliat Support Care 17(4):441–447. https://doi.org/10.1017/S1478951518000652

Nissen RD (2019) In that most secular of rooms—the religious patient in secular psychiatry. PhD Thesis. University of Southern Denmark, Odense

Nissen RD, Gildberg FA, Hvidt NC (2018) Psychiatry, a secular discipline in a Postsecular world? A Review Religions 9(1):32. https://doi.org/10.3390/rel9010032

Nissen RD, Falkø E, Toudal DV, Assing-Hvidt E, Büssing A, Søndergaard J, Walin JA, Hvidt NC (2020) The catalogue of spiritual care instruments: a scoping review. Religions 11:252. https://doi.org/10.3390/rel11050252

Nolan S, Saltmarsh P, Leget C (2011) Spiritual care in palliative care: working towards an EAPC task force. Europena Journal of Palliative Care 18(2):86–89

O'Brien ME (1993) Spiritual assessment scale. In: O'Brien ME sixth edition 2018. Spirituality in nursing. Standing on holy ground. Jones and Bartlett Publishers, pp 49–56. ISBN: 9781284121001

Østergaard Steenfeldt V (2018) Understanding and optimization of spiritual care for the dying in nursing homes. Post-Doc Post-Doc. Institute of Public Health, University of Southern Denmark/University College Absalon, Odense/Sorø

Otuzoglu M, Talas MS (2019) Development of a scale to identify spiritual care needs of oncology patients. International Journal of Medical Research & Health Sciences 8(4):39–53

Pedersen CS, Post RC (2012) Åndelig omsorg—Et litteraturstudie af de eksisterende barrierer. MA Thesis, Professionshøjskolen Metropol, København

Peterman AH, Fitchett G, Brady MJ, Hernandez L, Cella RD (2002) Measuring spiritual well-being in people with Cancer: the functional assessment of chronic illness therapy—spiritual well-being scale (FACIT-Sp). Ann Behav Med 24(1):49–58

Puchalski C, Ferrell B, Virani R, Otis-Green S, Baird P, Bull J, Chochinov H, Handzo G, Nelson-Becker H, Prince-Paul M, Pugliese K, Sulmasy D (2009) Improving the quality of spiritual care as a dimension of palliative care: the report of the consensus conference. J Palliat Care 12(10):885–904. https://doi.org/10.1089/jpm.2009.0142

Ramezani M, Ahmadi F, Mohammadi E, Kazemnejad A (2014) Spiritual care in nursing: a concept analysis. Int Nurs Rev 61(2):211–219

Rushton L (2014) What are the barriers to spiritual care in a hospital setting? Br J Nurs 23(7):370–374

Seddigh R, Keshavarz-Akhlaghi AA, Azarnik S (2016) Questionnaires measuring patients' spiritual needs: a narrative literature review. Iran J Psychiatry Behav Sci 10(1):e4011. https://doi.org/10.17795/ijpbs-4011

Selman L, Siegert RJ, Higginson IJ, Agupio G, Ninat N, Downing J, Gwyther L, Mashao T, Mmoledi K, Moll Y, Sebuyira LM, Ikin B, Harding R (2012) The "Spirit 8" successfully captured spiritual well-being in African palliative care: factor and Rasch analysis. J Clin Epidemiol 65:434–443. https://doi.org/10.1016/j.jclinepi.2011.09.014

Sharma RK, Astrow AB, Texeira K, Sulmasy DP (2012) The spiritual needs assessment for patients (SNAP): development and validation of a comprehensive instrument to assess unmet spiritual needs. J Pain Symptom Manag 44(1):44–51

Slort W, Schweitzer BP, Blankenstein AH, Abarshi EA, Riphagen II, Echteld MA, Aaronson NK, van der Host H, Deliens L (2011) Perceived barriers and facilitators for general practitioner-patient communication in palliative care: a systematic review. Palliat Med 25(6):613–629. https://doi.org/10.1177/0269216310395987

Tae YS, Choi YS, Nam GH, Bae JY (2017) Development of the Hope scale for Korean Cancer patients. Korean J Adult Nurs 29(2):211–223. https://doi.org/10.7475/kjan.2017.29.2.211

Taylor EJ (2006) Prevalence and associated factors of spiritual needs among patients with cancer and family caregivers. Oncol Nurs Forum 33(4):729–735. https://doi.org/10.1188/06.ONF.729-735

Unsanit P, Sunsern R, Kunsongkeit W, O'Brien ME, McMullen PC (2012) Development and evaluation of the Thai spiritual well-being assessment tool for elders with a chronic illness. Pacific Rim Int J Nurs Res 16(1):13–28

Vilalta A, Valls J, Porta J, Vinas J (2014) Evaluation of spiritual needs of patients with advanced cancer in a palliative care unit. J Palliat Med 17(5):592–600. https://doi.org/10.1089/jpm.2013.0569

Vivat B, Young TE, Winstanley J, Arraras JI, Black K, Boyle F, Bredart A, Costantini A, Guo J, Irarrazaval ME, Kobayashi K, Kruizinga R, Navarro M, Omidvari S, Rohde GE, Serpentini S, Spry N, Van Laarhoven HWM, Yang GM, EORTC Quality of Life Group (2017) The international phase 4 validation study of the EORTC QLQ-SWB32: a stand-alone measure of spiritual well-being for people receiving palliative care for cancer. Eur J Cancer Care (Engl) 26(6). https://doi.org/10.1111/ecc.12697

Wu LF, Koo M, Liao YC, Chen YM, Yeh DC (2016) Development and validation of the spiritual care needs inventory for acute care hospital patients in Taiwan. Clin Nurs Res 25(6):590–606. https://doi.org/10.1177/1054773815579609

Yong J, Kim J, Han SS, Puchalski CM (2008) Development and validation of a scale assessing spiritual needs for Korean patients with Cancer. J Palliat Care 24:240–246

CHAPTER 6

Application and Implementation of the Spiritual Needs Questionnaire in Spiritual Care Processes

Arndt Büssing

Background

Assessment of spiritual needs is foremost resource-oriented. When spiritual needs are the result of what is longed for in comparison to what is available, then this longing would indicate a source that is hoped for. When the need is met, then happiness, gratefulness, satisfaction and states of inner peace may be the result. When it is a desire, then the constant longing will persist (because it cannot be satisfied at all). When spiritual needs remain unmet over a long time, depressive resignation or emotional distancing from what is perceived as not available can be the consequence, too. Thus, it is essential to assess spiritual needs of persons, document the

A. Büssing (✉)
Professorship Quality of Life, Spirituality and Coping, Faculty of Health, Witten/Herdecke University, Herdecke, Germany

IUNCTUS—Competence Center for Christian Spirituality, Philosophical-Theological University of Münster, Münster, Germany
e-mail: arndt.buessing@uni-wh.de

A. Büssing (ed.), *Spiritual Needs in Research and Practice*,
https://doi.org/10.1007/978-3-030-70139-0_6

relevance and intensity of these needs and monitor changes over time during support processes.

Usage of the Instrument

The Spiritual Needs Questionnaire (SpNQ) (Büssing et al. 2010, 2018) can be used either as a diagnostic instrument to assess the strength of a person's unmet needs (and is thus a reason to start communication about these needs, how they can be supported, etc.) or as a research instrument to measure spiritual needs in different cohorts in a standardized way. The diagnostic instrument uses 27–30 items (and three free text fields to encourage a reflection on additional specific needs of importance), while the research instrument uses 20 items. Persons rate whether they currently have the respective needs (yes/no), and, if yes, how strong these needs are (0—not at all [the "no" answer]; 1—somewhat; 2—strong; 3—very strong).

The questionnaire can be either filled directly by the intended person (this approach is recommended to avoid biased responses) or interview-administered (either face to face or as a telephone interview). The required time is, depending on the age and abilities of the tested person, around five minutes.

There is a debate about whether spiritual concerns of patients should be proactively addressed as part of the routine or only when the person in need asks for spiritual support. Structured and short spiritual history tools such as the physician-developed FICA (Puchalski and Romer 2000) or HOPE (Anandarajah and Hight 2001) or the chaplain-developed FACT (Larocca-Pitts 2008) are intended to be applied routinely. When one waits for persons in need to signal that they would like to talk about these issues, one might miss all those who are not aware that one *could* talk about their spiritual needs, distress, resources and hopes, or who are too reluctant to talk about such "private" things. The proactive application of an assessment tool such as the SpNQ would clearly signal that these dimensions are valued as important and will, if necessary, be supported. If someone feels uncomfortable with these topics, one has the option to not respond, as its application should be understood as an offer from the spiritual/healthcare team which is interested in a person's spiritual concerns and intends to support these, and not as an obligation.

To facilitate use of the instrument by persons with different religious traditions and worldviews, it avoids exclusive religious terminology and is thus suited to both secular and religious societies. When a-religious persons do not have specific religious needs, they can state "not at all", and may find other (secular) needs which are of relevance to them.

Depending on participants' religious backgrounds, some of the religious items can be supplemented with explanations. Item N23, for example, asks for the need to "turn to a higher presence (i.e., God, Allah, Angels, Saints)". What such a "higher presence" may be to a specific person depends on their religious background. Therefore, the term God or Allah could be added where appropriate, but also "Angels and Saints" for specific Christian groups, or "Bodhisattvas" for persons with a Buddhist background.

Items of the Spiritual Needs Questionnaire

All items refer to the four main topics of the instrument (Fig. 6.1): *Religious* needs (Transcendence), *Existential* needs (Meaning/Purpose), *Inner Peace* needs (Peace) and *Giving/Generativity* needs (Connection) (Büssing et al. 2010). Several items refer to relational needs too (i.e., "talk with someone", "turn to someone", "give solace to someone", "pray with someone") which are integrated in the different factors.

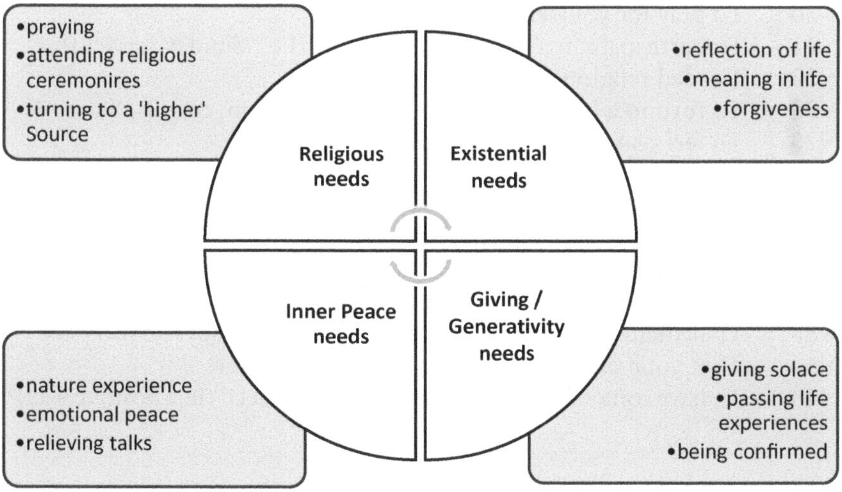

Fig. 6.1 Schematic representation of spiritual needs categories and related topics

The statements are formulated in short sentences and introduced with the phrase "During the last time, did you have needs …", followed by 27–30 statements and three free text fields for further needs:

N2	To talk with others about your fears and worries?
N3	That someone of your religious community (i.e., pastor) cares for you or comes to see you?
N4	To reflect back on your life?
N5	To dissolve/clarify open aspects of your life?
N6	To plunge into beauty of nature?
N7	To dwell at a place of quietness and peace?
N8	To find inner peace?
N10	To find meaning in illness and/or suffering?
N11	To talk with someone about the question of meaning in life?
N12	To talk with someone about the possibility of life after death?
N13	To turn to someone in a loving attitude?
N14	To give away something from yourself?
N15	To give solace to someone?
N16	To forgive someone from a distinct period of your life?
N17	To be forgiven?
N18	To pray with someone?
N19	That someone prays for you?
N20	To pray for yourself?
N21	To participate in a religious ceremony (i.e., Sunday service)?
N22	To read religious/spiritual books?
N23	To turn to a higher presence (i.e., God, Allah, Angels, Saints)?
N25	To feel connected with family?
N26	To pass own life experiences to others?
N27	To be assured that your life was meaningful and of value?
N28	To be re-involved by your family in their life concerns?
N29	To be invited by friends?
N30	To receive more support from your family?
N38	That there is someone there for you who is always at your side?
N43	That your situation is improving for the better?
N44	To have someone to assure you how to proceed (in a positive way)?

Spiritual Care Implementation

The spiritual needs assessment has to be implemented in spiritual/health-care processes (Fig. 6.2). When these needs are assessed (phase 1), the spiritual/health-care team has to consider which needs may have priority, who is available and competent to address specific needs and so forth (phase 2). This planning phase results in a *Support Plan*, which includes suggestions for concrete support options/interventions and a strategy of who takes responsibility (phase 3). Then starting communication with the patient is the crucial step for consent to the interventions or support options (phase 4). Next, the effects of these interventions have to be reevaluated and adapted when required (phase 5). The phases of this implementation process are in line with the recommendations of the 2009 Consensus Conference to improve the quality of spiritual care in palliative care (Puchalski et al. 2009).

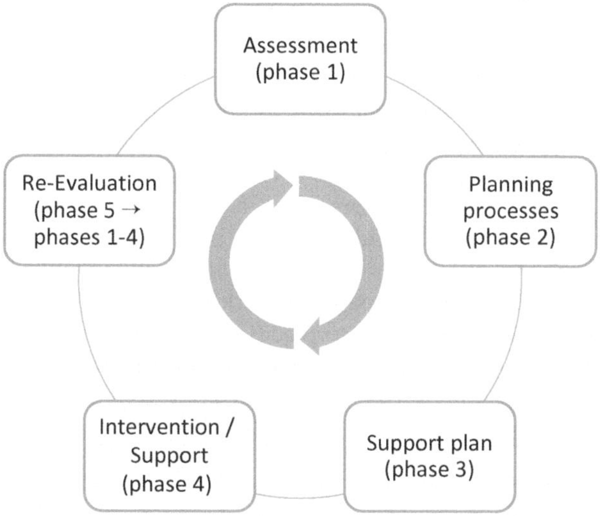

Fig. 6.2 Schematic representation of implementation processes and their different phases

Topics of a Support Plan

The support plan could be structured according to the main topics of the instrument (Fig. 6.1) or according to specific spiritual needs with strong relevance to the patient (intensity of unmet needs).

The following examples are intended as an open list of suggestions and can be part of a "spiritual tool box". These may be used variably by different professionals and according to the background and situation of the patient. These suggestions should be consented to by the patient to avoid encroachments. The spiritual tool box does not aim to *make* something, but to talk with patients and encourage them to choose the direction the process can take.

Religious needs: Provide formal prayer cards when the person is not able to pray any more (remembrance and reconnection); ask whether someone should come to pray for or with them or to send a specific blessing or the Holy Sacraments (the pastor for Christians); facilitate the performance of prescribed praying times (for Muslims); facilitate participation in religious ceremonies; provide a religious symbol that is important to the patient (hope and encouragement); invite for talks/conversations with pastoral care providers, pastors and so on.

Existential need: Facilitate life reviews and biographic history, provide (psychological) assistance to clarify conflicts, disappointments, ailing; facilitate processes of reconciliation (supervised by pastoral workers and psychologists), that is, writing letters when forgiveness or to be forgiven is crucial; facilitate phone calls and visits with the respective persons or with distant family members; invite for talks about meaning in life or fears and worries (with psychologists or pastoral workers).

Inner Peace needs: Reconnect to places or situations where inner peace was experienced (life story); introduce mindfulness meditation practices, if feasible in connection with, or conducive to, prayer/meditation; facilitate visits to beautiful places, gardens, forests (or pictures of these); play inspiring music which is of importance to the patient; encourage forgiveness and reconciliation processes; provide hope where possible.

Generativity needs: Connect persons in need with others (mutual support groups); facilitate creative art projects such as paining, writing, diaries (i.e., life history, peak experiences, peaceful situations, experiences of awe and gratefulness); establish intergenerational discussion groups; appreciate patients' intention to be able to give something away (e.g., a glass of honey); connect them with family members, facilitate visits (or phone calls) with friends.

Conclusions

The SpNQ was developed to assess patients' unmet spiritual, existential and psychosocial needs in a standardized way. It is first of all a resource-oriented diagnostic instrument that allows both communication and documentation. The process of implementation can be described in five phases, starting from assessment of a person's spiritual needs, planning of support options, consensus finding from the person in need and subsequent reevaluation processes of whether at all and how the respective spiritual needs are met.

References

Anandarajah G, Hight E (2001) Spirituality and medical practice: using the HOPE questions as a practical tool for spiritual assessment. Am Fam Physician 63:81–89

Büssing A, Balzat HJ, Heusser P (2010) Spiritual needs of patients with chronic pain diseases and cancer—validation of the Spiritual Needs Questionnaire. Eur J Med Res 15:266–273

Büssing A, Recchia DR, Koenig H, Baumann K, Frick E (2018) Factor structure of the Spiritual Needs Questionnaire (SpNQ) in persons with chronic diseases, elderly and healthy individuals. Religions 9:13. https://doi.org/10.3390/rel9010013

Larocca-Pitts MA (2008) FACT: taking a spiritual history in a clinical setting. J Health Care Chaplain 15(1):1–12. https://doi.org/10.1080/08854720802698350

Puchalski C, Romer AL (2000) Taking a spiritual history allows clinicians to understand patients more fully. J Palliat Med 3:129–137

Puchalski C, Ferrell B, Virani R, Otis-Green S, Baird P, Bull J, Chochinov H, Handzo G, Nelson-Becker H, Prince-Paul M, Pugliese K, Sulmasy D (2009) Improving the quality of spiritual care as a dimension of palliative care: the report of the Consensus Conference. J Palliat Med 12(10):885–904. https://doi.org/10.1089/jpm.2009.0142

CHAPTER 7

Structure of the Spiritual Needs Questionnaire in Patients with Chronic Diseases, Elderly and Healthy Persons and Their Association with Quality of Life Indicators

Arndt Büssing

Background

The Spiritual Needs Questionnaire (SpNQ) was developed to measure spiritual, existential and psychosocial needs of patients with chronic diseases (Büssing et al. 2009, 2010). The underlying topics refer to four core dimensions of spiritual needs, that is, Connection, Peace, Meaning/Purpose and Transcendence, which can be further attributed to the categories of social, emotional, existential and religious needs (Büssing

A. Büssing (✉)
Professorship Quality of Life, Spirituality and Coping, Faculty of Health, Witten/Herdecke University, Herdecke, Germany

IUNCTUS—Competence Center for Christian Spirituality, Philosophical-Theological University of Münster, Münster, Germany
e-mail: Arndt.buessing@uni-wh.de

A. Büssing (ed.), *Spiritual Needs in Research and Practice*,
https://doi.org/10.1007/978-3-030-70139-0_7

and Koenig 2010). According to Alderfer's model of *Relational*, *Existential* and *Growth* needs (Alderfer 1972), Connection needs and Religious needs refer to a *Relational* dimension (i.e., connection with concrete others in terms of love, belonging, alienation, partner communication, or connection with the Sacred in terms of spiritual resources, relationship with God, praying); Peace needs (i.e., inner peace, hope, balance, forgiveness, distress, fear of relapse) refer to the *Existential* dimension; and Meaning/Purpose needs (i.e., meaning in life, self-actualization, role function) refer to the *Growth* dimension (Büssing 2014). These needs have no hierarchy as their importance may vary interindividually.

The instrument has been so far applied to persons with chronic diseases, patients at a palliative care unit, patients at an emergency unit, healthy elderly living in retirement homes, persons with autism and dementia, and in stressed healthy persons (soldiers with and without posttraumatic stress disorders, relatives of sick people, mothers with newborns or with children born sick or of children with Down syndrome), and, in an adapted version (see Chap. 8), also to adolescents with chronic conditions or long treatments.

Factorial Structure of the Instrument

Since its first validation (Büssing et al. 2010) the SpNQ differentiated four main topics: *Religious* needs, *Existential* needs, *Inner Peace* needs, and *Giving/Generativity* needs. The latter factor was further supported with the introduction of two new items (N26 and N27) (Büssing et al. 2012). To optimize the content and underlying structure, several steps of deleting items (that could decrease the internal consistency) and adding items (to support the intended structure) were performed (Büssing et al. 2010, 2012, 2018).

In 2018, the four factors of the 20-item version (SpNQ-20) were verified in four large samples: (1) persons with chronic diseases ($n = 627$); (2) persons with chronic diseases plus the elderly ($n = 940$); (3) healthy persons (i.e., adults and the elderly; $n = 1468$); and (4) chronically ill, elderly, and healthy persons together ($n = 2095$) (Büssing et al. 2018). Here, structured equation modelling (SEM) confirmed the structure of the SpNQ-20 (CFI = 0.96, TLI = 0.95, RMSEA = 0.04, and SRMR = 0.03), with good reliability indices for the four factors (Cronbach's alpha varying from 0.71 to 0.81).

Table 7.1 shows the structure of the SpNQ-20, factor loadings, and mean values of items in a sample of 1200 persons with chronic diseases or the elderly living in retirement homes:

Table 7.1 Factor loading and mean values of items

	Mean (SD)	*Corrected item—scale correlation*	*Cronbach's alpha if item is deleted (alpha = 0.880)*	*Factor loading*			
				1	*2*	*3*	*4*
Religious needs (Eigenvalue: 6.2; Cronbach's alpha = 0.874)							
N20 pray for yourself	1.23 (1.27)	0.557	0.870	0.825			
N21 participate in a religious ceremony (i.e., service)	0.90 (1.17)	0.423	0.875	0.792			
N23 turn to a higher presence (i.e., God, Allah)	1.00 (1.24)	0.563	0.870	0.788			
N18 pray with someone	0.48 (0.93)	0.515	0.872	0.740			
N19 that someone prays for you	0.72 (1.07)	0.519	0.872	0.739			
N22 read religious/spiritual books	0.55 (0.98)	0.513	0.872	0.651			
Existential needs (Eigenvalue: 2.5; Cronbach's alpha = 0.771)							
N11 talk with someone about the question of meaning in life	0.68 (1.02)	0.568	0.870		0.646		
N10 find meaning in illness and/or suffering	0.79 (1.10)	0.451	0.874		0.620		
N2 talk with others about fears and worries	1.32 (1.17)	0.376	0.878		0.596		
N5 dissolve open aspects of your life	0.90 (1.16)	0.419	0.875		0.580		

(*continued*)

Table 7.1 (continued)

	Mean (SD)	*Corrected item—scale correlation*	*Cronbach's alpha if item is deleted (alpha = 0.880)*	*Factor loading*			
				1	*2*	*3*	*4*
N12 talk with someone about the possibility of life after death	0.55 (0.97)	0.518	0.872	0.385	0.551		
N17 be forgiven	0.59 (1.01)	0.507	0.872		0.515	0.412	
N16 forgive someone from a distinct period of your life	0.66 (1.05)	0.515	0.872		0.502	0.483	
Giving/generative needs (Eigenvalue: 1.2; Cronbach's alpha = 0.714)							
N15 provide solace to someone	1.25 (1.14)	0.499	0.872			0.709	
N14 give away something from yourself	1.11 (1.17)	0.536	0.871			0.696	
N26 pass own life experiences to others	1.32 (1.16)	0.439	0.874			0.669	
N27 be assured that your life is meaningful and of value	1.54 (1.24)	0.430	0.875			0.522	
Inner peace needs (Eigenvalue: 1.1; Cronbach's alpha = 0.718)							
N6 plunge into beauty of nature	1.91 (1.16)	0.399	0.876				0.742
N7 dwell at a place of quietness and peace	1.43 (1.25)	0.477	0.873		0.461		0.655
N8 find inner peace	1.38 (1.27)	0.533	0.871		0.582		0.553

Extraction method: principle components analysis (Varimax rotation with Kaiser normalization); rotation converged in 6 iterations; 5 factors explain 55% of variance; only loadings > 0.30 are depicted

Enrolled persons (N = 1200; 71% women, 29% men) with cancer (33%; mean age: 61 ± 12 years), chronic pain diseases (37%, mean age: 56 ± 13 years), other chronic diseases (1%; mean age: 64 ± 16 years), or elderly living in retirement homes (29%; mean age: 84 ± 7 years)

- The scale of *Religious* needs addresses needs to pray (either alone, with someone, or that someone prays for you), to participate in a religious ceremony, to read inspirational religious/spiritual books, and to be connected with a higher presence (i.e., God). The six respective items have good internal consistency (Cronbach's alpha = 0.87).
- The scale of *Existential* needs addresses three main topics: meaning finding with two items, clarification and forgiveness with three items, and relieving talks with others about fears and worries, meaning in life and in life after death. These seven items have acceptable internal consistency in this sample (Cronbach's alpha = 0.77).
- The scale of *Inner Peace* primarily had four items. However, in this sample item N2 (talking with someone about fears and worry) loads better on *Existential* needs, and also item N8 (find inner peace) would load strongly on that factor. The other two items address the intention to stay in the "beauty of nature" and to "dwell at a place of quietness and peace", both of which would result in states of inner peace. Both the 3-item subscale of this analysis and the primarily intended 4-item subscale have acceptable internal consistency (Cronbach's alpha = 0.72).
- The scale of *Giving/Generativity* needs addresses a relational and generative topic, that is, the intention to give away something of emotional worth to others, to give solace to someone (and thus to turn the role of a passive sufferer to an actively giving and participating person), and finally to be assured that one's own life is meaningful and of value, as one is also able to pass one's own life experiences to others and to guide the next generation. The four items of this subscale have acceptable internal consistency (Cronbach's alpha = 0.71).

The difficulty index (= mean values of items/3) of the SpNQ-20 is 0.34. All but three items are in the acceptable range of 0.2 to 0.8. These three items are N18, N22, and N12 with difficulty indexes of 0.16, 0.18, and 0.18, indicating bottom effects due to the low scores for these needs in the sample.

Relational Support Needs

The relational support items N28, N29, and N30 (which refer to the Connectedness dimension) were primarily intended to be used as additional information in studies with the elderly (Erichsen and Büssing 2013), and not as part of the SpNQ structure. However, if these three items were included, they would form an independent (fifth) factor with, however, less satisfying internal consistency (Cronbach's alpha = 0.65). Moreover, adding them would decrease the loading of the generativity items N26 (pass own life experiences to others), N2 (talk with others about fears and worries), and N12 (talking with someone about life after death), which were all regarded as essential. Thus, these three items should be seen as an option only to get additional information, but not as a structural element of the SpNQ.

Switching Items in Different Samples

In this sample, item N2 (talk with others about fears and worries) switched completely to the *Existential* scale, and item N8 (find inner peace) would load strongly at that scale. The problem of switching items is depending on the persons in the test sample and their specific situation and view of illness.

In the subsample of persons with chronic pain diseases, items N8 and N2 loaded on *Inner Peace* needs and not on *Existential* needs, as it was primarily intended. Also in the subsample of the elderly, items N8 and N2 loaded on *Inner Peace* needs and not on *Existential* needs. However, in the subsample of persons with cancer, item N8 loaded on *Inner Peace* needs and only weakly on the *Existential* scale, while item N2 loaded on *Existential* needs and not on *Inner Peace* needs. Focusing on palliative cancer patients revealed the same loading for items N2 and N8. It might be that for some patients with cancer, talking with others about fears and worries (N2) is an existential matter, and responding to these needs could lead to states of inner peace. In line with this, needs to find inner peace (N8) can thus also be related to the intention to clarify difficult situations from the past, to talk with others, to forgive and to be forgiven, finally resulting in states of inner peace.

Therefore, both items (N2 and N8) will be accounted to the *Inner Peace* scales, as was validated in the largest test sample so far of 2095 persons (see Büssing et al. 2018).

SpNQ-20 Mean Scores

To compare international data, switching items may be problematic. Moreover, the composition of some factors might vary, depending on the sample size, gender, age, and disease of enrolled persons, and cultural or religious contexts. To overcome this, one may use a mean score of all the 20 recommended items (see Table 7.1). This 20-item scale (SpNQ-20) has good internal consistency (Cronbach's alpha = 0.88).

Among the samples described earlier, the SpNQ-20 Mean Score is 1.01 ± 0.63 (median = 0.90; 25% percentile = 0.52, 75% percentile = 1.42).

Expression of Spiritual Needs in Different Samples of Persons

As shown in Fig. 7.1, *Religious* needs and *Existential* needs score lower than *Inner Peace* needs and *Giving/Generativity* needs. There were significant differences between patients with cancer or chronic pain diseases and the elderly living in retirement homes. With the exception of *Giving/*

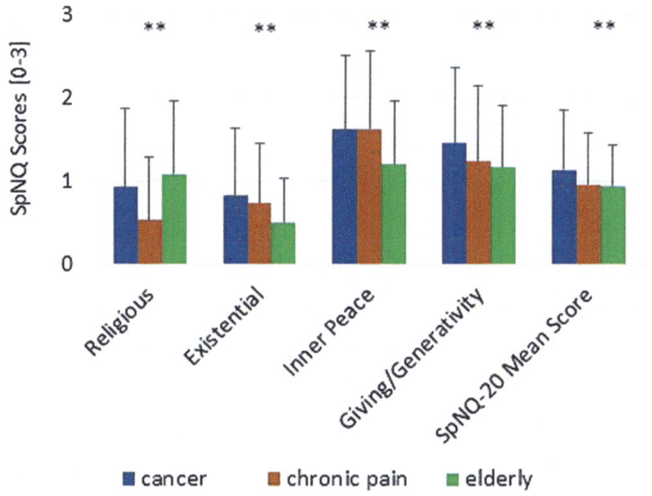

Fig. 7.1 Mean values of spiritual needs in the sample ($n = 1181$; without patients with "other" diagnoses); $^{**}p < 0.0001$ (Spearman rho)

Generativity needs, all other needs were significantly higher in women than in men ($F < 10.0$; $p < 0.0001$).

Age (in 10-year steps) had significant effect on the expression of spiritual needs ($p < 0.0001$): *Religious* needs were highest in the elderly (>80 years of age; $F = 11.9$), while *Existential* needs (>80 years; $F = 9.9$) and *Inner Peace* needs were lowest in the elderly (>80 years; $F = 17.6$). *Giving/Generativity* needs were highest in the mid-age range (60–70 years; $F = 5.6$).

Univariate analyses with these three variables revealed that for *Religious* needs gender was more relevant than the other variables. For *Existential* needs there were no clear hints, while for *Inner Peace* needs and *Giving/Generativity* needs a combination of gender, age, and sample had the strongest influence compared to gender or sample alone.

Spiritual Needs in Persons Without a Religious Affiliation

In a sample of 351 persons with chronic diseases (65.5% women, 34.5% men; mean age 56 ± 14 years; 85% chronic pain diseases, 15% cancer), patients stated whether they had a religious affiliation or not. Here 36% had no religious affiliation and 64% had one (61% Christians and 3% other). Persons without a religious affiliation had significantly lower *Religious needs* (0.20 ± 0.45 versus 0.76 ± 0.87; $p < 0.001$, Mann-Whitney-U test), *Existential* needs (0.64 ± 0.74 versus 0.83 ± 0.70; $p = 0.013$, Mann-Whitney-U test) compared to persons with a religious affiliation, while their *Inner Peace* needs and their *Giving/Generativity* needs did not significantly differ. Further, their SpNQ-20 mean score was significantly lower, too (0.76 ± 0.58 versus 1.03 ± 0.69; $p < 0.001$, Mann-Whitney-U test).

Within the subgroup of persons without a religious affiliation, strong to very strong needs to pray with someone (N18: 15%), that someone pray for them (N19: 22%), and to pray by themselves (N20: 37%) were observed. Participating in a religious ceremony (N21) was strongly to very strongly important for 25% and turning to a higher presence (N23) for 29%. However, that someone from a religious community cares (N3) was of relevance for 9%. This means that even among those patients who may not have a religious affiliation (either they have turned away from institutional religiosity or they were never affiliated), several will nevertheless have specific religious needs that may require attention. It might be that there is a chance to reconcile with religious disappointments they may have experienced in their life. To them, talking about their fears and worries was of strong or even very strong importance (N2: 54%), to be assured that their life was meaningful (N27: 51%), to connect with the beauty of nature (N6: 59%), and to find inner peace (N8: 56%). Their strongest need was to connect with the family (N25: 71%).

Intercorrelations Between SpNQ Subscales

As was obvious in previous analyses, in this sample also *Existential* and *Inner Peace* needs are strongly interconnected ($r = 0.58$). Among the *Inner Peace* needs, the intention to "plunge into beauty of nature" (N6) scored highest among all other items of the SpNQ, followed by the need to "dwell at a place of quietness and peace" (N7). Both items indicate a wish to find peace in distinct places and to escape from the burdening situation of illness in order to find inner peace and harmony (as ideally found in the nature).

Interestingly, both forgiveness items (N16, N17) from the *Existential* needs scale loaded onto the *Giving/Generativity* scale, and thus one may find that both scales are strongly associated, too ($r = 0.53$). This *Giving/Generativity* scale was moderately related with *Inner Peace* needs ($r = 0.48$) as well.

Among the *Religious* needs, praying for oneself scored the highest, while praying with someone scored the lowest (Table 7.1). *Religious* needs correlated moderately with *Existential* needs ($r = 0.40$) and *Giving/Generativity* needs ($r = 0.36$), and weakly only with *Inner Peace* needs ($r = 0.28$).

Spiritual Needs and Spirituality as a Resource to Cope

When patients have access to their spirituality (faith), they may use it as a resource to cope with their life situation. An indicator of this could be a person's *Search* for access to spirituality as a resource to cope, their *Trust* in such a higher source, and their ability to *Reflect* their life concerns in terms of a positive interpretation of disease (Büssing 2010).

In patients with chronic diseases (n = 392) their search for access was strongly associated with *Religious* needs (r = 0.56), moderately with *Existential* needs (r = 0.42) and *Giving/Generativity* needs (r = 0.31), and weakly with *Inner Peace* needs (r = 0.27) (Büssing et al. 2013). Their religious Trust was strongly related with *Religious* needs (r = 0.69), moderately with *Existential* needs (r = 0.37), and weakly with *Inner Peace* needs (r = 0.21) and *Giving/Generativity* needs (r = 0.25). Reflection was moderately related with *Religious* needs (r = 0.49), *Existential* needs (r = 0.39), *Inner Peace* needs (r = 0.32), and *Giving/Generativity* needs (r = 0.33).

In the elderly living in retirement homes (n = 100), religious trust was strongly related with *Religious* needs (r = 0.76), weakly with *Inner Peace* needs (r = 0.29), and not significantly with *Existential* needs (r = 0.11) or *Giving/Generativity* needs (r = 0.24) (Erichsen and Büssing 2013).

Thus, *Religious* needs are an indicator that persons have religious trust and may rely on this resource in times of need.

Spiritual Needs and Spiritual Well-being

Are high spiritual needs an indicator of lacking spiritual well-being? This question was addressed in a sample of palliative treatment patients with cancer, in patients with chronic pain diseases, and in healthy stressed mothers. Spiritual well-being was measured with the 12-item Functional Assessment of Chronic Illness Therapy—Spiritual Well-Being Scale (FACIT-Sp), which differentiates well-being in the dimensions of Faith, Meaning, and Peace (Peterman et al. 2002; Bredle et al. 2011).

In patients with chronic pain diseases (n = 82), *Existential* needs were moderately inversely related with Meaning well-being (r = -0.32) and Peace well-being (r = -0.31), *Inner Peace* needs were moderately negatively correlated with Peace well-being (r = -0.36) and weakly negatively also with Meaning well-being (r = -0.25), while *Religious* needs were strongly positively associated with Faith well-being (r = 0.65). *Giving/Generativity* needs were weakly positively related to the Meaning component of spiritual well-being (r = 0.23) (Büssing et al. 2013).

In patients with cancer (n = 118), *Religious* needs were strongly positively associated with Faith well-being (r = 0.56), *Existential* needs were marginally negative (and not significantly) related with Meaning well-being (r = -0.15), while *Inner Peace* needs were marginally negative (and not significantly) related with Peace well-being, and *Giving/Generativity* needs neither with Peace (r = 0.09) nor with Meaning (r = 0.08) well-being (Büssing et al. 2020). None of the spiritual needs were significantly related with patients' life satisfaction, their perceived health status, or satisfaction with the support received (Büssing et al. 2020). In these palliative care patients, their Faith well-being was rather low, their Peace well-being in the mid-range, and their Meaning well-being quite high.

In healthy young mothers with sick newborns or premature children (n = 125), *Religious* needs were positively and strongly related with Faith well-being (r = 0.74), *Existential* needs were not significantly related with Meaning (r = 0.03) or Peace well-being (r = -0.05), *Inner Peace* needs were marginally negatively related with Peace well-being (r = -0.19), and *Giving/Generativity* needs weakly positively related with Faith well-being (r = 0.24) (Büssing et al. 2017).

One would expect negative associations between spiritual well-being and spiritual needs as lack of well-being could theoretically trigger the intensity of spiritual needs. These inverse associations were found indeed for the secular needs, while Faith well-being and *Religious* needs were strongly positively associated. The latter association might be explained by the fact that religiosity plays a less important role in the German society and thus *Religious* needs might simply indicate that persons do have this resource, and thus stating these needs would be positively associated with Faith well-being when this resource is available. This may further mean that spiritual needs are not simply the opposite of spiritual well-being, as both address different dimensions which are not strongly related.

Spiritual Needs and Mental Health Indicators

One may assume that spiritual needs are the product of expectations (which might be high) and comparisons with the current situation (which might be less satisfying). Therefore, all stressors (i.e., chronic illness) which would permanently restrict a person's quality of life and abilities to participate would increase the intensity of specific needs.

In patients with fibromyalgia (n = 141), particularly *Inner Peace* needs correlated moderately with anxiety (r = 0.47), the intention to escape from illness (r = 0.41), catastrophizing (r = 0.36), and depressive symptoms (r = 0.30) (Offenbaecher et al. 2013). With respect to SF36's quality-of-life components, moderately negative associations between *Inner Peace* needs and the subscales mental health (r = -0.42), social functioning (r = -0.32), and emotional role (r = -0.32) were found. *Existential* needs were moderately related with HADS' anxiety scale ($r = 0.35$), negatively with SF36's mental health component ($r = -0.32$), and weakly ($r < 0.30$) positively with escape from illness, catastrophizing, and depressive symptoms. *Giving/Generativity* needs were best related with SF36's bodily pain component ($r = -0.26$) and not significantly with the aforementioned mental health indicators. None of the described mental health indicators were significantly related with *Religious* needs. Further, none of the SpNQ scales correlated significantly with SF36's physical health component (Offenbaecher et al. 2013).

In outpatients with cancer ($n = 285$), Höcker et al. (2014) found that anxiety was the best predictor of *Existential* needs and *Inner Peace* needs. For *Religious* needs, neither depression, nor hopelessness, nor distress was a significant predictor, but weakly coherence as an attitude in life.

In the elderly living in retirement homes ($n = 100$), *Inner Peace* needs were moderately associated with grief ($r = 0.41$) and emotional tiredness ($r = 0.36$), and weakly ($r < 0.30$) with reduced quality of life and reduced life satisfaction (Erichsen and Büssing 2013). *Existential* needs were significantly associated with emotional tiredness ($r = 0.40$), but not with grief, quality of life, or life satisfaction. Both *Religious* needs and *Giving/Generativity* needs were weakly ($r < 0.30$) related to emotional tiredness, but not significantly with grief, quality of life, or life satisfaction.

In healthy soldiers ($n = 1092$), stress perception was moderately related with *Inner Peace* needs ($r = 0.39$), *Existential* needs ($r = 0.33$), and weakly with *Giving/Generativity* needs ($r = 0.23$) and marginally only with *Religious* needs ($r = -0.13$) (Büssing and Recchia 2016). Similarly, their posttraumatic stress disorder (PTSD) symptoms were moderately related with *Inner Peace* needs ($r = 0.37$), *Existential* needs ($r = 0.33$), and weakly with *Giving/Generativity* needs ($r = 0.27$) and marginally only with *Religious* needs ($r = 0.17$). In that sample, life satisfaction was moderately negatively associated with *Inner Peace* needs ($r = -0.34$), weakly with *Existential* needs ($r = -0.29$), marginally with *Giving/Generativity* needs ($r = -0.17$), and not significantly with *Religious* needs ($r = -0.05$).

In contrast, in healthy young mothers with sick newborns or premature children ($n = 125$), *Inner Peace* needs were moderately related with stress perception ($r = 0.34$) and weakly with grief ($r = 0.23$), while *Religious* needs, *Existential* needs, or *Giving/Generativity* did not show any significant association with stress perception or mood states (Büssing et al. 2017). Further, in these healthy mothers, none of the spiritual needs were related to life satisfaction.

This means, indicators of reduced mental health or negative mood states were related especially with *Inner Peace* needs and *Existential* needs, while *Religious* needs or *Giving/Generativity* did not show similar correlations. Depending on the sample of enrolled persons, their life satisfaction is either not at all or weakly to moderately related with their spiritual needs, particularly with *Inner Peace* needs.

Spiritual Needs and Interpretation of Illness

How patients interpret their life situation and illness might be crucial for their coping processes. According to Lipowski's meaning of illness (Lipowski 1970), one may differentiate between positive interpretations (i.e., Challenge, Value), strategy-associated interpretations (i.e., Relieving break from life, Call for help), guilt-associated interpretations (i.e., Punishment, Weakness/Failure), and fatalistic negative interpretations (i.e., Threat/Enemy, Interruption of life).

In patients with chronic diseases ($n = 392$), *Religious* needs were associated with illness seen as a Call for help ($r = 0.36$) and something of Value ($r = 0.33$), indicating that praying to God as an external instance of help is addressed (Büssing et al. 2013). *Existential* needs were related to illness as something of Value ($r = 0.42$), but also as a Relieving break ($r = 0.30$). *Inner Peace* needs were weakly ($r < 0.30$) related to illness as an Interruption and nevertheless also as Value. *Giving/Generativity* needs were weakly ($r < 0.30$) associated with Call for help, Value, and Threat.

The positive interpretation of illness as something of Value indicates a matter of hope that the situation may improve and that own attitudes and behaviors could be changed (Büssing and Fischer 2009). This positive interpretation was associated with all SpNQ subscales, particularly with *Existential* needs and *Religious* needs, while guilt-associated negative interpretations were not at all or only marginally associated (Büssing et al. 2013). Having such needs may thus mean that patients' intention to find meaning in their life, to clarify open processes from their past and to forgive, and also their need to communicate (with others or with God in prayer) are indicators that life is still seen as something of value, that it is worth all the efforts to fight against disease.

Conclusions

The SpNQ was developed to assess patients' unmet spiritual, existential, and psychosocial needs in a standardized way. It was finally validated with 20 items and four main scales: *Religious* needs, *Existential* needs, *Inner Peace* needs, and *Giving/Generativity* needs. The internal consistency of the SpNQ-20 is good (Cronbach's alpha = 0.88); the internal consistency of the subscales with four to six items per scale ranges from Cronbach's alpha 0.71 to 0.87. The factorial structure was confirmed by structured equation modelling (SEM). Depending on the enrolled group of persons with chronic diseases, some items may switch from the *Inner Peace* topic to *Existential* issues, depending on patients' interpretation of their situation and their expectations. Thus, apart from reporting differentiated findings with the subscales, the SpNQ-20 Mean Score (which uses all 20 items as a single scale) should also be reported to make data internationally comparable.

In different groups of persons one may see positive associations particularly between *Inner Peace* needs and *Existential* needs on the one hand and indicators of reduced mental health, negative mood states, and positive interpretations of illness such as Value on the other hand. Spiritual needs are not simply the opposite of spiritual well-being, as both are not consistently negatively associated—with the exception of *Religious* needs and Faith well-being, which are positively related. Thus, to provide spiritual care one has to assess spiritual needs, too, because patients with mid-range scores of spiritual well-being may nevertheless have specific unmet spiritual needs which should be addressed and supported. These dimensions are not that closely related as one would expect.

Therefore, with the SpNQ-20 a standardized, valid, and reliable instrument is available to be used in different samples and international studies.

Acknowledgments Thanks a lot to all who have helped to recruit the participants, particularly Hans-Joachim Balzat, Gerhild Becker, Jens Büntzel, Eckhard Frick, Andreas Kopf, and Jochen Rentschler.

References

Alderfer CP (1972) Existence, relatedness, and growth; human needs in organizational settings. Free Press, New York

Bredle JM, Salsman JM, Debb SM, Arnold BJ, Cella D (2011) Spiritual well-being as a component of health-related quality of life: the functional assessment of chronic illness therapy—spiritual well-being scale (FACIT-Sp). Religions 2:77–94. https://doi.org/10.3390/rel2010077

Büssing A (2010) Spirituality as a Resource to Rely on in Chronic Illness: The SpREUK Questionnaire. Religions 1:9–17

Büssing A (2014) Spiritual needs of those with chronic diseases. In: Michalos AC (ed) Encyclopedia of quality of life and well-being research. Springer, Dordrecht, pp 6269–6274

Büssing A, Fischer J (2009) Interpretation of illness in cancer survivors is associated with health-related variables and adaptive coping styles. BMC Womens Health 9:2. http://www.biomedcentral.com/1472-6874/9/2

Büssing A, Koenig HG (2010) Spiritual needs of patients with chronic diseases. Religions 1:18–27. https://doi.org/10.3390/rel1010018

Büssing A, Recchia DR (2016) Spiritual and Non-spiritual Needs Among German Soldiers and their Relation to Stress Perception, PTDS Symptoms, and Life Satisfaction – Results from a Structural Equation Modeling Approach. Journal of Religion and Health 55(3):747–764

Büssing A, Balzat HJ, Heusser P (2009) Spirituelle Bedürfnisse von Patienten mit chronischen Schmerz- und Tumorerkrankungen. Perioperative Medizin 1:248

Büssing A, Balzat HJ, Heusser P (2010) Spiritual needs of patients with chronic pain diseases and cancer – validation of the spiritual needs questionnaire. Eur J Med Res 15:266–273

Büssing A, Janko A, Kopf A, Lux EA, Frick E (2012) Zusammenhänge zwischen psychosozialen und spirituellen Bedürfnissen und Bewertung von Krankheit bei Patienten mit chronischen Erkrankungen. Spiritual Care 1:57–73

Büssing A, Janko A, Baumann K, Hvidt NC, Kopf A (2013) Spiritual Needs among Patients with Chronic Pain Diseases and Cancer Living in a Secular Society. Pain Med 14:1362–1373

Büssing A, Wassermann U, Hvidt NC, Längler A, Thiel M (2017) Spiritual needs of mothers with sick new born or premature infants. Woman and Birth 31(2):e89–e98. https://doi.org/10.1016/j.wombi.2017.08.002

Büssing A, Recchia DR, Koenig H, Baumann K, Frick E (2018) Factor structure of the spiritual needs questionnaire (SpNQ) in persons with chronic diseases, elderly and healthy individuals. Religions 9:13. https://doi.org/10.3390/rel9010013

Büssing A, Baumann K, Rentschler J, Becker G (2020) Spirituelle Bedürfnisse von Tumorpatienten verändern sich während der palliativmedizinischen Betreuung kaum. Deutsche Zeitschrift für Onkologie. Online first: https://doi.org/10.1055/a-1135-3566

Erichsen NB, Büssing A (2013) Spiritual needs of elderly living in retirement / nursing homes. Evid Based Complement Alternat Med 2013:Article ID 913247. https://doi.org/10.1155/2013/913247

Höcker A, Krüll A, Koch U, Mehnert A (2014) Exploring spiritual needs and their associated factors in an urban sample of early and advanced cancer patients. Eur J Cancer Care 23:786–794. https://doi.org/10.1111/ecc.12200

Lipowski ZJ (1970) Physical illness, the individual and the coping processes. Psychiatry Med 1:91–102

Offenbaecher M, Kohls N, Toussaint LL, Sigl C, Winkelmann A, Hieblinger R, Walther A, Büssing A (2013) Spiritual needs in patients suffering from fibromyalgia. Evid Based Complement Alternat Med 2013:Article ID 178547. https://doi.org/10.1155/2013/178547

Peterman AH, Fitchett G, Brady MJ, Hernandez L, Cella D (2002) Measuring spiritual well-being in people with cancer: the functional assessment of chronic illness therapy – spiritual well-being scale (FACIT-Sp). Ann Behav Med 24:49–58

CHAPTER 8

Adapted Spiritual Needs Questionnaire for Adolescents with Chronic Diseases

Arndt Büssing

Background

It was the intention to adapt and shorten the conventional Spiritual Needs Questionnaire (SpNQ) in order to assess spiritual needs of adolescents with chronic states/diseases. There are several studies underlining that the topic of spirituality is also of importance in younger persons (Damsma Bakker et al. 2018), even when several of them would regard themselves as nonreligious (Büssing et al. 2012). While a qualitative meta-synthesis by Damsma Bakker et al. (2018) would argue that their spirituality is related to "identity focusing on normalcy" and refers to a "supportive God," in rather secular healthy adolescents, religiosity is of low relevance (Büssing et al. 2012). Instead, conscious dealings with others and the nature, compassion and intentions to help others were more relevant to them. Bull and Gillies (2007) investigated the spiritual needs of five

A. Büssing (✉)
Professorship Quality of Life, Spirituality and Coping, Faculty of Health, Witten/Herdecke University, Herdecke, Germany

IUNCTUS—Competence Center for Christian Spirituality, Philosophical-Theological University of Münster, Münster, Germany
e-mail: arndt.buessing@uni-wh.de

A. Büssing (ed.), *Spiritual Needs in Research and Practice*,
https://doi.org/10.1007/978-3-030-70139-0_8

hospitalized school-age children using pictures to facilitate storytelling. Interview data revealed that relationships were an important need, and also coping with the invasive treatments, their attitudes toward their health and belief system, as well as influences of the hospital environment. Petersen (2013) argued that for children spirituality is particularly relevant at the end of life, as it gives "comfort; support; and a sense of connection." In her concept analysis of spiritual care she identified six attributes: "assessing spiritual needs; assisting the child to express feelings; guiding the child in strengthening relationships; helping the child to be remembered; assisting the child to find meaning; and aiding the child to find hope." However, this was in reference to dying children. In a study by Feudtner et al. (2003) pastors assessed the spiritual care needs of children (one-third were chronically ill and one-fifth were dying); however, the children themselves were not interviewed; this was the pastoral care provider's perception. A qualitative study by Cai et al. (2020) assessed spiritual needs among families in pediatric palliative care, but not the needs of the children. In fact, so far there is no validated assessment instrument available that focuses on adolescents' spiritual needs, particularly those who either have to live with a chronic condition or have to cope with longer courses of treatment.

Development of a Shortened and Adapted Version

To generate a shortened and adapted version we referred to the standardized SpNQ used for adults (Büssing et al. 2018). Items that focus too much on problematic aspects were not used (i.e., life review, confrontation with death). Deleted items were the existential items: N5 (dissolve open aspects of life), N12 (talk with someone about the possibility of life after death) and N17 (be forgiven). Further deletions were the generative items N15 (give solace to someone), N26 (pass own life experiences to others) and the optional item N4 (reflect back on your life). Instead we added three items that address receiving attention and positive confirmation: N38 (there is someone for you who is always at your side), N43 (your situation is improving for the better) and N44 (have someone to assure you how to proceed [in a positive way]). Thus, building from the findings of Petersen (2013) and Bull and Gillies (2007), we included the topics finding meaning, finding hope, relationships between concrete persons, intentions to relate to the Sacred through prayer and finding inner peace.

The 18 primary items have the same 4-option scoring to assess the strength of spiritual needs like the SpNQ-20: 0—none, 1—somewhat,

2—moderate, 3—strong. These items were tested first in a pilot study among 16 adolescents (mean age: 14 ± 2 years). The respective questions were understood well and could be adequately answered; the resulting response patterns were comprehensible and consistent in themselves. Then we tested the instrument on a sample of 200 adolescents (62% female, 38% male; mean age: 16 ± 2 [11–22] years) recruited from various treatment centers in Germany. Respondents were adolescents with either physical diseases (52%) or with psycho-emotional diseases (46%); 2% had unclear diagnoses.

Exploratory Factor Analysis of the Shortened Instrument

Exploratory factor analysis indicated four main components (Table 8.1), which would explain 68% of variance. Two items loaded too weakly on factor 3 and were thus eliminated (N25, feel connected with family; N16, forgive someone from a distinct period of life). Further, item N10 (find meaning in illness and/or suffering) was eliminated because it weakened the internal consistency of the scale. The shortened 15-item version for adolescents has the following structure:

- Factor 1 addresses primarily praying needs and the intention to turn to a higher presence of monotheistic religious traditions. The four respective items have good internal consistency (Cronbach's alpha = 0.89).
- Because four items from the *Giving/Generativity* and *Existential Needs* factors of the adult version (SpNQ-20) were not used here, factor 2 combines four items from both topics with acceptable internal consistency (Cronbach's alpha = 0.76). The focus is on a relational aspect (turn to someone in a loving attitude, and giving solace to someone) on the one hand, and on a communicative aspect (someone assures that your life is meaningful and of value and someone is there to talk about meaning in life in general) on the other.
- Factor 3 includes the three new items that address receiving attention and positive confirmation, and the need to talk with someone about fears and worries. The relational aspect with a solving and assuring motif is at the forefront of this factor. The four items have good internal consistency (Cronbach's alpha = 0.82). Item N38 (there is someone there for you who is always at your side) strongly

Table 8.1 Exploratory factor and reliability analyses

	Mean (SD)	*Corrected item—scale correlation*	*Cronbach's alpha if item is deleted (alpha = 0.872)*	*Factor loading*			
				1	*2*	*3*	*4*
Factor 1: Religious/praying needs (eigenvalue: 5.4; alpha = 0.892)							
N20 pray for yourself	0.64 (0.99)	0.396	0.869	0.894			
N23 turn to a higher presence (i.e., God, Allah)	0.76 (1.08)	0.399	0.870	0.878			
N18 pray with someone	0.35 (0.75)	0.389	0.869	0.858			
N19 that someone prays for you	0.54 (0.91)	0.465	0.866	0.810			
Factor 2: Existential/giving needs (eigenvalue: 2.7; alpha = 0.763)							
N13 turn to someone in a loving attitude	1.69 (1.10)	0.603	0.860		0.743		
N27 be assured that your life is meaningful and of value	1.46 (1.19)	0.654	0.857		0.684		
N11 talk with someone about the question of meaning in life	1.19 (1.18)	0.520	0.864		0.670		
N15 provide solace to someone	1.56 (1.04)	0.544	0.863		0.662		
Factor 3: Attention/positive confirmation needs (eigenvalue: 1.1; alpha = 0.819)							
N43 that your situation is improving for the better	2.16 (1.09)	0.526	0.863			0.831	
N44 have someone to assure you how to proceed (in a positive way)	1.85 (1.16)	0.669	0.856		0.341	0.708	

(*continued*)

Table 8.1 (continued)

	Mean (SD)	*Corrected item—scale correlation*	*Cronbach's alpha if item is deleted (alpha = 0.872)*	*Factor loading 1*	*2*	*3*	*4*
N38 that there is someone there for you who is always at your side	2.14 (1.08)	0.651	0.857		0.523	0.672	
N2 talk with someone about your fears and worries	1.65 (1.01)	0.584	0.861		0.407	0.580	
Factor 4: Inner peace needs (eigenvalue: 1.0; alpha = 0.719)							
N6 plunge into beauty of nature	1.45 (1.02)	0.379	0.870				0.782
N7 dwell at a place of quietness and peace	1.75 (1.04)	0.404	0.869				0.749
N8 find inner peace	1.88 (1.13)	0.578	0.861			0.461	0.663
Excluded items							
N25 feel connected with family	1.48 (1.15)	–	–			–	
N16 forgive someone from a distinct period of your life	1.10 (1.06)	–	–			–	
N10 find meaning in illness and/or suffering	1.15 (1.17)	–	–		–		

Extraction method: principle components analysis (Varimax rotation with Kaiser normalization); rotation converged in five iterations; five factors explain 68% of variance; only loadings > 0.30 are depicted

cross-loads on *Existential/Giving* needs, but fits much better with the intention of the needs for *Attention/Positive Confirmation*.

- The topic of factor 4 is *Inner Peace* needs which are measured with three items and acceptable internal consistency (Cronbach's alpha = 0.72). Here, inner peace is found in nature and at special places of "quietness and peace" to result in states of inner peace.

In this group of adolescents, the praying needs scored quite low, particularly for praying with someone. Among the *Existential/Giving* needs, the stabilization aspect of a loving relation (turn to someone in a loving attitude) scored the highest, followed by the intention to provide solace to someone, which is again a relational aspect. Within the *Inner Peace* needs factor, the need to find inner peace scored the highest, as well as the wish to dwell at a place of quietness and peace. The highest scores were found for the needs for *Attention/Positive Confirmation*, particularly the confirmation that your situation is improving for the better and that there is someone for you who is always at your side. Here, the hope aspect is at the forefront.

Associations of Subscales with External Measures

The life satisfaction of persons investigated herein (as measured with the BMLSS-10) was significantly ($p < 0.001$; Spearman rho) and moderately inversely related to *Attention/Positive Confirmation* needs ($r = -0.30$), and weakly negatively to *Inner Peace* needs ($r = -0.29$) and *Existential/Giving* needs ($r = -0.20$), but not significantly with *Religious* needs ($r = -0.08$). Similarly, perceived impairment through symptoms of the underlying disease was moderately positively associated with *Attention/Positive Confirmation* needs ($r = 0.40$), weakly with *Inner Peace* needs ($r = 0.22$) and *Existential/Giving* needs ($r = 0.24$), and also with *Religious/ Praying* needs ($r = 0.23$). This means perceived impairment of quality of life and well-being is related particularly to *Attention/Positive Confirmation* needs, indicating that adolescents with chronic conditions call for help to support them and to assure a positive outcome.

Attention/Positive Confirmation needs were moderately related also to *Inner Peace* needs ($r = 0.47$), and one may assume that sick adolescents were awaiting that attention and were given hope by external persons which resulted in states of inner peace. Moreover, *Attention/Positive Confirmation* needs were strongly associated with *Existential/Giving* needs ($r = 0.61$); this effect was mainly related to the meaning-finding component (N27; $r = 0.52$) and the relational aspect (N13: $r = 0.49$).

However, *Religious/Praying* needs were moderately related to *Existential/Giving* needs ($r = 0.33$); here, the relational topic was only weakly associated (N13: $r = 0.27$; N15: $r = 0.26$). This could be explained because relations can either have a horizontal (concrete persons) or vertical (God) direction—and both are important when the symptom burden is too high. Moreover, *Religious/Praying* needs were strongly related to the frequency of one's own prayers and church attendance ($r = 0.67$), while all other needs were only marginally or not at all related to religious practices ($r < 0.20$).

Thus, these correlations are plausible from a theoretical point of view and would underline the relevance of this shortened instrument.

Conclusions

The adapted 15-item version for adolescents with chronic states or long-lasting treatments (SpNQ-Ad) has a similar structure to the SpNQ-20 for adults. The factors *Religious* needs and *Inner Peace* needs were retained, while, due to the shortening process, the formerly separate topics of existential and giving needs were now condensed into one factor termed *Existential/Giving* needs. Because of the introduction of three new items with a new topic, an additional factor emerged, termed needs for *Attention/Positive Confirmation*, which showed the highest scores. The internal consistency of these four factors is good (ranging from Cronbach's alpha 0.72 to 0.89), and the correlations with external measures such as life satisfaction, symptom burden and religious practices are sound from a theoretical point of view. The standardized SpNQ-Ad can thus be used in future studies with adolescents.

Acknowledgments Thanks a lot to all who have helped to recruit the participants, particularly Laura Sieber, Justine Hussong, Alexander von Gontard, Charlotte Roch and Jörg Große-Onnebrink.

References

Bull A, Gillies M (2007) Spiritual needs of children with complex healthcare needs in hospital. Pediatr Nurs 19:34–38

Büssing A, Kerksieck P, Föller-Manici A, Baumann K (2012) Aspects of spirituality and ideals to help in adolescents from Christian academic high schools. International Journal of Children's Spirituality 17(2):99–116

Büssing A, Recchia DR, Koenig H, Baumann K, Frick E (2018) Factor structure of the Spiritual Needs Questionnaire (SpNQ) in persons with chronic diseases, elderly and healthy individuals. Religions 9:13. https://doi.org/10.3390/rel9010013

Cai S, Guo Q, Luo Y, Zhou Y, Abbas A, Zhou X, Peng X (2020) Spiritual needs and communicating about death in nonreligious theistic families in pediatric palliative care: a qualitative study. Palliat Med 23:269216319896747

Damsma Bakker AA, van Leeuwen RRR, Roodbol PFP (2018) The spirituality of children with chronic conditions: a qualitative meta-synthesis. J Pediatr Nurs 43:e106–e113

Feudtner C, Haney J, Dimmers MA (2003) Spiritual care needs of hospitalized children and their families: a national survey of pastoral care providers' perceptions. Pediatrics 111:e67–e72

Petersen CL (2013) Spiritual care of the child with cancer at the end of life: a concept analysis. J Adv Nurs 70:1243–1253

CHAPTER 9

Structures of Spiritual Needs Questionnaire Versions in Countries with Different Cultural and Religious Backgrounds

Olga Riklikienė, Wilson Correia de Abreu, Tânia Cristina de Oliveira Valente, Maryam Rassouli, Janusz Surzykiewicz, and Arndt Büssing

BACKGROUND

Although the terms *health* and *salvation* have the same root in several languages such as Sanskrit, the Anglo-Saxon languages, Latin and Hebrew, and although healing has been associated with religiosity since ancient times, until recently the religious and spiritual aspects were the least considered and those that most generated doubts and discomfort for

O. Riklikienė (✉)
Faculty of Nursing, Medical Academy, Lithuanian University of Health Sciences, Kaunas, Lithuania
e-mail: olga.riklikiene@lsmuni.lt

W. C. de Abreu
Porto School of Nursing, Porto, Portugal CINTESIS (Center for Health Technology and Services Research), University of Porto, Porto, Portugal
e-mail: wjabreu@esenf.pt

A. Büssing (ed.), *Spiritual Needs in Research and Practice*,
https://doi.org/10.1007/978-3-030-70139-0_9

health care (Backes et al. 2012). This scenario has changed in the last 20 years with the increase of research on religion/spirituality and health. Between 2001 and 2010, research in the area almost tripled, going from 1200 to over 3000 studies (Moreira-Almeida 2010; Koenig 2012), and has aroused great interest from professionals and researchers and the emergence of many discoveries about the health–spirituality–religiosity triad (Koenig 2015).

Research in this field, particularly the assessment of spiritual needs, makes it necessary to better understand the cultural factors (i.e., value systems) for public mental health (Forsman et al. 2015; Oman 2018). There is another interest in assessing spirituality resulting from growing acceptance of the strengths perspective which posits one's personal and environmental needs and strengths as important to cope with health challenges or healing processes through the use of ones' own capabilities in everyday life and in times of sickness.

The multidimensional definition of spirituality as "the aspect of humanity that refers to the way individuals seek and express meaning and purpose and the way they experience their connectedness to the moment, to self, to others, to nature, and to the significant or sacred" (Puchalski et al. 2014, p. 643) poses significant difficulty in measuring the spirituality

T. C. de Oliveira Valente
Interdisciplinary Medical Anthropologic Studies and Research Laboratory, Rio de Janeiro State Federal University, Rio de Janeiro, Brazil

M. Rassouli
Cancer Research Center, Shahid Beheshti University of Medical Sciences, Tehran, Iran

J. Surzykiewicz
Faculty of Philosophy and Education, Katholische Universität Eichstätt-Ingolstadt, Eichstätt, Germany

Faculty of Education, Cardinal Stefan Wyszynski University in Warsaw, Warsaw, Poland
e-mail: Janusz.Surzykiewicz@ku.de

A. Büssing
Professorship Quality of Life, Spirituality and Coping, Faculty of Health, Witten/Herdecke University, Herdecke, Germany

IUNCTUS—Competence Center for Christian Spirituality, Philosophical-Theological University of Münster, Münster, Germany
e-mail: Arndt.buessing@uni-wh.de

phenomenon. In the context of the spiritual needs assessment, this complexity became critical.

Spiritual needs can be defined as *the need of connection to the moment, the self, others, nature and the significant or sacred* (Seddigh et al. 2016, p. 6). The author highlighted the main problems for spiritual needs research: the diversity of spiritual needs according to the severity of the patients; the variety of needs expressed in the results of qualitative studies, covering transcendental, mystical and other needs that involve conceptual aspects; the challenge to include it in research instruments, in addition to the need for a reductionist approach so that the instruments can be used in daily life routines by health professionals.

Importantly, for rigorous spirituality assessment, well-prepared, valid and reliable measurement tools are needed. The development of new research tools is always a time-consuming process requesting the involvement of competent investigators and experts in the field. For this reason, instead of developing their own study instruments, researchers more often search and select the most appropriate existing tool to perform its linguistic, cultural and practical adaptation. The biggest obstacle in the validation process, however, is linked to cultural issues.

The Spiritual Needs Questionnaire (SpNQ), initially developed in Germany and published in English (Büssing et al. 2010), whose model was proposed in 2009, has been translated and validated so far in the languages and used in the following countries: Germany (Büssing et al. 2010, 2018), Brazil (Oliveira da Silva et al. 2020), China (Büssing et al. 2013), Croatia (Glavas et al. 2017), Indonesia (Nuraeni et al. 2015), Iran (Moeini et al. 2018; Hatamipour et al. 2018), Lithuania (Riklikienė et al. 2019), Pakistan (Kashif and Kanwal 2018), Poland (Büssing et al. 2015), Portugal (Valente et al. 2018), Italy (accomplished by Renata Spalek and Janusz Surzykiewicz), France (Marion Trousselard), Greece (Fradelos et al. 2020), Denmark (Niels Christian Hvidt), Spain (Japcy Margarita Quiceno and Stefano Vinaccia Alpi), Japan (Hoshina Uehara) and Korea (Kyeonga Yoon).

However, depending on the cultural and religious background on the one hand and the selected sample (i.e., patients with chronic diseases, the elderly, healthy persons), cognitive abilities (i.e., persons with dementia), and sample size on the other hand, the structure of multifactorial instruments, particularly those focusing on spiritual issues, may change (Table 9.1). Moreover, when specific items are deleted from a subscale or new items are added which were so far not regarded as 'spiritual' (i.e., family concerns), the structure will change, too. With respect to the SpNQ, there is an interchange of some of the 'existential' items because

Table 9.1 The structure of SpNQ when adapting it for different cultural and religious backgrounds and in various samples

	Germany	*Poland*	*Lithuania*	*Portugal*	*Brazil 1*	*Brazil 2*	*Iran 1*	*Iran 2*	*China*
N20 pray for yourself	Re	Re	Re	Re	Re	Re	Re	Re	Re
N21 participate in a religious ceremony (i.e., service)	Re	Re	Re	Re	Re	RR	Re	Re	–
N23 turn to a higher presence (i.e., God, Allah)	Re	Re	Re	Re	Re	Re	Re	Re	Re
N18 pray with someone	Re	Re	Re	RR	Re	Re	Re	–	Re
N19 that someone prays for you	Re	Re	Re	RR	Re	Re	Re	Re	Re
N22 read religious/ spiritual books	Re	Re	Re	Re	Ex	RR	Re	Re	Re
N3 someone from the religious community cares for you	(Re)	–	Re	–	Re	RR	–	–	–
N11 talk with someone about the question of meaning in life	Exe	Exe	GF	ExC	Ex	Ex	Ex	Ex	–
N10 find meaning in illness and/or suffering	Ex	Ex	(GF)	ExC	Ex	Ex	Ex	Ex	IP
N2 talk with others about fears and worries	Ex	Ex	(Re)	ExC	–	Ex	IPAG	Em	–
N4 reflect on previous life	(Ex)	–	IP	–	–	ExC	Ex	Ex	Ex
N5 dissolve open aspects of your life	Ex	Ex	(IP)	ExC	–	ExC	Ex	Em	Ex

N12 talk with someone about the possibility of life after death	Ex	Ex	Re	ExC	Ex	Ex	Ex	Ex	Ex
N17 be forgiven	Ex	–	(GF)	IPG	GG	–	–	–	–
N16 forgive someone from a distinct period of your life	Ex	Ex	GF	IPG	GG	–	–	GF	GG
N15 provide solace to someone	GG	GG	GF	IPG	–	(Re)	IPAG	GF	GG
N14 give away something from yourself	GG	–	GF	IPG	–	Re	IPAG	–	–
N26 pass own life experiences to others	GG	GG	ExF	IPG	(Ex)	(Re)	–	GF	GG
N27 be assured that your life is meaningful and of value	GG	GG	ExF	IPG	–	–	–	GF	GG
N13 turn to someone in a loving attitude	(GG)	–	GG	–	Ex	–	IPAG	Em	GG
N6 plunge into beauty of nature	IP	IP	IP	IPG	IP	IPF	IPAG	IP	IP
N7 dwell in a place of quietness and peace	IP	IP	IP	IPG	IP	IPF	IPAG	IP	IP
N8 find inner peace	IP	IP	IP	IPG	IP	IPF	IPAG	IP	IP
N24 be complete and safe	–	–	(ExF)	Extra	–	–	–	–	–
N25 feel connected with family	–	–	ExF	NP	FF	IPF	–	–	–

(*continued*)

Table 9.1 (continued)

	Germany	*Poland*	*Lithuania*	*Portugal*	*Brazil 1*	*Brazil 2*	*Iran 1*	*Iran 2*	*China*
N28 be re-involved by your family in their life concerns	–	–	ExF	NP	FS	(IPF)	–	–	–
N30 receiving more support from family	–	–	–	NA	FS	(IPF)	–	–	–

Abbreviations: Re—Religious needs; RR—Religious Recognition needs; Ex—Existential needs; ExF—Existential/Family needs; Family Support needs; IP—Inner Peace needs; IPF—Inner Peace/Family Support needs; GG—Giving/Generativity needs; GF—Giving/Forgiveness needs; ExC—Existential Reflection/Clarification needs; RR—Religious recognition need; NP—Need for participating; NA—Need for attention; IPAG—Inner Peace /Active Giving; IPG—Inner Peace/Generativity needs; Em—Emotional needs; Extra—the item was not used in primary version some of them address clarification and resolving issues, which are related to states of inner peace as a result, and can thus be both *Inner Peace* items and *Existential* needs items. In other cases, Catholic persons will see needs to forgive as a *Religious* need, while nonreligious people will interpret it as an existential issue with the consequence of clarifying open aspects in their life.

The primary version of the SpNQ is described in Chap. 7. In the following sections we will present and discuss findings from international studies using either the same structure or adapted variant versions.

The SpNQ in Different Cultural and Practical Contexts

Lithuanian Version of SpNQ

The SpNQ was selected based on the analysis of the literature and review of similar tools to assess spiritual needs of individuals in Lithuania. Keeping in mind the complexity of the Lithuanian language, cultural sensitivity and ambiguity in understanding the research construct (i.e., spiritual needs), a priority for the European-based instrument was assigned initially. The previous translations and validations of SpNQ into many languages created promising expectations for researchers to successfully transfer the instrument into the Lithuanian language, culture and practice.

The important aspect was the fact that the SpNQ was designed for use in adults with chronic diseases. Further, the researchers anticipated that traditional self-reported survey type of data collection will not work easily for hospitalized older adult cancer patients and face-to-face interviews might be an option, too. The SpNQ was recognized as an easy and suitable tool for interview administration. Moreover, the SpNQ is simple in language with short statements to start communication with patients about their spirituality and their unmet needs. Finally, the data from the first qualitative phase of study mentioned earlier revealed that the main spiritual concerns of cancer patients match the four core dimensions of spiritual needs: connection, peace, meaning/purpose and transcendence (Büssing and Koenig 2010).

The Lithuanian version of the SpNQ was culturally tested in a sample of 247 patients hospitalized in nursing and supportive treatment units at public hospitals (Riklikienė et al. 2019). There were more female patients (61%) than male. The age of patients varied from 32 years to 96 years, and the mean age was 67.1 ± 11.6 years. Two-thirds (78%) identified themselves as religious, 10% as nonreligious and 12% were undecided (Riklikienė et al. 2019).

The structure of the SpNQ in its Lithuanian version was confirmed during the factor analysis process. Following the Varimax rotation, items loaded significantly on four factors: *Religious* needs (eight items; factorial loads between 0.46 and 0.84), *Giving/Generativity* (including Forgiveness) needs (four items; factorial loads ranging from 0.61 to 0.78), *Existential* needs (five items; factorial loads between 0.42 and 0.71) and *Inner Peace* needs (three items; factorial loads ranging from 0.65 to 0.85). In total, 18 items out of 20 of the consented SpNQ-20 version had a loading range higher than 0.5 and explained 64% of variance.

For non-terminally ill cancer patients ($N = 227$) in Lithuania, the most important needs were *Inner Peace* needs (1.75 ± 0.66) and *Giving/Generativity and Forgiveness* needs (1.64 ± 0.68), followed by *Existential* needs (1.33 ± 0.67) and *Religious* needs (1.26 ± 0.79) (Riklikienė et al. 2020).

Validation of the SpNQ-20 in the Lithuanian language and clinical practice revealed that the domain of *Religious* needs was the most stable and complied with the original German version the best. The same six items (N18, N19, N20, N21, N22, N23) on the *Religious* needs domain were found in the German language version of SpNQ (Büssing et al. 2010) and the Polish version of SpNQ (Büssing et al. 2015). The Lithuanian version of SpNQ-20 had two additional items included for the *Religious* domain: the *Inner Peace* need to talk with others about your fears and worries (N2) and the *Existential* need to talk with someone about the possibility of life after death (N12). The latter need could indeed be interpreted as a religious issue, particularly for Christians who belief in some kind of resurrection.

The validation process revealed that *Existential* needs as well as *Giving/Generativity and Forgiveness* needs domains in the Lithuanian version of SpNQ-20 lost their original structure to the maximum extent. The Lithuanian SpNQ-20 domain of *Giving/Generativity and Forgiveness* needs consists of four items: two giving ones (N14: give away something from yourself; N15: give solace to someone), and the two forgiveness items N16 and N17. These four items have in common the topic of relational connections. Three *Existential* needs items were the same as in the original German version (N5, N10 and N11), addressing meaning in life and suffering, and dissolving open aspects in life. However, the other two items (N26: pass own life experiences to others; N27: be assured that your life was meaningful and of value) included here were originally derived from the *Giving/Generativity* needs scale in the Lithuanian version. In the original SpNQ-20 version the *Inner Peace* domain had four items (N2, N6, N7, N8), while in the Lithuanian SpNQ-20 version, one item (N2) about sharing fears and worries with someone loaded better to the *Religious* needs domain. However, because of very low loading, it did not fit any of the four factors (Riklikienė et al. 2019).

Polish Version of the SpNQ

To assess spiritual needs in Poland, the SpNQ was selected based on the analysis of the literature and review of similar tools. The items of the German version were translated by a bi-language scientist and then critically discussed with a group of Polish psychologists, theologians and medical doctors, and the primary author of the SpNQ. To guarantee linguistic equivalence, critical phrases were discussed in the team and adjusted with respect to cultural specifics. An important aspect was the fact that the SpNQ was designed for use in adults with chronic diseases and was identified as an easy and suitable tool for interview administration.

The Polish version was then validated in a sample of 275 patients with chronic diseases (35% with cancer, 10% with chronic pain diseases, 16% with diabetes mellitus, and 40% with other chronic diseases (Büssing et al. 2015). They were recruited consecutively by a psychologist and educators in the Oncology Hospital in Wieliszew and in the Department of Social Welfare in the province of Warsaw. Among 74% women and 26% men with a mean age of 56 ± 16 years, where all were Christians, 78% regard themselves as religious and spiritual, 7% as religious but not spiritual, 2% as not religious but spiritual, and 13% as neither religious nor spiritual.

During the process of factorial analyses (Oblimin rotation) with the 20-item pool, two items were deleted, either due to a weak factor loading (N4W: reflect back on life) or strong side loadings (N6W: plunge into beauty of nature). Explorative factor analysis indicated five factors which would explain 68% of variance and internal consistency coefficients (Cronbach's alpha) ranging from 0.59 to 0.91. These were with the factors of the original version of the SpNQ. However, the existential items were split into two factors: Meaning (Cronbach's alpha = 0.80) and Relief (a = 0.59). Particularly, the latter factor had an unsatisfactory internal consistence and thus a 4-factor solution was tested. Here, the internal consistency coefficients ranging from 0.71 to 0.91 were more satisfying and were in line with the intended structure (Büssing et al. 2015).

Religious needs with six items (N18, N19, N20, N21, N22, N23; Cronbach's alpha = 0.91), *Existential* needs: Meaning with six items (N5, N10, N11, N12, N16, N2; Cronbach's alpha = 0.79), *Giving/Generativity* needs with four items (N13, N15, N26, N27; Cronbach's alpha = 0.78), *Inner Peace* needs with three items (N6, N7, N8; Cronbach's alpha = 0.71). Here all items fit onto the intended loadings, with the exception of item N2 (talk about fears and worries), which is primarily an *Inner Peace* item that nevertheless fits in this context. This structure was underlined by confirmatory factor analysis (Büssing et al. 2015).

Part of the validation study was to verify the instrument's convergence accuracy. In Polish patients with chronic diseases, *Religious* needs were not a matter of high or low life satisfaction. *Religious* needs can be predicted best by Religious Attitudes (SQS), spiritual Search (SpREUK) and SpREUK's Reflection (Positive Interpretation of Illness) scale. The strongest predictor of *Existential* needs was the interpretation of illness as a Threat/Enemy (IIQ), while the ability to also see illness as a Challenge was a negative predictor. *Giving/Generativity* needs were predicted best by Ethical Sensitivity (SQS), while the best predictors of the *Inner Peace* scale were illness interpretations such as Call for help, Punishment and Threat/Enemy, and further by Ethical Sensitivity/SQS).

Thus, the 18-item Polish version of the SpNQ has a similar structure as the primary version and good internal consistency of the four underlying factors, and can thus be used for further research in a predominantly Catholic population such as Poland.

Portuguese Version of SpNQ

Given the history of Portugal, whose nationality was conquered a thousand years ago due to the Christian identity, the values, traditions and beliefs are closely linked to religion and spirituality, especially in the North of the country. The influence of spirituality as an adjustment to the chronic disease, preservation of hope and acceptance of the therapeutic regime is very present in chronic diseases and cannot be devalued when studying health needs and defining treatment. The SpNQ was selected based on the analysis of the literature, debates with health professionals and evaluation of similar tools to assess spiritual needs of individuals in the country. The validation process took into account the nature of Portuguese as a Latin language, Portuguese culture and the religious identities of the population. Before the validation in Portugal, the validation processes of SpNQ in other cultural contexts were analyzed. The previous translations and validations of SpNQ into many languages created promising expectations for researchers/experts to successfully validate the instrument into Portuguese language, culture and practice to be used in Portugal, because the version in Portuguese from Brazil has some sentences that could raise doubts in Portuguese reality as experts concluded.

The SpNQ was developed to be used in people of different ages and health conditions, including people with chronic diseases. There is a long version with 27 items to be used as a clinical instrument and a reduced version for research purposes with 20 items with research proposals. Here we will refer to the 20-item version (SpNQ-20). Participants of the study filled out the tool (self-administration) with the support of the researchers whenever necessary. The confidence in the tool was based on the simple language it uses and the perspective on spirituality that underpins the tool. In general, our participants, as part of the Portuguese population, are close to the four core dimensions of spiritual needs: connection, peace, meaning/purpose and transcendence (Büssing and Koenig 2010).

The Portuguese version of the SpNQ was culturally tested in a sample of 379 patients (in hospitals and in the community), all of them with chronic diseases (neurocognitive, cardio-circulatory, endocrine, skeletal, oncological and hematological). The age of the patients was on average 62.2 ± 23.7 [18–97] years; 60% were male. The majority (88%) identified themselves as religious and 12% as nonreligious.

The structure of the SpNQ-20 in its Portuguese version was confirmed during the factor analysis process. Following the Varimax rotation, items loaded significantly on four factors: *Inner Peace/Generativity* needs (nine items: N6; N7; N8; N14; N15; N16; N17; N26; N27; factorial loads between 0.46 and 0.84), *Religious* needs (four items: N20; N21; N22; N23; factorial loads ranging from 0.38 to 0.74), *Existential Reflection/Clarification* needs (five items: N2; N5; N10; N11; N12; factorial loads between 0.46 and 0.82) and *Religious Recognition* needs (two items: N18; N19; factorial loads ranging from 0.53 to 0.77). In total, 15 items out of 20 of the consented SpNQ-20 version had a loading range higher than 0.5 and explained 75% of variance.

Validation of the SpNQ-20 in the Portuguese language to Portugal revealed some differences compared to the factors of the original version, which can be considered usual. There were no problems with the translation from English to Portuguese (and back) and the terms or expressions in the original document were easily understood by both experts and the population. The most substantive difference occurred in terms of the domains and the valuation that people gave to each issue. More than one-third of the population had dementia as an associated chronic disease, which implies the presence of memory problems and cognitive decline. Anyway, the presence of *Religious* needs domain was found as it was in the German version of the SpNQ (Büssing et al. 2010) and the Polish version of SpNQ (Büssing et al. 2015). There are some variants in the Portuguese version validated so far in patients with dementia. *Inner Peace/Generativity* needs comprise nine items (N6: plunge into beauty of nature; N7: dwell at a place of quietness and peace; N8: find inner peace; N14: give away something from yourself; N15: provide solace to someone; N16: forgive someone from a distinct period of your life; N17: be forgiven; N26: pass own life experiences to others; N27: be assured that your life is meaningful and of value) and combines *Inner Peace* items, but also the primary four *Giving/Generativity* items (N14, N15, N26, N27) and two *Existential* and forgiveness items (N16, N17) which are related to states of inner peace, of course. The *Religious* needs items are split in two factors: *Religious* needs with four items (N20: pray for yourself; N21: participate in a religious ceremony; N22: read religious/spiritual books; N23: turn to a higher presence (i.e., God)), and a second one termed *Religious Recognition* needs with two items (N18: pray with someone; and N19: that someone prays for you). The factor *Existential Reflection/Clarification* needs has five items and combines four of the *Existential* items (N5: dissolve open aspects of your life; N10: find meaning in illness and/or suffering; N11: talk with someone about the question of meaning in life; N12: talk with someone about the possibility of life after death) with one *Inner Peace* item (N2: talk with others about fears and worries) which nevertheless fits well with the other items. Three items which were not used in the primary German language version are not present in the Portuguese version, too (N3: someone from the religious community cares for you, N4: reflect on previous life; and N13: turn to someone in a loving attitude), while they were used in the Brazilian version.

Brazilian Version of SpNQ

Concerning Brazil, the country is a vast mosaic, both from the historical point of view, reflecting a social formation that combined the knowledge of the Amerindian, African populations and the Portuguese, French and Dutch colonizers, and because of the large territorial extension where these elements have manifested in different ways. Moreover, the fact that most instruments present in the literature addressing spiritual needs have Christianity as a religious reference makes it challenging to apply standardized tools in countries where religious hybridity is the main characteristic, such as in Brazil. Bearing this in mind, the challenges of conducting research on spiritual needs was evidenced.

One of the main characteristics of the Brazilian identity is the highlight on the relationship between religiosity and health (Andrade 2009). Caretakers, shamans, mediums and saints, among other elements, have always inhabited the imagination, being frequently present in the cultural manifestations, such as in books, films and popular festivals. Most of the population believes that the transcendent interferes with the evolution and cure of illnesses and values religious/spiritual treatments to solve health problems, with issues related to diseases being among the main reasons that lead people to seek religious help in Brazil (Mello 2020). Such aspects are associated with the differences in the role attributed to religiosity in the different regions of Brazil. All of this attributes very peculiar characteristics to spiritual needs, which would hardly be covered by any single instrument.

During the SpNQ adaptation to the Portuguese language and validation process the questionnaire was applied to a sample of people living with HIV in Rio de Janeiro, located in southeast Brazil, and in João Pessoa, located in the northeast of the country. The validation results in both samples were different.

In Rio de Janeiro, the final SpNQ structure presented a composition of four factors: *Religious* needs (N3, N18, N19, N20, N21, N22, N23), *Giving/Generativity and Forgiveness* needs (N10, N11, N12, N13, N14, N17), *Inner Peace* needs (N4, N6, N7 and N8) and *Family Support* needs (N25, N28, N30) (Valente et al. 2018). The last three items were primarily not a part of the factorial structure of the original SpNQ, and used as 'informative' items only. By adding these items, further factors appeared in the Brazil sample. In the mainly Catholic sample from João Pessoa, the final structure presented a new composition, with five factors (or domains): *Religious* needs (N13, N14, N15, N18, N19, N20, N23 and N26); *Inner Peace and Family Support* needs (N6, N7, N8, N25, N28 and N30); *Existential* needs (N2, N10, N11 and N12); *Social Recognition* needs (N3, N21 and N22) and *Time Domain: Reflection and Clarification* needs

(N4 and N5) (Oliveira da Silva et al. 2020). Here, the items addressing family support needs would load together with the *Inner Peace* needs, while two items addressing reflection on life and subsequent needs to clarify certain aspects (N4 and N5) form an independent factor. Item N3 (someone of your religious community (i.e., pastor) cares for you or comes to see you) was not used in the primary version, while it is included in both samples from Brazil. In both Brazilian cities it is a religious needs item, while in João Pessoa it will load together with participating in a religious ceremony (N21) and reading spiritual/religious books (N22) as an independent factor termed *Social Recognition* needs.

Thus, the configuration of the factors also had a distinct distribution of items, demonstrating that cultural differences within a country of territorial dimensions like Brazil can lead to differences in spiritual needs between individuals. It might be more relevant to combine heterogeneous data sets from different cultural and religious regions of Brazil and revalidate them together to make data comparable.

Iranian Version of SpNQ

In the studies conducted in Iran with mainly Shiite Muslims, spirituality is introduced as a relationship with God and trust in Him, the source of hope and the cause of immunity, and leads to reduced pressures and tensions. On the contrary, its absence is associated with losing the meaning of life (Farahani et al. 2019; Zamanzadeh et al. 2014).

Studies have shown that people experience spiritual distress when they face difficult challenges such as cancer, and their spiritual needs increase (Zamanzadeh et al. 2014). Therefore, spiritual coping is the most powerful approach through which patients can deal with diseases (Lim and Yi 2009). However, many patients do not receive the spiritual care they seek. The spiritual needs of cancer patients are either addressed minimally or ignored (Büssing and Koenig 2010). These unmet spiritual needs will result in reduced quality of care, decreased patient satisfaction and poor quality of life (Zamanzadeh et al. 2014).

Accordingly, the identification of patients' spiritual needs is of great significance due to the religious nature of Iranians and the prevalence of religious beliefs due to which the underlying religious rules and values are considered an inevitable part of life and even end-of-life moments. Therefore, a qualitative research conducted by Hatamipour et al. (2015) in this regard revealed that the spiritual needs of Iranian cancer patients, including connection, peace, meaning and purpose, and transcendence, consist of the subclasses of social support, normal behavior, inner peace, seeking forgiveness, hope, acceptance of reality, seeking meaning, ending well, change of life meaning, strengthening spiritual belief, communication with God and prayer (Hatamipour et al. 2015).

The next step in assessing the spiritual needs of persons and addressing them was accessing the right tool. Based on a qualitative study that approved the consistency of the obtained themes with the SpNQ subscales and using the Consensus-based Standards for the Selection of health status Measurements Instruments (COSMIN), it was discovered that among the available tools, the SpNQ has psychometric properties that are appropriate for use in Iranian cancer patients. Therefore, in a methodological research done by Hatamipour et al. (2018), the SpNQ was translated and its Farsi version was validated in a sample of 400 cancer patients visiting Tehran Cancer Institute. The tool was first translated into Farsi and then back-translated. After the translated version was ready the tool was approved by its developer, the content validity was examined through measuring the Content Validity Index (CVI) by ten experts in the fields of instrument development, cancer and spirituality, which was reported to be 0.98. In addition, for face validity, ten cancer patients were asked to rate the items in terms of clarity and simplicity.

Confirmatory factor analysis (CFA) was performed to evaluate the construct validity and the model fitness. In the initial 4-factor model, the fit indices of the model were undesirable. Therefore, in order to modify the model, Exploratory Factor Analysis (EFA) was performed. First, the samples were divided into two groups of 200 samples. Thus, EFA was performed with 200 samples. Latent variables in the tool were extracted using screen plot and according to the load factor. There were three factors with eigenvalue of above 1 that explained 54.3% of the total variance. These factors were respectively named need for *Peace and Active Giving* with 8 items (N1, N2, N6, N7, N8, N13, N14, N15), *Religious* needs with 6 items (N18, N19, N20, N21, N22, N23) and *Existential* needs with 5 items (N4, N5, N10, N11, N12). After performing EFA and determining the dimensions of the questionnaire, CFA was performed on the sample with 200 subjects to verify the model. CFA indicated a good fit for the 3-factor model of the questionnaire. So it can be said that three factors of the questionnaire have been confirmed.

Cronbach's alpha was 0.91 for the whole questionnaire and 0.76–0.86 for its subscales. In order to examine the Intra-class Correlation Coefficient

(ICC) through test–retest, the questionnaire was completed by 15 cancer patients on two occasions with a 3-week time interval. The ICC was reported to be 0.82.

Psychometric results showed that the modified Farsi version of the SpNQ, with three subscales and 19 items, can be used to assess the spiritual needs of Iranian cancer patients. Obviously, there are some differences between the Iranian version and the original version of the scale, due to the cultural and religious context of the Iranian society, because of which religion and religious needs have a strong relationship with the spiritual needs of patients (Hatamipour et al. 2018).

Another translation is the 19-item SpNQ Persian Version (SpNQ-PV) which was validated with a sample of 100 persons with chronic diseases at two university hospitals in Qom, Iran (Moeini et al. 2018). Here five factors were differentiated: *Religious* needs with 5 items (N19, N20, N21, N22, N23), *Existential* needs with 4 items (N4, N10, N11, N12), *Forgiveness/Generativity* needs with 4 items (N15, N16, N26, N27), *Inner Peace* needs with 3 items (N6, N7, N8) and *Emotional* needs with 3 items (N2, N5, N13). Cronbach's alpha ranged from 0.56 (the 3-item scale *Emotional* needs) to 0.78 (*Religious* needs) and the test-retest reliability ranged from 0.72 to 0.91.

Both versions from Iran have similarities with respect to *Religious* needs and *Inner Peace* needs, but differ particularly with respect to *Giving/Generativity* needs (Table 9.1). The version of Hatamipour et al. (2018) uses three factors (and does not include the forgiveness items N16 and N17, and the generativity items N26 and N27) and the version of Moeini et al. (2018) uses five factors (and does not include the forgiveness item N17 and the praying item N18).

Chinese Version of the SpNQ

Talking about own 'weakness' (i.e., depression) and health difficulties is problematic in China's cultural context. Mental health problems are often less acceptable than physical health problems or work-related stress. Therefore, it was interesting to see whether a standardized (self-reported) assessment of spiritual needs would be applicable in patients from Shanghai. For that purpose, the items of the SpNQ were translated by a team of medical doctors from China and checked for consistency by a bilingual colleague living in Germany. Unclear phrasings were discussed with the developer of the instrument and adjusted where needed.

To validate the Chinese version, 168 patients from Shanghai with a mean age of 51 ± 16 years (61% men and 39% women) were enrolled (Büssing et al. 2013). Their diagnoses were cancer (63%), chronic pain diseases (10%) or other chronic conditions (23%); 5% did not provide information. Most had no religious affiliation (68%), while 13% were Buddhist, 5% Christians and 2% with other religious affiliations; 11% did not provide information.

During the process of validation, item N21 (participate in a religious ceremony) was not used because it was too weak an item to scale correlation, while item N5 (dissolve open aspects of life) from a previous version (SpNQ 1.0) was included. Further, the *Inner Peace* needs item N2 (talk about fears and worries), the *Existential* needs item N11 (talk about the meaning in life) and the *Giving/Generativity* needs item N14 (give away something from yourself) had to be eliminated due to weak factor loading. Using the remaining 17 items, exploratory factor analyses revealed five main factors, which would explain 64% of variance. The scale *Inner Peace* needs (Cronbach's alpha = 0.76) used the intended three items (N6, N7, N8) and the existential item N10 (finding meaning in illness and suffering). The scale *Giving/Generativity* needs (Cronbach's alpha = 0.78) used five items, three of the intended items (N16, N26, N27), one from a previous version of this scale (N13: turn to someone in a loving attitude) and the Forgiveness item N16. *Religious* needs were split into two subconstructs: one with the three *Praying* items N18, N19 and N20 (Cronbach's = 0.81) and one with the two *Sources* items N22 and N23 (Cronbach's alpha = 0.72). The *Existential/Reflection* needs scale (Cronbach's alpha = 0.51) used two Existential items (N5 and N12) and one Reflection item from a previous version of the scale (N4: reflect back on your life). Due to the switch of *Inner Peace* item N10 to the *Inner Peace* scale, the truncated 3-item *Existential/Reflection* scale's internal consistency is less satisfactory.

Most spiritual needs scored rather low in this sample from Shanghai. The strongest need was to know that your life was meaningful and of value (N27: 1.52 ± 0.96) and to be connected with the family (N25: 1.71 ± 0.93), which was used as a control item. The lowest scoring need was to read religious/spiritual books (N22: 0.28 ± 0.58).

The resulting spiritual needs factors differed significantly between nonreligious and religious persons only with respect to both *Religious* needs factors, but not for the other needs (Büssing et al. 2013). Thus, the SpNQ in its Chinese version was applicable in persons from Shanghai and showed similar mean scores compared to those of persons with chronic diseases from secular Germany.

Conclusions

Comparison of the different language versions of the SpNQ (Table 9.1) revealed that *Religious* needs an *Inner Peace* needs prove to be the most stable domains. With the inclusion of items which were primarily intended to be used as informational items only, the factorial structure of the tool will change and the items will load differently. The item switch in different language versions is also related to cultural differences and the way things are interpreted by populations in various contexts. Even in one and the same country, large territorial dimensions and religious hybridity (i.e., Brazil) can lead to different spiritual concerns and interpretations among individuals and slightly modified structure of the measurement applied. For this reason, careful attention should be paid to contextual features more generally in the translation and validation process of the SpNQ.

Nevertheless, application of the different language versions of SpNQ-20, which keeps items from the original structure, allows international comparison of the results and identification of cultural peculiarities in individuals' perception of their spiritual needs. For this purpose, the additional usage of the SpNQ-20 mean score is recommended, which uses the consented 20 items without weighting the underlying items. This allows accounting for cultural and religious specificities on the one hand when the culturally adapted versions are used, and enables intercultural/interreligious comparisons with the SpNQ-20 mean score on the other hand.

References

Andrade MO (2009) A religiosidade brasileira: o pluralismo religioso, a diversidade de crenças e o processo sincrético. Revista Eletrônica de Ciências Sociais 14:106–118

Backes D, Backes M, Medeiros H, Siqueira DFD, Pereira SB, Dalcin CB, Rupolo I (2012) Oficinas de espiritualidade: alternativa de cuidado para o tratamento integral de dependentes químicos. Rev Esc Enferm USP 46:1254–1259. https://doi.org/10.1590/s0080-62342012000500030

Büssing A, Balzat HJ, Heusser P (2010) Spiritual needs of patients with chronic pain diseases and cancer - validation of the spiritual needs questionnaire. Eur J Med Res 15:266–273

Büssing A, Koenig H (2010) Spiritual needs of patients with chronic diseases. Religions 1:18–27. https://doi.org/10.3390/rel1010018

Büssing A, Zhai X, Peng W, Ling C (2013) Psychosocial and spiritual needs of patients with chronic diseases: validation of the Chinese version of the spiritual needs questionnaire. J Integr Med 11:106–115. https://doi.org/10.3736/jintegrmed2013020

Büssing A, Pilchowska I, Surzykiewicz J (2015) Spiritual needs of polish patients with chronic diseases. J Relig Health 54:1524–1542. https://doi.org/10.1007/s10943-014-9863-x

Büssing A, Recchia D, Koenig H, Baumann K, Frick E (2018) Factor structure of the spiritual needs questionnaire (SpNQ) in persons with chronic diseases, elderly and healthy individuals. Religions 9:13. https://doi.org/10.3390/rel9010013

Farahani AS, Rassouli M, Salmani N, Mojen LK, Sajjadi M, Heidarzadeh M, Masoudifar Z, Khademi F (2019) Evaluation of health care providers' perception of spiritual care and the obstacles to its implementation. Asia Pac J Oncol Nurs 6:122. https://doi.org/10.4103/apjon.apjon_69_18

Forsman AK, Wahlbeck K, Aarø LE, Alonso J, Barry MM, Brunn M, Cardoso G, Cattan M, de Girolamo G, Eberhard-Gran M, Evans-Lacko S, Fiorillo A, Hansson L, Haro JM, Hazo JB, Hegerl U, Katschnig H, Knappe S, Luciano M, Miret M, Nordentoft M, Obradors-Tarragó C, Pilgrim D, Ruud T, Salize HJ, Stewart-Brown SL, Tómasson K, van der Feltz-Cornelis CM, Ventus DBJ, Vuori J, Värnik A, ROAMER Consortium (2015) Research priorities for public mental health in Europe: recommendations of the ROAMER project. Eur J Public Health 25(2):249–254

Fradelos EC, Prapa P, Alikari V, Papathanasiou IV, Lavdaniti M, Tzavella F, Platis Ch, Theofilou P (2020) Investigation of the Psychometric Properties of the Greek Version of the Spiritual Needs Questionnaire (SpNQ) Hellenic Journal of Nursing 59(4):360–368

Glavas A, Jors K, Büssing A, Baumann K (2017) Spiritual needs of PTSD patients in Croatia and Bosnia-Herzegovina: a quantitative pilot study. Psychiatr Danub 29:282–290. https://doi.org/10.24869/psyd.2017.282

Hatamipour K, Rassouli M, Yaghmaie F, Zendedel K, Majd H (2015) Spiritual needs of cancer patients: a qualitative study. Indian J Palliat Care 21:61. https://doi.org/10.4103/0973-1075.150190

Hatamipour K, Rassouli M, Yaghmaie F, Zendedel K (2018) Psychometric properties of the Farsi version of "spiritual needs questionnaire" for Cancer patients in Iran: a methodological study. Asian Pac J Cancer Prev 19:989–995. https://doi.org/10.22034/APJCP.2018.19.4.989

Kashif A, Kanwal Z (2018) Translation, cultural adaptation of spiritual needs questionnaire in Pakistan. Religions 9:163. https://doi.org/10.3390/rel9050163

Koenig HG (2012) Religion, spirituality, and health: the research and clinical implications. ISRN Psychiatry:278730. https://doi.org/10.5402/2012/278730

Koenig HG (2015) Religion, spirituality, and health: a review and update. Adv Mind Body Med 29(3):19–26

Lim J, Yi J (2009) The effects of religiosity, spirituality, and social support on quality of life: a comparison between Korean American and Korean breast and gynecologic Cancer survivors. Oncol Nurs Forum 36:699–708. https://doi.org/10.1188/09.onf.699-708

Mello M (2020) Práticas terapêuticas populares e religiosidade afro-brasileira em terreiros no Rio de Janeiro: um diálogo possível entre saúde e antropologia. In: Arca.fiocruz.br. https://www.arca.fiocruz.br/handle/icict/13795

Moeini B, Zamanian H, Taheri-Kharameh Z, Ramezani T, Saati-Asr M, Hajrahimian M, Amini-Tehrani M (2018) Translation and psychometric testing of the Persian version of the spiritual needs questionnaire among elders with chronic diseases. J Pain Symptom Manag 55:94–100. https://doi.org/10.1016/j.jpainsymman.2017.08.024

Moreira-Almeida A (2010) O crescente impacto das publicações em espiritualidade e saúde e o papel da Revista de Psiquiatria Clínica. Arch Clin Psychiatry 37:41–42. https://doi.org/10.1590/s0101-60832010000200001

Nuraeni A, Nurhidayah I, Hidayati N, Sari M, Mirwanti R (2015) Kebutuhan Spiritual pada Pasien Kanker. Jurnal Keperawatan Padjadjaran 3:57–66. https://doi.org/10.24198/jkp.v3n2.1

Oliveira da Silva C, Rodrigues Cavalcanti A, da Silva Lima K, Macêdo Cavalcanti CA, de Oliveira Valente TC, Büssing A (2020) Spiritual needs questionnaire (SpNQ): validity evidence among HIV+ patients in Northeast Brazil. Religions 11:234. https://doi.org/10.3390/rel11050234

Oman D (2018) Elephant in the room: why spirituality and religion matter for public health. In: Oman D (ed) Why religion and spirituality matter for public health evidence, implications, and resources, vol 2. Springer International, Basel, pp 1–16

Puchalski C, Vitillo R, Hull S, Reller N (2014) Improving the spiritual dimension of whole person care: reaching national and international consensus. J Palliat Med 17:642–656. https://doi.org/10.1089/jpm.2014.9427

Riklikienė O, Spirgienė L, Kaselienė S, Luneckaitė Ž, Tomkevičiūtė J, Büssing A (2019) Translation, cultural, and clinical validation of the Lithuanian version of the spiritual needs questionnaire among hospitalized Cancer patients. Medicina 55:738. https://doi.org/10.3390/medicina55110738

Riklikienė O, Tomkevičiūtė J, Spirgienė L, Valiuliene Ž, Büssing A (2020) Spiritual needs and their association with indicators of quality of life among non-terminally ill cancer patients: cross-sectional survey. Eur J Oncol Nurs 44:101681. https://doi.org/10.1016/j.ejon.2019.101681

Seddigh R, Keshavarz Akhlaghi A, Azarnik S (2016) The spiritual needs of patients and the procedure to measure them: a literature review. Iran J Psychiatry Behav Sci 10(1):e4011. https://doi.org/10.17795/ijpbs-4011

Valente T, Cavalcanti A, Büssing A, Costa Junior C, Motta R (2018) Transcultural adaptation and psychometric properties of Portuguese version of the spiritual needs questionnaire (SpNQ) among HIV positive patients in Brazil. Religions 9:135. https://doi.org/10.3390/rel9040135

Zamanzadeh V, Rassouli M, Abbaszadeh A, Nikanfar A, Alavi-Majd H, Ghahramanian A (2014) Factors influencing communication between the patients with cancer and their nurses in oncology wards. Indian J Palliat Care 20:12–20. https://doi.org/10.4103/0973-1075.125549

PART III

Findings in Different Populations: Persons with Chronic Diseases

CHAPTER 10

Spiritual Needs of Patients with Chronic Pain Diseases

Arndt Büssing and Simon Peng-Keller

Background

Persons facing chronic pain, which is a negative experience with different causes and various aggravating factors (physical, cognitive, emotional, social, and spiritual), have to find ways to cope. Patients' pain perception which starts with a sensory stimulus is related to strong emotions, fears, and worries about the future, as they may also lose their social functioning, experience physical decline, lack abilities to participate in the social networks, struggle with their faith, experience loss of meaning in life, and thus aggravating hopelessness and depressive states (Fig. 10.1). According to Cicely Saunders' concept of total pain (1993), several dimensions might be influenced by the primarily sensory pain (as a perception), which finally

A. Büssing (✉)
Professorship Quality of Life, Spirituality and Coping, Faculty of Health, Witten/Herdecke University, Herdecke, Germany

IUNCTUS—Competence Center for Christian Spirituality, Philosophical-Theological University of Münster, Münster, Germany
e-mail: Arndt.buessing@uni-wh.de

S. Peng-Keller
Faculty of Theology, University of Zürich, Zürich, Switzerland

A. Büssing (ed.), *Spiritual Needs in Research and Practice*,
https://doi.org/10.1007/978-3-030-70139-0_10

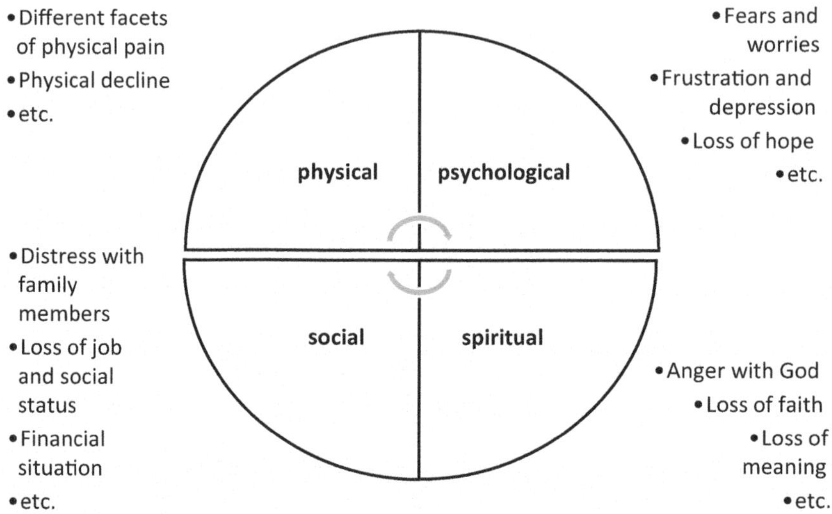

Fig. 10.1 Principles of the concept of total pain according to Cicely Saunders (1993) with its four basic, interacting components. Here, pain is understood multidimensionally and not restricted as a bodily experience only

becomes a multidimensional 'pain disease'. According to Saunders, physical pain, emotional suffering, social isolation, and spiritual distress may be mutually reinforcing. The existential suffering in chronic pain raises questions similar to those in end-of-life situations. Persistent and seemingly inexplicable pain not only impairs daily living but also gnaws at the human need for meaning in life.

Chronic pain as a stressor in life may result in patients' attempts to cope, either by problem-solving and thus attempts to control it, or by finding social support, or by accepting the situation as it is in terms of adapting to the situation (Lazarus and Folkman 1984; van Damme et al. 2008). Prayer and hope are among the positive coping strategies (Fernandez and Turk 1989), while avoidance and escape are among the negative strategies related to mood affections, pain severity, functional impairment, and low self-efficacy, indicating uncontrollability of the situation (Brown and Nicassio 1987).

For American patients, praying and religious coping seems to be highly relevant (McCaffrey et al. 2004; Moreira-Almeida and Koenig 2008), while in rather secular societies such as Germany the prevalence of religious activities (inclusively praying) is rather low (Büssing et al. 2009) but nevertheless relevant (Zwingmann et al. 2006, 2008; Rettke et al. 2020). Baetz and Bowen (2008) surprisingly reported that "religious persons were less likely to have chronic pain and fatigue"; they were found to be praying more often and using their spirituality to cope. However, their statement is rather questionable: as though being religious is a buffer against the experience of suffering and pain. The general experience is rather that religious persons also become ill, suffer from pain, and are anxious and depressed, even when it is true that they may use their spirituality as a resource to cope.

For healthy persons it was found that meditation increases their pain tolerance and spiritual well-being (Sollgruber et al. 2018), implying that meditation is an indicator of spirituality. However, this study refers to a short-term pain experience with a defined end. For patients with chronic pain conditions the situation is different, as their pain is difficult to control (which makes them dependent on medical doctors, physiotherapists, etc.) and reappears. Nevertheless, practices of mindful meditation might be somewhat helpful to cope with pain conditions, as at least small decreases were found in a recent meta-analysis (Hilton et al. 2017). In these studies, mindful meditation was used as a psychotherapeutic approach rather than a 'spiritual practice'. However, secular forms of meditation may be reframed spiritually by participants, as Wachholtz and Pargament (2005) showed, and the effects of secular meditation can be enhanced when their spiritual dimension is made explicit.

Dedeli and Kaptan (2013) underlined that spiritual and religious variables may have an impact on pain perception and experience of illness. Spiritual struggles and the perception of being abandoned by God (in terms of negative religious coping) may aggravate the total pain experience (Wachholtz and Pearce 2010). Baetz and Bowen (2008) reported that religious persons, in contrast to spiritual ones, may have less pain and less fatigue. Their coping strategies were different: Both religious and spiritual persons were using more positive coping strategies than nonreligious or non-spiritual persons, while spiritual patients were more often using negative coping strategies (Baetz and Bowen 2008). However, religious persons were defined by their worship attendance only (which is a good indicator for very strict religious persons, but not for all believers), while spiritual persons were defined by the single statement as to whether "spiritual values play an important role" in their lives. One is defined by values (attitude) and the other by an active participation (activity), and thus these findings are biased by methodological problems.

Another approach is to ask patients what they need instead of how they think they are (i.e., religious, spiritual, neither). For that purpose, the Spiritual Needs Questionnaire (SpNQ) was developed and applied in various groups of patients with chronic diseases. As shown in Chap. 7 (Fig. 7.1), outpatients with chronic pain diseases have a similar pattern of spiritual needs compared to patients with cancer. Nevertheless, their *Religious* needs and *Giving/Generativity* needs scored significantly lower compared to tumor patients, while their *Existential* needs and *Inner Peace* needs were not significantly different. Further, enrolled patients with chronic pain diseases were about 5 years younger than tumor patients ($p < 0.0001$; Mann-Whitney-U test) and had a much lower life satisfaction (BMLSS: 55.6 ± 18.9 vs 65.9 ± 16.8; $p < 0.0001$, Mann-Whitney-U test). One would expect that a lower life satisfaction would result in higher needs. However, there might be some other aspects that could interpret these findings.

Interpretations of Illness and Their Association with Spiritual Needs

Patients with cancer, particularly women, regard their illness mostly as a challenge, but also as something of value to grown from, but nevertheless as a threat (Büssing and Fischer 2009). Instead, patients with chronic pain diseases would rather reject the positive interpretations (Büssing et al. 2006). Focusing on womens' interpretation only (to avoid gender-related effects), it became clear that particularly the interpretation of illness as a disturbing interruption was of relevance, but also the view of illness as a threat, but nevertheless a challenge and as something of value (Büssing 2017). Here, the negative interpretations were more relevant, but the possibility that chronic pain could be a challenge to overcome—which is a matter of hope—was of relevance. Interestingly, particularly the positive interpretations (Challenge and Value) were related to patients' spiritual/religious self-perception, with higher positive scores in spiritual (R+S+ and R-S+) persons compared to non-spiritual (R+S- and R-S-) women (Büssing 2017). This means, the underlying spiritual attitude was of relevance to how persons with chronic pain conditions experience their illness and its impact on their life concerns. Further, the negative views were moderately related with patients' intention to escape from their life situation (which is an avoidance coping strategy) and weakly with low life satisfaction, while the positive views were not significantly or marginally related. The best predictors of womens' positive interpretations of illness were their ability to reflect on their life concerns (which is a reappraisal coping strategy) and intentions to change (which means to fight and keep hopes high) (Büssing 2017). Patients with chronic pain diseases suffer from their illness and this influences how they see their life with the intention to escape from their situation (and their pain). In most cases, the pain medication reduces the pain perceptions for a while, but the pain is quite difficult to effectively treat all the time and to be 'cured' completely. Therefore, depressive states, anxiety, alcohol misuse, hopelessness, and suicide risk are prevalent among them (Ishak et al. 2018; Racine 2018).

In another study among German patients with chronic pain diseases (including 14% with cancer), *Religious* needs were moderately associated with the view of illness as a call for help or as something of value, and weakly with illness seen as a challenge (Büssing et al. 2013). *Existential* needs were moderately related to the view of illness as something of value and as a relief from the demands of life, and weakly with illness as an interruption, a challenge, or a call for help. *Inner Peace* needs were weakly associated with illness as an interruption, as something of value, or as a call for help. *Giving/Generativity* needs were weakly related only with a call for help. Thus, different views of illness may have a differential impact on the spiritual needs that patients might express. In most cases, the call for help was prevalent (either in terms of concrete contacts or praying to God as an external source) with the hopeful view that the illness may nevertheless have some value and has thus meaning—even when this 'meaning' might be difficult to understand in the current situation.

In Polish patients with chronic diseases, *Existential* needs were weakly associated with the view of illness as a threat or as an interruption, while *Inner Peace* needs were weakly related with the view of illness as a call for help (Büssing et al. 2015). *Religious* needs were only marginally related with illness as a call for help, while *Giving/Generativity* needs were moderately related with illness as something of value. Thus, both the cultural background and the more religious background of Polish patients may result in different attributions to what their illness may mean to them—and this may further influence their coping with the chronic pain condition.

Gender- and Age-Related Differences in Spiritual Needs of Persons with Chronic Pain Diseases

Among patients with chronic diseases, women had significantly higher *Religious* needs, *Existential* needs, and *Inner Peace* needs than men did, while they did not differ in their *Giving/Generativity* needs (Büssing et al. 2013). In a sample of 408 patients (data source: Büssing et al. 2018) with chronic pain diseases, this difference could be underlined as women having significantly stronger *Religious* needs ($F = 13.3, p < 0.0001$), *Existential* needs ($F = 13.3, p < 0.0001$), and *Inner Peace* needs ($F = 7.7, p = 0.006$) than men, while again their *Giving/Generativity* needs did not differ ($F = 1.0$, n.s.). The SpNQ-20 mean score for women was significantly higher than that for men (1.03 ± 0.64 vs 0.77 ± 0.58; $F = 13.9, p < 0.0001$).

As shown in Fig. 10.2, *Religious needs* and *Giving/Generativity* needs differ with respect to the age cohorts, with the lowest scores in younger patients and the highest in the older ones, while *Existential* needs and

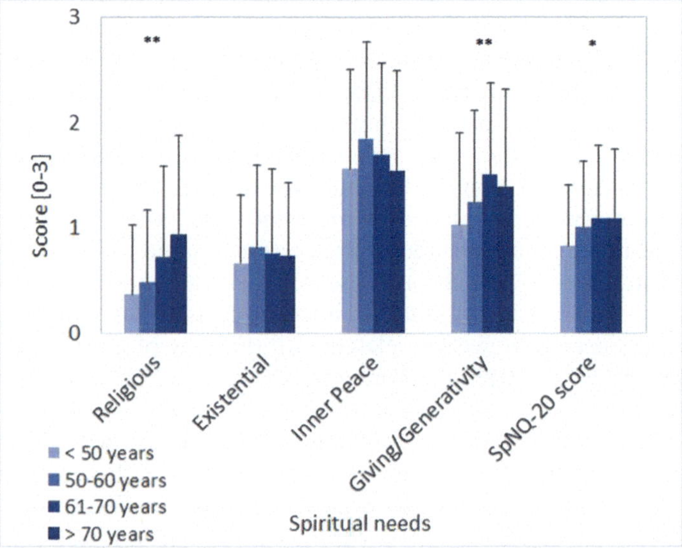

Fig. 10.2 Spiritual needs of patients with chronic pain conditions who reported on their age ($n = 339$; 73% women, 27% men; mean age: 56 ± 13 years). (Data source: Büssing et al. (2018); $^{**}p < 0.01$; $^{*}p < 0.05$ (ANOVA))

Inner Peace needs are not significantly different with respect to the age cohorts. Univariate analyses with age and gender as influencing variables revealed that for *Religious* needs gender had a stronger influence than age, while for *Existential* needs gender alone had a significant influence; in contrast, *Inner Peace* needs and *Giving/Generativity* needs were influenced mostly by gender and by the combination of gender and age, while age alone had a weak influence only on *Inner Peace* needs, but no influence on *Giving/Generativity* needs (data not shown). It seems that the intention to guide the next generation with their experiences in life (and maybe also to cope with illness) and to be assured that life has meaning (which are the main topics of the *Giving/Generativity* domain) are more relevant for the elderly as compared to younger patients with chronic pain conditions. Similarly, the resource of one's own faith and the ability to pray is more prevalent in older persons compared to younger ones. This might be due to a different religious socialization in the older age cohorts.

Which needs were of particular importance to the aforementioned patients with chronic pain conditions? Talking about fears and worries was important for 56%, but not to talk with someone about meaning in life (important for 21%) or that someone from a religious community comes for such talks (important for 5% only). To reflect on life was important for 40%, but less relevant was to forgive others (important for 27%) or to be forgiven (important for 22%). Finding external and internal peace was of outstanding relevance: To plunge into the beauty of nature, finding a place of quietness and peace; and finding inner peace was important for 65%, 60%, and 57%, respectively. Turning to someone in a loving attitude was seen as important by 56%, to give solace to someone by 44%, and to be connected with the family by 69%. To pass one's own life experiences to others was relevant for 53% and to be assured that one's own life was meaningful for 51%. In contrast, praying was important for 28% and participating in a religious ceremony (i.e., Sunday service) for 18% only.

All these needs were regarded as important by the patients, and required a reaction. Not all unmet needs can be fulfilled, but they are an opportunity to start communication about how health-care professionals, psychologists, social workers, pastoral workers, and others can help.

Spiritual Needs and Their Association with Mental Health Conditions

Fibromyalgia is a chronic pain condition with symptoms such as tenderness on pressure (tender points), widespread pain, but also fatigue, disturbed, and unrefreshed sleep, along with psychological distress (Wolfe et al. 2010). In a sample of 141 patients with fibromyalgia (95% women, mean age 58 ± 10 years), *Inner Peace* needs scored the highest, followed by *Giving/Generativity* needs, while *Existential* needs and *Religious* needs scored the lowest (Offenbaecher et al. 2013). Additional items addressing needs for participation (i.e., being more involved in family business, invited by friends, and more connected with family) scored relatively high, indicating that concrete contacts and participation is required (Offenbaecher et al. 2013).

In these patients, tender points were not significantly related to their spiritual needs, while the fibromyalgia impact was weakly related to *Inner Peace* needs. Instead, mental health indicators were more relevant: *Inner Peace* needs were moderately positively associated with anxiety, depressive symptoms, the intention to escape from illness, and catastrophizing, and with reduced emotional and social functioning (Offenbaecher et al. 2013). This means, there is a cluster of variables which may trigger patients' need for inner peace, and they all indicate that the situation of life with chronic pain conditions exceeds the capacity to cope, resulting in fears, worries, and catastrophizing, and thus a depressive intention to escape from the situation. Interestingly, catastrophizing as a negative coping strategy is a strong predictor of worsening pain conditions, greater disability, low quality of life, and discontinuation of pharmacotherapy (Toth et al. 2013). These indicators can be regarded as primarily negative coping strategies related to a poor life situation (Brown and Nicassio 1987), and thus needs to find states of inner peace and emotional stability are comprehensible.

Existential needs were moderately positively related to anxiety and reduced mental health scores. As this factor addresses the need to find meaning in illness and suffering, and intentions to talk about the question of meaning in life on the one hand, and to reflect back on life with intentions to clarify open aspects in life and to forgive and be forgiven on the other hand, the topic of anxiety as a relevant trigger is obvious.

Religious needs were not at all related to these mental health indicators, which means that some may utilize this resource to cope and others may not. In fact, this resource was utilized primarily by persons with religious and spiritual self-perception (R+S+: 18%), but not by nonreligious/non-spiritual patients (R-S-: 39% in that sample).

Giving/Generativity needs were at least weakly negatively associated with bodily pain (Offenbaecher et al. 2013), indicating that bodily pain perception may negatively interfere with their intentions to help others and be assured of meaning in life despite disease symptoms.

To analyze which of these various related variables can be regarded as the best predictors of spiritual needs, Offenbaecher et al. (2013) performed stepwise regression analyses. The findings showed that *Religious* needs were predicted best by religious trust and search for a spiritual source of help on the one hand and by fibromyalgia impairment (which includes reduced physical functioning, number of days felt good, pain, fatigue, morning tiredness, stiffness, anxiety, and depression) on the other. *Existential* needs were predicted best by anxiety, search for a source, and having trust. *Inner Peace* needs were predicted best by anxiety and a reflection of life concerns in terms of a reappraisal coping strategy. *Giving/Generativity* needs were predicted best by low depression and catastrophizing. Thus, the underlying causes and triggers of patients' spiritual needs are complex and involve both spiritual resources and negative mental health indicators. Impaired mental health can be either the result of the chronic pain perception and/or an aggravating modulator.

Conclusions

Whether the support of patients' spiritual needs will really change their situation remains unclear. At least addressing these needs is the signal that talking about their fears, worries, and unmet needs is possible. In a recent study conducted in Switzerland, a majority of patients wished to include spiritual aspects in pain therapy (Hasenfratz et al. submitted). Optimal pain management, psychological support, and spiritual care interventions are seen as core elements of a comprehensive and patient-centered treatment of patients who have experienced the limitations of modern medicine, as their pain is still a chronic condition that affects different areas of life. According to the concept of total pain (Fig. 10.1), an optimal treatment addresses the physical, psychological, social, and spiritual aspects of pain, which may all interact, and thus one cannot ignore to ask about patients' spiritual needs. The central concern is the patients' perception of pain and its subjective interpretation, and thus an individual assessment of pain in its complexity of related health affections (including mood disturbances, loss of hope, and spiritual struggles) is important. This implies a multidimensional treatment plan that involves multi-professional care concepts.

Acknowledgments We are grateful to all who have helped to enroll the patients, particularly Annina Janko, Andreas Kopp, and Hans-Joachim Balzat, and all the patients who have filled the questionnaire.

References

Baetz M, Bowen R (2008) Chronic pain and fatigue: associations with religion and spirituality. Pain Res Manag 13:383–388

Brown GK, Nicassio PM (1987) Development of a questionnaire for the assessment of active and passive coping strategies in chronic pain patients. Pain 31:53–64

Büssing A (2017) Krankheitsbewertungen von Personen mit chronischen Schmerzerkrankungen und ihr Zusammenhang mit Indikatoren der Spiritualität. Spiritual Care 6:303–313

Büssing A, Fischer J (2009) Interpretation of illness in cancer survivors is associated with health-related variables and adaptive coping styles. BMC Womens Health 9(2). https://doi.org/10.1186/1472-6874-9-2

Büssing A, Keller N, Michalsen A, Moebus S, Dobos G, Ostermann T, Matthiessen PF (2006) Spirituality and adaptive coping styles in German patients with chronic diseases in a CAM health care setting. J Complement Integr Med 3. https://doi.org/10.1186/1471-2458-10-507

Büssing A, Michalsen A, Balzat HJ, Grünther RA, Ostermann T, Neugebauer EAM, Matthiessen PF (2009) Are spirituality and religiosity resources for patients with chronic pain conditions? Pain Med 10:327–339

Büssing A, Janko A, Baumann K, Hvidt NC, Kopf A (2013) Spiritual needs among patients with chronic pain diseases and cancer living in a secular society. Pain Med 14:1362–1373

Büssing A, Pilchowska I, Surzykiewicz J (2015) Spiritual needs of polish patients with chronic diseases. J Relig Health 54:1524–1542

Büssing A, Recchia DR, Koenig H, Baumann K, Frick E (2018) Factor structure of the spiritual needs questionnaire (SpNQ) in persons with chronic diseases, elderly and healthy individuals. Religions 9:13. https://doi.org/10.3390/rel9010013

Dedeli O, Kaptan G (2013) Spirituality and religion in pain and pain management. Health Psychol Res 1:e29. https://doi.org/10.4081/hpr.2013.e29

Fernandez E, Turk DC (1989) The utility of cognitive coping strategies for altering pain perception: a meta-analysis. Pain 38:123–135

Hasenfratz K, Peng-Keller S, Rufer M (submitted for publication) Do Chronic Pain Patients in Switzerland Want Spiritual Issues to be Considered in Treatment? – A Multicentred Cross-Sectional Study with over 200 Chronic Pain Patients in Switzerland.

Hilton L, Hempel S, Ewing BA, Apaydin E, Xenakis L, Newberry S, Colaiaco B, Maher AR, Shanman RM, Sorbero ME, Maglione MA (2017) Mindfulness meditation for chronic pain: systematic review and meta-analysis. Ann Behav Med 51:199–213

IsHak WW, Wen RY, Naghdechi L, Vanle B, Dang J, Knosp M, Dascal J, Marcia L, Gohar Y, Eskander L, Yadegar J, Hanna S, Sadek A, Aguilar-Hernandez L, Danovitch I, Louy C (2018) Pain and depression: a systematic review. Harv Rev Psychiatry 26:352–363

Lazarus R, Folkman S (1984) Stress, appraisal and coping. Springer, New York

McCaffrey AM, Eisenberg DM, Legedza AT, Davis RB, Phillips RS (2004) Prayer for health concerns: results of a national survey on prevalence and patterns of use. Arch Intern Med 164:858–862

Moreira-Almeida A, Koenig HG (2008) Religiousness and spirituality in fibromyalgia and chronic pain patients. Curr Pain Headache Rep 12:327–332

Offenbaecher M, Kohls N, Toussaint LL, Sigl C, Winkelmann A, Hieblinger R, Walther A, Büssing A (2013) Spiritual needs in patients suffering from fibromyalgia. Evidence-based Complementary and Alternative Medicine 2013; Article ID 178547

Racine M (2018) Chronic pain and suicide risk: a comprehensive review. Prog Neuropsychopharmacol Biol Psychiatry 87(Pt B):269–280

Rettke H, Naef R, Mörgeli HP, Rufer M, Peng-Keller S (2020) Spiritualität und Behandlung. Die Perspektive von Patienten mit chronischen Schmerzen. Der Schmerz. https://doi.org/10.1007/s00482-020-00524-3

Saunders C (1993) Introduction: history and challenge. In: Saunders C, Sykes N (eds) The Management of Terminal Malignant Disease. Hodder and Stoughton, London, pp 1–14

Sollgruber A, Bornemann-Cimenti H, Szilagyi IS, Sandner-Kiesling A (2018) Spirituality in pain medicine: a randomized experiment of pain perception, heart rate and religious spiritual well-being by using a single session meditation methodology. PLoS One 13(9):e0203336

Toth C, Brady S, Hatfield M (2013) The importance of catastrophizing for successful pharmacological treatment of peripheral neuropathic pain. J Pain Res 7:327–338

Van Damme S, Crombez G, Eccleston C (2008) Coping with pain: a motivational perspective. Pain 139:1–4

Wachholtz AB, Pargament KI (2005) Is spirituality a critical ingredient of meditation? Comparing the effects of spiritual meditation, secular meditation, and relaxation on spiritual, psychological, cardiac, and pain outcomes. J Behav Med 28:369–384

Wachholtz AB, Pearce MJS (2010) Shaking the blues away: energizing spiritual practices for the treatment of chronic pain. In: Plante TG (ed) Contemplative practices in action. Spirituality, meditation, and health. Praeger, Santa Barbara

Wolfe F, Clauw DJ, Fitzcharles MA, Goldenberg DL, Katz RS, Mease P, Russell AS, Russell IJ, Winfield JB, Yunus MB (2010) The American College of Rheumatology preliminary diagnostic criteria for fibromyalgia and measurement of symptom severity. Arthritis Care Res 62:600–610

Zwingmann C, Wirtz M, Müller C, Körber J, Murken S (2006) Positive and negative religious coping in German breast cancer patients. J Behav Med 29:533–547

Zwingmann C, Müller C, Körber J, Murken S (2008) Religious commitment, religious coping and anxiety: a study in German patients with breast cancer. Eur J Cancer Care 17:361–370

CHAPTER 11

Spiritual Needs of Non-terminally Ill Cancer Patients from Lithuania

Olga Riklikienė

Introduction

The modern methods of treatment, state-of-the-art technology and pharmaceutical advancements help in the diagnosis and treatment of oncological diseases, although the well-being of the oncological patient is not only a matter of I am sick/I am not sick, there are symptoms/no symptoms or good symptom control/bad control. The important questions arise in the background of a complex psychological process, spiritual transformation and social change: "Why does a person live?", "Does life make sense?", "Are other people something more than themselves?", "Is there any higher power than God?", "Why does man suffer?", "Why do people die?", "What is the meaning of death?", "Why does this happen to me?" (Rousseau 2000). To find the answers to these questions and to continue to live with them, patients need the support of health professionals, family, friends and others, for their needs assessment and satisfaction.

O. Riklikienė (✉)
Faculty of Nursing, Medical Academy, Lithuanian University of Health Sciences, Kaunas, Lithuania
e-mail: olga.riklikiene@lsmuni.lt

A. Büssing (ed.), *Spiritual Needs in Research and Practice*,
https://doi.org/10.1007/978-3-030-70139-0_11

Lithuania is a unique crossroad of the East and the West with the centuries-old heritage of many different faiths (Žemaitis 2020). The freedom of faith had returned with the restoration of independence in 1991. Nowadays Lithuania may be called a very religious nation and state: during the 2011 census, 84% of the Lithuanian population identified themselves as following a religion; 77.2% of the population indicated they were Roman Catholics; and Orthodoxy was the second largest faith of Lithuania with 4.1%. Other inhabitants attribute themselves to Old Believers, Evangelical Lutherans, Reformed Evangelicals and other faiths; 6.1% did not attribute themselves to any religious community; 10.1% did not answer the question (Statistics Lithuania 2020).

Like in other countries, in Lithuania, there are intentions to expand duties and competences of health-care staff to spiritual care provision, to intensify pastoral care and spiritual advising in hospitals. Health-care professionals and clergy are expected to work as a team within the context of interdisciplinary holistic patient care (Riklikienė et al. 2020a). Kirshbaum and Rodriguez (2018) note that holistic care addresses the individual's worldview, inclusive of life experience, background, culture and religious orientation. All these result in determining what is meaningful to the patient.

Spiritual Needs of Non-terminally Ill Cancer Patients

In 2017, a multi-professional group of young multidisciplinary researchers at the Lithuanian University of Health Sciences, Faculty of Nursing, initiated a national two-year research project fostering spirituality in nursing (Riklikienė 2019). The researchers expected that evidence-based information about non-terminally ill oncology patients' unmet spiritual needs may result in a better understanding of how the disease and treatment may influence their well-being. Previously, no significant empirical research on the spirituality and spiritual needs of cancer patients had been developed in Lithuania. To date, there have been no validated tools to assess spiritual aspects of care for healthy or illness-affected Lithuanian people in a standardized way.

In total, 247 non-terminally ill cancer patients participated in the study in 2018. There were more females (60.7%) than males. The age varied from 32 years to 96 years with a mean of 66.7 ± 11.65 years. Most of the patients were married (70.6%), with an urban residence (59.5%) and with higher education (40.8%). The majority (68.0%, $n = 168$) answered that they were religious persons, of which 95.8% were affiliated with the Roman Catholic religion, two patients were Russian Orthodox, three patients were Russian Orthodox Old Believers, one patient was Evangelical Lutherans and one neo-pagan.

The average duration of hospitalization for cancer patients was 25.62 ± 36.05 and the oncological illness lasted 3.78 ± 4.69 years. The majority of patients were diagnosed with a stage III (36.9%) or stage II or IV tumor (27.8% each). The spiritual needs of patients were assessed with the Lithuanian version of SpNQ-27 (Riklikienė et al. 2019). Additionally, to assess patients' satisfaction with life and subjective feeling of their happiness, the Brief Multidimensional Life Satisfaction Scale (BMLSS) (Büssing et al. 2009) and the Oxford Happiness Questionnaire (OHQ) were applied (Hills and Argyle 2002).

Inner Peace needs (1.75 ± 0.66) and *Giving/Generativity and Forgiveness* needs (1.64 ± 0.68) were expressed as the most important for non-terminally ill cancer patients, while *Existential* (1.33 ± 0.67) and *Religious* needs (1.26 ± 0.87) were slightly lower but nevertheless high (Riklikienė et al. 2020b).

Spiritual needs such as to be healthy and feel safe (N24), to feel connected with a family (N25), to be involved by family members in their life concerns (N28), to dwell in a place of quietness and peace (N7) and to receive more support from the family (N29) were expressed as very or extremely important needs for the majority of non-terminally ill cancer patients while in hospital. Family is a core value in Lithuanian society explaining its dominance during the health crisis of an individual. Connectedness with family members and their assistance and support in a difficult situation were the most expected and valued by study respondents.

There were significant differences between the spiritual needs of non-terminally ill oncology patients in terms of gender and religiosity. The SpNQ-20 mean scores were significantly higher in women compared to those in men, and higher in religious persons compared to those who are either not religious or undecided about it (Table 11.1). Younger patients, if compared with those 70 years and older, expressed the need to talk with others about their fears and worries (N2) ($p = 0.025$), to reflect back on their life (N4) ($p = 0.001$), to dissolve open aspects of life (N5) ($p = 0.021$) to find meaning in illness and/or suffering (N10) ($p = 0.011$) and to

Table 11.1 Spiritual needs of non-terminally ill cancer patients in relation to their importance (very strong or strong need) and gender and religiosity

Spiritual Needs	*Strong to very strong need (%)*	*Gender*		*Religiosity*	
		Male N (%)	*Female* N (%)	*Yes* N (%)	*No* N (%)
N24—For being completely healthy and safe	93.4	90 (92.8)	137 (91.9)	180 (93.8)	46 (86.8)
N25—To feel connected with family	90.7	85 (87.6)	138 (93.2)	180 (94.2)*	42 (79.2)
N28—To be re-involved by your family in their life concerns	83.1	80 (83.3)	126 (84.6)	162 (84.8)	43 (81.1)
N7—To dwell in a place of quietness and peace	80.1	72 (74.2)*	125 (83.9)	161 (83.9)*	35 (66.0)
N29—To receive more support from your family	74.3	73 (75.3)	111 (75.0)	147 (77.0)	36 (67.9)
N8—To find inner peace	73.7	62 (65.3)*	118 (79.2)	151(78.6)*	28(54.9)
N26—To pass own life experiences to others	65.6	59 (60.8)	106 (70.7)	134(69.4)	31(58.5)
N27—To be assured that your life was meaningful and of value	65.0	59 (61.5)	103 (68.7)	131(68.2)	31(58.5)
N6—To plunge into beauty of nature	61.6	53 (55.8)	95 (63.8)	126(65.6)*	24(46.2)
N16—To forgive someone from a distinct period of your life	60.9	53 (55.2)	98 (65.8)	124(64.6)*	23(45.1)
N13—To turn to someone in a loving attitude	59.8	45 (47.4)*	102 (68.5)	121(63.7)*	26(49.1)
N17—To be forgiven	59.6	48 (50.0)*	95 (63.8)	124(64.9)*	21(39.6)

(*continued*)

Table 11.1 (continued)

Spiritual Needs	*Strong to very strong need (%)*	*Gender*		*Religiosity*	
		Male *N (%)*	*Female* *N (%)*	*Yes* *N (%)*	*No* *N (%)*
N15—To give solace to someone	59.1	49 (51.0)*	97 (65.1)	120(62.5)*	22(42.3)
N14—To give away something from yourself	55.3	43 (44.8)*	95 (63.3)	121(63.0)*	16(30.2)
N20—To pray for yourself	51.1	37 (38.5)*	94 (63.9)	122(63.5)*	9(18.0)
N23—To turn to a higher presence (i.e., God, Angels, Saints)	49.1	28 (29.8)*	96 (64.9)	116(60.4)*	26(49.1)
N5—To dissolve open aspects of your life	47.6	45 (46.9)	78 (52.3)	99(51.6)	21(39.6)
N10—To find meaning in illness and/or suffering	47.6	35 (36.5)*	86 (57.7)	102(53.1)*	18(34.6)
N4—To reflect back on your life	46.5	35 (36.1)*	83 (55.7)	100(52.1)*	17(32.1)
N21—To participate in a religious ceremony (i.e., service)	45.3	30 (30.9)	85 (57.4)	122(58.2)*	3(5.8)
N11—To talk with someone about the question of meaning in life	44.0	34 (35.1)*	77 (52.0)	92(48.2)	19(35.8)
N2—To talk with others about your fears and worries	40.6	29 (30.5)*	76 (51.0)	91(47.9)*	13(24.5)
N19—That someone prays for you	38.4	22 (23.2)*	80 (53.7)	94(49.0)*	7(13.7)
N18—To pray with someone	36.2	22 (23.2)*	70 (47.0)	84(43.8)*	7(13.7)

(*continued*)

Table 11.1 (continued)

Spiritual Needs	*Strong to very strong need (%)*	*Gender*		*Religiosity*	
		Male N (%)	*Female* N (%)	*Yes* N (%)	*No* N (%)
N3—That someone of your religious community cares for you	32.3	19 (20.0)*	61 (41.2)	75(39.5)*	5(9.6)
N22—To read religious/spiritual books	28.1	14 (14.6)*	57 (38.5)	69(35.9)*	2(3.9)
N12—To talk with someone about the possibility of life after death	22.2	15 (15.8)*	41 (27.3)	47(24.6)	9(17.0)
SNQ-20 mean score (± SD)		**1.58 ± 0.61**	**1.27 ± 0.56**	**1.57 ± 0.58**	**1.10 ± 0.57**
F value, P value		**17.12, <0.0001**		**29.80, <0.0001**	

*$p < 0.05$, the Chi-square test.

restore significantly more Inner Peace. The latter sought more strongly to participate in religious ceremonies ($p = 0.027$).

In relation to the family structure, cancer patients who were married or lived with a partner had higher unmet spiritual needs and needed to be assured that their life was meaningful (N27) ($p = 0.032$) and to talk with someone about their fears and worries (N2) ($p = 0.021$) than single, divorced or widowed patients.

In addition, other health- and illness-related variables also had correlation with spiritual needs. Patients who were less satisfied with their life, in particular health status ($r = -0.229$, $p = 0.001$) and possibilities to overcome life difficulties ($r = -0.228$, $p = 0.001$), expressed higher *Religious* needs. Cancer patients who were dissatisfied with their life (BMLSS score < 50 points), in comparison with those who were satisfied (BMLSS score ≥ 50 points), expressed certain more important spiritual needs: the need that someone of their religious community will care about them (N3) ($p = 0.002$), to pray with someone (N18) ($p = 0.021$) and that someone pray for them (N19) ($p = 0.025$), to read religious/spiritual books (N22) ($p = 0.041$), to talk with someone about personal fears and worries (N2) ($p = 0.016$) and about the possibility of life after death (N12) ($p = 0.001$), to plunge into beauty of nature (N6) ($p < 0.001$) and to be assured that their life was meaningful (N27) ($p = 0.017$).

Spiritual needs and the subjective feeling of happiness showed a significant relationship with the Inner Peace domain: these spiritual needs were expressed as more important for 'unhappy' patients (1.85 ± 0.62) than happy patients (1.61 ± 0.70).

Discussion

The Lithuanian version of SpNQ-20, which retains elements of the original structure, was applied to assess spiritual needs according to their four domains. This enabled international comparisons of results and the identification of cultural differences in patients' perceptions of their spiritual needs.

Inner Peace needs (1.75 ± 0.66) and *Giving/Generativity and Forgiveness* needs (1.64 ± 0.68) were expressed as the most important for Lithuanian cancer patients to find the strength in coping with and living in changing life and health situations. Nowadays an oncological disease is no longer viewed as having an ultimately fatal diagnosis, but as a condition that requires prolonged treatment and constant support from relatives, health-care providers and others with similar experiences. These findings corresponded to the German study where needs for *Inner Peace* and *Giving/Generativity* emerged to be of greatest importance (Höcker et al. 2014).

Despite the fact that *Religious* needs among Lithuanian cancer patients were least expressed, they were much stronger as compared to the German (Büssing et al. 2013a; Höcker et al. 2014) or Chinese samples (Büssing et al. 2013b) and rather similar to Polish patients (Büssing et al. 2015) from the neighbor country with historically strong cultural, political, social and economic links. Patients who are 70 years and older were more interested in participating in religious ceremonies than the younger participants as the former were more dedicated to traditions, well-established value systems and rituals. Another explanation of this difference in younger and older cancer patients may be related to the loneliness of older adults with broken social and family connections. Other studies confirm that religion and faith are helpful for symptom management, to cope with the experience of illness and suffering, to decrease loneliness and social isolation (Cheng et al. 2018).

Interestingly, the majority of patients, although being Roman Catholics and traditionally believing in afterlife, were at least interested in addressing the theme of death through talking about this, praying or reading spiritual literature. Findings suggested that during the nonterminal phase of cancer, health-care providers and family members should be very sensitive to these personal and private aspects. It is more important for the patients to focus their attention primarily on positive perspectives of life. Those who still prefer the reflection on death and dying must be very carefully addressed.

Lithuanian patients with a wide belonging to faith expressed a strong need to be forgiven (59.6%) and to forgive others (60.9%). These unmet spiritual needs in this group of patients were more strongly expressed than in German fibromyalgia patients where 38% stated needs to be forgiven and nearly half to forgive someone from their past life (Offenbaecher et al. 2013).

Similar (like for single items) significant differences in gender and religiosity groups of cancer patients were revealed in relation to four SpNQ-20 domains. For female patients the spiritual needs of four domains were significantly stronger than for males. Similarly, those patients who considered themselves as religious had stronger spiritual needs in all SpNQ-20 domains than nonreligious patients or those who were not able to identify their religiosity. The place of residence or marital status did not make any difference to cancer patients' spiritual needs. *Religious* needs at the domain level did not differ with respect to patients' age and education although the importance of three other spiritual needs domains were graded significantly higher by younger patients (<70 years) and those with higher education (Riklikienė et al. 2020b).

All four spiritual needs domains were interconnected among nonterminally ill cancer patients with the strongest association between Existential needs and the other three domains, showing that spiritual concerns are related and should be addressed as a patient's integral health and care issue. On the other hand, illness- and treatment-related factors, such as duration of illness, tumor stage or duration of hospitalization, did not demonstrate relevant associations with spiritual needs and should be treated adequately in the care process (Riklikienė et al. 2020b).

Lithuanian patients' life satisfaction (Riklikienė et al. 2020b) was slightly lower than in Polish patients of chronic disease (Büssing et al.

2015) and at the domain level was marginally ($r = -0.19$, $p = 0.01$) associated with the Religious needs only. In the German study (Offenbaecher et al. 2013) the relationship of spiritual needs and life satisfaction was not found.

In this study 'happiness' was not operationalized as gladness and joy, but as mental well-being. Spiritual needs items from the Inner Peace domain reflect on searching peace of mind and feeling connection with nature and its beauty. Such a need is essential for cancer patients and does not require extraordinary efforts to fulfill. The connection with nature is characteristic of Lithuanian people since ancient times because entire generations grew in the environment of nature, worked on the land and enjoyed the goodness of nature. Furthermore, the old Lithuanian religion included paganism, in which natural beings were worshipped and prayed to.

Spiritual needs as a multidimensional phenomenon which is also dependent on the religious and cultural background of patients (Büssing and Koenig 2010) have to be assessed and supported by the whole team relying on the competences of each member and on agreed national standards of practice and assistance protocols (Riklikienė et al. 2020a). Still one of the greatest challenges for Lithuanian nurses is to assess and to satisfy patients' spiritual needs in their clinical practice due to the impersonate and private nature of these needs.

Practical Implications

As a result of the project, a Protocol of Spiritual Care was developed and distributed to the units involved in the study as an opportunity to improve the quality of spiritual care. It must refer to the legal documents governing nursing practice, but spiritual competence in nursing is not included in the nurse's medical norm. Authorities have the freedom to develop the Protocol and use it in a way they feel comfortable to do so. The Spiritual Needs Questionnaire SpNQ-20 is recommended for clinicians and nurses to identify patients' spiritual needs and plan their holistic care.

The SpNQ as a valid and reliable tool is currently applied in Lithuania for research purposes with different populations: children and adolescents with cancer, oncohematological patients and palliative care patients.

Conclusions

The first ever Lithuanian study on non-terminally ill cancer patients' spirituality aspects and spiritual needs provided the evidence and new insights that may be of relevance and importance for surrounding Eastern and Central European and former Soviet Union countries with similar developmental histories, enforced atheism and religious suppression in the past, and medicalization of health care with a strongly dominated biomedical model that inhibited a holistic approach to the sick person.

Inner Peace needs were expressed most by non-terminally ill cancer patients, followed by *Giving/Generativity and Forgiveness* needs. Gender, age and religiosity of these patients made a difference in the expression of unmet spiritual needs. Certain spiritual needs were associated with life satisfaction and needs for inner peace were related to the subjective feeling of happiness.

Although spirituality and religion are very personal and private matters, they should be taken into account by a multi-professional team during a cancer patient's comprehensive assessment, care planning and care implementation in hospital. A Protocol of Spiritual Care is an opportunity for practitioners to improve the quality of spiritual care.

References

Büssing A, Koenig H (2010) Spiritual needs of patients with chronic diseases. Religions 1:18–27. https://doi.org/10.3390/rel1010018

Büssing A, Fischer J, Haller A, Heusser P, Ostermann T, Matthiessen P (2009) Validation of the brief multidimensional life satisfaction scale in patients with chronic diseases. Eur J Med Res 14:171. https://doi.org/10.1186/2047-783x-14-4-171

Büssing A, Janko A, Baumann K, Hvidt NC, Kopf A (2013a) Spiritual needs among patients with chronic pain diseases and cancer living in a secular society. Pain Med 14:1362–1373. https://doi.org/10.1111/pme.12198

Büssing A, Zhai X, Peng W, Ling C (2013b) Psychosocial and spiritual needs of patients with chronic diseases: validation of the Chinese version of the spiritual needs questionnaire. Journal of Integrative Medicine 11:106–115. https://doi.org/10.3736/jintegrmed2013020

Büssing A, Pilchowska I, Surzykiewicz J (2015) Spiritual needs of polish patients with chronic diseases. J Relig Health 54:1524–1542. https://doi.org/10.1007/s10943-014-9863-x

Cheng Q, Xu X, Liu X, Mao T, Chen Y (2018) Spiritual needs and their associated factors among cancer patients in China: a cross-sectional study. Support Care Cancer 26:3405–3412. https://doi.org/10.1007/s00520-018-4119-z

Hills P, Argyle M (2002) The Oxford happiness questionnaire: a compact scale for the measurement of psychological well-being. Personal Individ Differ 33:1073–1082. https://doi.org/10.1016/s0191-8869(01)00213-6

Höcker A, Krüll A, Koch U, Mehnert A (2014) Exploring spiritual needs and their associated factors in an urban sample of early and advanced cancer patients. Eur J Cancer Care 23:786–794. https://doi.org/10.1111/ecc.12200

Kirshbaum M, Rodriguez A (2018) Spirituality in western multicultural societies. In: Curran WS, Rogers M (eds) Spirituality competent practice in health care. Taylor and Francis, Boca Raton, FL

Offenbaecher M, Kohls N, Toussaint L, Sigl C, Winkelmann A, Hieblinger R, Walther A, Büssing A (2013) Spiritual needs in patients suffering from fibromyalgia. Evid Based Complement Alternat Med 2013:1–13. https://doi.org/10.1155/2013/178547

Riklikienė O (2019) The restoration of holistic approach to nursing Care in Lithuania. Nursing education, research, & practice 9:31–32. Available at http://nerp.lsmuni.lt/the-restoration-of-holistic-approach-to-nursing-care-in-lithuania/

Riklikienė O, Spirgienė L, Kaselienė S, Luneckaitė Ž, Tomkevičiūtė J, Büssing A (2019) Translation, cultural, and clinical validation of the Lithuanian version of the spiritual needs questionnaire among hospitalized cancer patients. Medicina 55:738. https://doi.org/10.3390/medicina55110738

Riklikienė O, Harvey C, Spirgienė L, Luneckaitė Ž, Karosas L (2020a) Perceptions of clergy regarding the provision of spiritual Care in Lithuanian Hospitals for cancer patients. J Relig Health 59:1494–1509. https://doi.org/10.1007/s10943-019-00899-3

Riklikienė O, Tomkevičiūtė J, Spirgienė L, Valiulienė Ž, Büssing A (2020b) Spiritual needs and their association with indicators of quality of life among non-terminally ill cancer patients: cross-sectional survey. Eur J Oncol Nurs 44:101681. https://doi.org/10.1016/j.ejon.2019.101681

Rousseau P (2000) Spirituality and the dying patient. J Clin Oncol 18:2000–2002. https://doi.org/10.1200/jco.2000.18.9.2000

Statistics Lithuania (2020) Tautybė, gimtoji kalba ir tikyba | Ethnicity, mother tongue. http://statistics.bookdesign.lt/esu_04.htm?lang=en. Accessed 12 Aug 2020

Žemaitis A (2020) Religions (Faiths) In Lithuania: Extensive Guide | True Lithuania. http://www.truelithuania.com/topics/culture-of-lithuania/religions-faiths-in-lithuania. Accessed 12 Aug 2020

CHAPTER 12

Spiritual Needs of Cancer Patients in Iran

Maryam Rassouli, Azam Shirinabadi Farahani, and Khadijeh Hatamipour

Background

Spirituality as one of the dimensions of human existence is common to all human beings (Memaryan et al. 2016a). This concept is influenced by cultural, religious and even ethnic and environmental background and is rooted in education and the effects of culture on society (Memaryan et al. 2016b; Forouzi et al. 2017; Torabi et al. 2018; Lepherd 2015). Studies show that spirituality has positive impacts on quality of life–related health in human life (De Campos et al. 2020; Akbari et al. 2020).

M. Rassouli (✉)
Cancer Research Center, Shahid Beheshti University of Medical Sciences, Tehran, Iran

A. Shirinabadi Farahani
Pediatric Nursing Department, School of Nursing and Midwifery, Shahid Beheshti University of Medical Sciences, Tehran, Iran

K. Hatamipour
Department of Nursing, Tonekabon Branch, Islamic Azad University, Tonekabon, Iran

A. Büssing (ed.), *Spiritual Needs in Research and Practice*,
https://doi.org/10.1007/978-3-030-70139-0_12

In Iran, due to the dominance of Iranian and Islamic culture, patients somehow try to protect themselves from diseases by relying on spiritual resources. Some patients see the disease as a divine test and believe that they will be saved if their faith is strong. Others think that they have been punished by God for their past immoral behavior (Zand and Rafiei 2016), while others rely on transcendental spiritual resources through worship, prayers, recourse, faith, saying mantras and seeking refuge in God and His saints, charity, repentance, showing gratitude to God, patience and reciting the Qur'an and try to adapt to the disease and minimize the damage caused by it (Forouzi et al. 2017; Torabi et al. 2018; Nikseresht et al. 2016a).

Although there are various degrees of spiritual needs in all human beings, the types of needs differ from patient to patient, and cancer patients may feel a greater need for spiritual care than people with other diseases (Zhao et al. 2019; Shirinabadi Farahani et al. 2019b). Therefore, spiritual needs and identifying them has always been an issue in cancer patients (Memaryan et al. 2015). When cancer patients are aware of their disease or are faced with treatments, their needs, including spiritual needs, change during the course of the disease and at the end of their lives (Hatamipour et al. 2015b).

In various studies conducted in Iran, spirituality and spiritual needs in cancer patients and also at the end-of-life stages are regarded as similar to the relationship with and trust in God, and as a source of hope, guide in making decisions, the optimistic factor and the contributor to hope and immunity against uncertainty and confusion (Nikseresht et al. 2016a, b; Shirinabadi Farahani et al. 2016; Sajjadi et al. 2016; Rahnama et al. 2012).

Despite the importance of spirituality and spiritual care, many cancer patients and their families do not receive the spiritual care they seek from caregivers (Rassouli et al. 2019; Sandor et al. 2006). These unmet spiritual needs are associated with a decrease in the quality of care, patient satisfaction and their quality of life (Sharma et al. 2012). Spiritual needs of cancer patients are mostly ignored or addressed minimally (Büssing and Koenig 2010).

A cross-sectional study on the spiritual needs in elderly patients with cancer or other chronic diseases in Iran showed that these patients have at least one unmet spiritual need, mostly related to "*asking God for help*" and least frequently related to "*discussing afterlife*" (Ramezani et al. 2019). Moreover, 70% of mothers who have children with cancer at advanced stages have many unmet spiritual needs (Javedanpour et al. 2017).

The Conceptual Framework for Spiritual Needs in Cancer Patients

Büssing and Koenig (2010) presented a model for Spiritual Needs of Patients with the four major dimensions of connection, peace, meaning/purpose and transcendence (Büssing and Koenig 2010). These dimensions are at the center of psychosocial, emotional, existential and religious needs. This model is a framework for further research and clinical practice. Caregivers and patients' relatives can help patients fight a chronic and serious disease by identifying the spiritual needs of patients.

Considering the fact that spiritual needs are influenced by the cultural and religious situations of each society, Hatamipour et al. (2015a) conducted a qualitative study performing a directed content analysis based on Büssing and Koenig's model with the aim of determining the spiritual needs of cancer patients in Iran.

These needs are categorized into the dimensions of *connection* (associated with the social dimension of spirituality and in the form of the patient's communication with others, and receiving inspiring support), *finding meaning and purpose* (by accepting the reality, finding the causes and changing the meaning of life for the patient), *seeking peace* (achieving inner peace, seeking forgiveness and inspiring hope in the patient), and *transcendence* (an inner way for the patient, including worshipping and the relationship with God as major components) (Hatamipour et al. 2015b).

Spiritual Needs in Cancer Patients

Spiritual needs are considered as important predictors of health outcomes in patients with cancer and other chronic diseases, as well as individuals' ability to cope with spiritual distress (Hatamipour et al. 2015b). Obviously, considering that 98% of Iranians are Muslims, the dimensions of spiritual needs in Iranian patients, including cancer patients, may vary. The results of a qualitative content analysis that evaluated the views of Iranian experts and scholars to provide a definition for spirituality showed that "spirituality is the sublime aspect of human existence bestowed on all humans in order for them to traverse the path of transcendence that is closeness to God (Allah) (Memaryan et al. 2016a).

Knowing Him is considered as the first step on the path of a meaningful and spiritual life. Nearness to Him is the main objective for the creation of man. God is the most perfect being, and man instinctively seeks and moves toward perfection. For this reason, the ultimate goal of spiritual activities and behaviors is closeness to Him (Zibad et al. 2017).

According to Islam, however, justice is one of the five principles of religion and denying it is synonymous with leaving the faith as God is the source of justice and all He does (including being affected by cancer) is a manifestation of justice. He has, therefore, envisioned a way of reaching transcendence for every creature through trust in God, resorting to praying and appealing to the Infallible Imams (Nemati et al. 2017).

In addition, due to the fact that religion is interwoven with spirituality, part of the spiritual needs may be expressed in the form of religious needs. In their qualitative study with a hermeneutic approach, Yousefi and Abedi (2011) differentiated spiritual needs of patients in the three categories: *hopefulness*, *comprehensive relations* and *performing religious practices* (Yousefi and Abedi 2011). The need for hopefulness was associated with subjects such as the need for support, becoming acquainted with different people and encouragement. The second need—comprehensive relations—was defined as the necessity for building trust, establishing verbal relationships, empathy and attention. Moreover, the final category was determined as the relationship with God, preparing for worship, becoming acquainted with the religious rules of the ward and respecting the patients' beliefs.

More specifically, in a qualitative study, Hatamipour et al. (2015a) examined cancer patients' experiences of religious needs. These needs were defined in the three categories of *religious beliefs* (belief, recourse), *relationship with God* (closeness to God, having faith in God) and *the need to worship* (prayers, performing religious practices). The dimension *transcendental needs* (with the two sub-themes *religious needs* and *epistemology needs*) and the dimension *pleasurable needs* (with the two sub-themes *psycho-spiritual needs* and *spiritual support needs*) are other categorizations of the dimensions of spiritual needs among Iranian cancer patients (Moghimian et al. 2019).

Furthermore, Ghahramanian et al. (2016) regarded *thinking about God, trusting God, seeing others happy, trying for life beside the disease, being prayed for by others, and the need for kindness* and *helping others* as different dimensions of spiritual needs among Iranian cancer patients (Ghahramanian et al. 2016).

On the other hand, the studies conducted in Iran referred to the relationship of some variables with the spirituality and spiritual needs of cancer patients. For example, as the patient grows older, his/her spiritual needs may change (Rassouli and Sajjadi 2016; Forouzi et al. 2017).

The results of the study by Ramezani et al. (2019) on these variables showed that all elderly cancer patients have spiritual needs, and that depression and the duration of the disease are related to the extent of their spiritual needs. The quality of life can also be impacted by spiritual needs and the extent to which they are addressed (Ramezani et al. 2019).

Another study shows that the score of spiritual needs in cancer patients is positively related to their quality of life, and that in order to meet spiritual needs, the quality of life in these patients should be enhanced (Forouzi et al. 2017). However, the causality as well as direction of effects is not clear. Heidarzadeh et al. (2014) showed that in the post-traumatic growth phenomenon occurring in cancer patients, the dimension *spiritual changes* has the highest mean score among the various dimensions of post-traumatic growth. In a study investigating uncertainty in Iranian cancer patients, Sajjadi et al. (2016) identified the need for spiritual peace as the most important dimension that leads to the patient's adaptation to the uncertainty following the incidence of cancer.

But what matters concerning the spiritual needs of cancer patients is how they are objectively defined, why patients and family members have difficulties expressing them, and why health-care providers are unable to identify them (Büssing and Koenig 2010). Therefore, answering these questions requires measuring spiritual needs.

Spiritual Needs Assessment

In each country, the scale for the measurement of spiritual needs in patients is developed according to the dominant culture of that country. In Iran, to assess the spiritual needs of patients, various researchers have developed or psychometrically evaluated different tools (Hatamipour et al. 2015b, 2018b; Forouzi et al. 2017, Zand and Rafiei 2016; Javedanpour et al. 2017; Moeini et al. 2018; Nejat et al. 2016; Taheri-Kharameh and Moeini 2017).

Due to the importance of understanding and identifying the spiritual needs of cancer patients and the need to investigate them, an Iranian study was conducted on the development and psychometric evaluation of the spiritual needs assessment scale for cancer patients.

First, a qualitative study was done to explore the spiritual needs of cancer patients, and each dimension was defined theoretically (according to the model of Spiritual Needs) as well as practically (according to the findings of the qualitative study). According to the model, spiritual needs include the essential needs of human life such as connection, seeking peace, finding meaning and purpose, and achieving transcendence. According to the results of the qualitative research, spiritual needs are generally the basic human need in the spiritual dimension and the need of cancer patients in particular, which increases during the disease. These needs are caused by the shortage or lack of factors that are lost due to the disease, including effective connection, seeking peace, finding the meaning of life and the need for transcendence (Hatamipour et al. 2015b).

Then the scale items were extracted from the results of the qualitative section. In the quantitative part, the scale was validated. According to the exploratory factor analysis of 400 questionnaires, the developed scale had five factors. Finally, a 38-item scale was obtained with five subscales which was called "Spiritual Needs Assessment Scale of Patients with Cancer". Cronbach's alpha was 0.81 for the whole scale, 0.88 for the religious dimension, 0.77 for meaning and purpose, 0.70 for peace, 0.74 for connection, and 0.67 for support and independence. With regard to the result of the retest, ICC was found to be 0.89. The results showed that this spiritual needs scale in cancer patients can differentiate various dimensions of spiritual needs. The correlation (r) between the score of "Spiritual Needs Assessment Scale of Patients with Cancer" and the score of the "Spiritual Need Questionnaire" (SpNQ) which was developed by Büssing et al. in 2010 was determined to be 0.74, $p < 0.001$.

The SpNQ translated and validated by Hatamipour et al. (2018b) was to be used for patients with cancer in Iran. The findings by Hatamipour et al. (2018b) showed that a scale with 19 terms and the three subscales of needs for *Peace and Active Giving* (eight items), *Religious* needs (six items) and *Existential* needs (five items) is appropriate for these patients. Moeini et al. (2018) validated the SpNQ in a sample of patients with chronic pain diseases and found five factors (SpNQ-Persian Version): *Religious* needs, *Existential* needs, *Forgiveness/Generativity* needs, *Inner peace* needs and *Emotional* needs.

Considering the fact that the "Spiritual Needs Assessment Scale of Patients with Cancer" by Hatamipour et al. is also based on Büssing and Koenig's conceptual framework of spiritual needs developed for Iranian patients, similarities and differences with respect to the SpNQ are studied and compared (Table 12.1).

In some cases, the approach a person takes to express his/her spirituality may not be common among others or to those in other societies. In other words, some approaches are acquired and are strongly influenced by

Table 12.1 A comparison of the SpNQ (Büssing et al. 2010, 2018) with the "Spiritual Needs Assessment Scale of Patients with Cancer" (SNAS) by Hatamipour et al. (2018).

Common items	*SNAS*	*SpNQ*
N10 find meaning in illness and/or suffering[a] Understanding the meaning of the disease	Meaning & Purpose	Existential
N4 reflect back on your life[a] Reviewing my life and deeds[b]	Meaning & Purpose	Existential
N5 dissolve open aspects of your life[a] Finishing my unfinished businesses[b]	Meaning & Purpose	Existential
Being hopeful[b]	Peace	–
N19 that someone prays for you[a] Being prayed for by others[b]	Religion	Religious
N20 pray for yourself[a] Praying for yourself[b]	Religious	Religious
Your physical needs are addressed respectfully[b]	Peace	–
N21 participate in a religious ceremony[a] Perform religious practices such as performing Salah, reciting the Quran, reading religious prayers and participating in religious ceremonies more than before[b]	Religion	Religious
Have faith in god[b]	Religion	–
N12 talk with someone about the possibility of life after death[a] Discuss the afterlife with a clergyman[b]	Meaning & Purpose	Existential
N28 re-involved by your family in their life concerns[a] Be among friends and family members[b]	Connecting	Connection
My opinions are respected[b]	Support & Independence	–
N7 dwell in a place of quietness and peace[a] Like to be in a peaceful and quiet place[b]	Support & Independence	–
Have high spirits[b]	Peace	–
N2 talk with others about fears and worries[a]	Connecting	Connection
N38 that there is someone there for you who is always at your side[a] Like others to be by my side[b]		

[a]Büssing et al. (2010); [b]Hatamipour et al. (2018)

the deeds of those around and the dominant customs and traditions of the society. In some cases, these approaches were not initially expressed by patients as a major and important need (items such as "listen to music and enjoy", "experience and understand the nature", "think about afterlife", "think of death", "your life should be purposeful", "talk to a clergyman about your fears and worries").

In the Islamic culture, death is considered as presence before the throne of God and a return to Him. However, with regard to the two items on the acceptance of death by the patient ("think of afterlife", "think about death"), the taboo in Iranian culture prevents patients from thinking about death in any way possible and somehow causes them to unconsciously suppress it (Rassouli and Sajjadi 2014). Death is a major concept well addressed in Islam. In Iranian Islamic folklore, death is a time for reporting to God and being held accountable for one's own deeds in this world, which has caused death and dying to be considered a frightening experience that people try to avoid (Rassouli and Sajjadi 2016).

In addition, the scale developed in the present study takes into account some characteristics that are important to Iranian cancer patients according to their experiences, feelings, perception and religion, but do not exist in other scales ("have a good fate", "have access to the necessary facilities for religious practices", "have recourse to religious leaders", "strengthen your religious beliefs").

The Scores of Spiritual Needs Among Iranian Cancer Patients Compared to Patients in Other Countries

In 2018, the SpNQ was validated in Iran, showing that the spiritual needs in Iranian patients are mostly associated with *Existential* needs, *Peace and Active Giving* needs and *Religious* needs (Hatamipour et al. 2018a). It was found that *Existential* needs was the strongest one among patients with cancer (1.6 ± 1.28). The next need was *Peace and Active Giving* needs (0.82 ± 0.96) and the lowest need reported was *Religious* needs (0.57 ± 0.74).

In the validation study by Büssing et al. (2010) the sequence of intensity of spiritual needs was *Inner Peace*, *Giving/Generativity*, *Existential* and *Religious* needs. In 2013, the SpNQ was used in China to determine the spiritual needs of the patients with chronic diseases. In this study, the strongest need among Chinese patients was stated as *Giving/Generativity* (1.30 ± 0.64). The next need was the need for *Inner peace* (1.16 ± 0.69). The lowest of all was *Religious* needs (0.69 ± 0.74). Among Polish Catholics the major need of patients was reported to be the need for *Inner peace* and the lowest, *Existential* needs (Büssing et al. 2014). In the study of Höcker et al. (2014) among Germany cancer patients, the major need was related to *Giving/Generativity* and *Inner Peace*, while the lowest need was associated with the *Religious* need dimension.

The existential dimension of life consists in finding meaning and purpose. Finding meaning can be considered an essential and central component of spirituality. Every person has incentives that give meaning and purpose to their life, and helps them enjoy their existence. If, for any reason, the incentives are removed, life will become empty and meaningless for them. They may even question what they are living for (Hatamipour et al. 2018a).

In many studies, the strongest need among patients with cancer and chronic diseases was the need for *Inner Peace* (Hatamipour et al. 2018b, Büssing et al. 2013, 2014). According to Büssing and Koenig's model, peace is the emotional dimension of spiritual needs that includes inner peace, hopefulness, balance, forgiveness, tension and the fear of recurrence. It seems that due to the fact that the need for inner peace is common among all studies, this need should be given more attention.

What is common in various studies is the high need for inner peace among patients, which shows that patients, before anything else, seek a bubble of hope to achieve peace. The evidence of this claim is the quotations from the qualitative study by (Hatamipour et al. 2015b) reflecting their tendency to solitude in order to achieve peace.

Religious needs are the lowest need among cancer patients in the Iranian Muslim community. Religion is the supportive force in reducing stress as well as increasing life satisfaction (Shirinabadi Farahani et al. 2019a). Religious practices can help one feel well, prevent some health issues and assist to easily cope with illness and death (Hatamipour et al. 2018a). Praying, reading holy books or attending religious ceremonies, faith and recourse are some of the resources through which some religious people may undergo less harm in the face of stressful life events.

According to Rassouli and Sajjadi (2014), in order to deal with the tensions caused by the disease and possible death, most patients turn to religion to improve their psychological and mental health (Rassouli and Sajjadi 2014). In the study by Büssing et al. (2014) which was conducted in Poland, all the patients were Christians. The study showed that the second need of patients is the religious need. However, in the study by Büssing et al. (2013) in China, religious need was reported to be low due to the lack of a religious environment, which is not uncommon in a secular community (Büssing et al. 2013). A 2014 study by Höcker et al. (2014)

in Germany shows that although there is less interest in performing traditional and formal religious practices among the research population, spiritual needs moderately exist, reflecting human's innate tendency toward spirituality (Höcker et al. 2014).

Conclusion

Iranian cancer patients seek help from spirituality, and specifically from religion, to accept or deal with their disease. Religion is an effective and inspiring variable among cancer patients. Religious orders play an effective role in empowering patients and improving their conditions. Turning to religious practices creates peace and hopefulness and promotes the level of personal social connection and increases hope in patients. According to the opinions on the provision of holistic care in the health-care system, it is necessary to address all the needs of cancer patients, including their spiritual needs, which necessitates a spiritual needs assessment among patients. Therefore, the spiritual needs scale in Iranian patients with cancer was developed by Hatamipour et al., and the SpNQ was translated and validated in Iran. Due to the psychometric properties of these two scales, both are suitable for assessing the spiritual needs of Iranian cancer patients and it is recommended to validate them in patients with other chronic diseases.

References

Akbari S, Pazokian M, Shirinabadi Farahani A, Nasiri M, Rajab A (2020) Investigating the effect of spiritual care on the hope of diabetic patients referred to the Iranian Diabetes Association: a clinical trial. Arch Pharma Pract 11:124–130

Büssing A, Koenig HG (2010) Spiritual needs of patients with chronic diseases. Religions 1:18–27. https://doi.org/10.3390/rel1010018

Büssing A, Balzat HJ, Heusser P (2010) Spiritual needs of patients with chronic pain diseases and cancer: Validation of the Spiritual Needs Questionnaire. Eur J Med Res 15(6):266–273

Büssing A, Zhai X, Peng W, Yuan H (2013) Psychosocial and spiritual needs of patients with chronic diseases: validation of the Chinese version of the Spiritual Needs Questionnaire. J Integr Med 11:106–115

Büssing A, Pilchowska I, Surzykiewicz J (2014) Spiritual needs of polish patients with chronic diseases. J Relig Health 54:1524–1542

Büssing A, Recchia DR, Koenig H, Baumann K, Frick E (2018) Factor structure of the Spiritual Needs Questionnaire (SpNQ) in persons with chronic diseases, elderly and healthy individuals. Religions 9:13. https://doi.org/10.3390/rel9010013

De Campos RJDS, Lucchetti G, Lucchetti ALG, Da Rocha Ribeiro TC, Chebli LA, Malaguti C, Gaburri PD, Pereira LMN, de Almeida JG, Chebli JMF (2020) The impact of spirituality and religiosity on mental health and quality of life of patients with active Crohn's disease. J Relig Health 59:1273–1286

Forouzi MA, Tirgari B, Safarizadeh MH, Jahani Y (2017) Spiritual needs and quality of life of patients with cancer. Indian J Palliat Care 23:437–444

Ghahramanian A, Markani AK, Davoodi A, Bahrami A (2016) Spiritual Needs of Patients with Cancer Referred to Alinasab and Shahid Ghazi Tabatabaie Hospitals of Tabriz, Iran. Asian Pac J Cancer Prev 17:3105–3109

Hatamipour K, Rassouli M, Yaghmaie F, Alavi Majd H, Zendedel K (2015a) Religious needs of cancer patients: a qualitative study. Medical Figh 20–21:141–170

Hatamipour K, Rassouli M, Yaghmaie F, Zendedel K, Alavi Majd H (2015b) Spiritual needs of cancer patients: a qualitative study. Indian J Palliat Care 21:61–67

Hatamipour K, Rassouli M, Yaghmaie F, Zendedel K (2018a) Psychometric properties of the Farsi version of 'Spiritual Needs Questionnaire' for cancer patients in Iran: a methodological study. Asian Pac J Cancer Prev 19:989–995

Hatamipour K, Rassouli M, Yaghmaie F, Zendedel K, Alavi Majd H (2018b) Development and psychometrics of a 'Spiritual Needs Assessment Scale of Patients with Cancer': a mixed exploratory study. Int J Cancer Manag e10083:11

Heidarzadeh M, Rassouli M, Mohammadi Shahbolaghi F, Alavi Majd H, Karam A-M, Mirzaee H, Tahmasebi M (2014) Posttraumatic growth and its dimensions in patients with cancer. Middle East J Cancer 5:23–30

Höcker A, Krull A, Koch U, Mehnert A (2014) Exploring spiritual needs and their associated factors in an urban sample of early and advanced cancer patients. Eur J Cancer Care 23:786–794

Javedanpour Z, Hossein iA, Cheraghi M, Mehran A (2017) Comparison of the spiritual care needs of mothers of less than 14-year-old children suffering from cancer in the diagnostic and terminal stages of the disease. Medical Ethics 11:45–56

Lepherd L (2015) Spirituality: everyone has it, but what is it? Int J Nurs Pract 21:566–574

Memaryan N, Rassouli M, Nahardani SZ, Amiri P (2015) Integration of spirituality in medical education in Iran: a qualitative exploration of requirements. Evid Based Complement Alternat Med:793085. https://doi.org/10.1155/2015/793085

Memaryan N, Ghanbari Jolfaei A, Ghaempanah Z, Shirvani A, Doos Ali Vand H, Ghahari SH, Bohari J (2016a) Spiritual care for cancer patients in Iran. Asian Pac J Cancer Prev 17:4289–4294

Memaryan N, Rassouli M, Mehrabi M (2016b) Spirituality concept by health professionals in Iran: a qualitative study. Evid Based Complement Alternat Med 8913870. https://doi.org/10.1155/2016/8913870

Moeini B, Zamanian H, Taheri-Kharameh Z, Ramezani T, Saati-Asr M, Hajrahimian M, Amini-Tehrani M (2018) Translation and psychometric testing of the Persian version of the spiritual needs questionnaire among elders with chronic diseases. J Pain Symptom Manage 55:94–100

Moghimian M, Irajpour A, Arzani H (2019) The inter-professional dimensions of spiritual care for chronically ill patients: a qualitative study. Nurs Midwifery Stud 8:34–39

Nejat N, Whitehead L, Crowe M (2016) Exploratory psychometric properties of the Farsi and English versions of the Spiritual Needs Questionnaire (SpNQ). Religions 7(7):84. https://doi.org/10.3390/rel7070084

Nemati S, Rassouli M, Ilkhani M, Baghestani AR (2017) The spiritual challenges faced by family caregivers of patients with cancer: a qualitative study. Holist Nurs Pract 31:110–117

Nikseresht RM, Torabi F, Farzinfard F, Mansouri S, Ilkhani M (2016a) The effect of spiritual care on mental health in mothers of children with cancer. Holist Nurs Pract 30:330–337

Nikseresht F, Torabi F, Shirinabadi Farahani A, Sajjadi M, Rassouli M (2016b) Spirituality measurement tools in Iranian nursing studies. Clin Exc 4:56–67

Rahnama M, Khoshknab MF, Maddah SSB, Ahmadi F (2012) Iranian cancer patients' perception of spirituality: a qualitative content analysis study. BMC Nursing 11:19. https://doi.org/10.1186/1472-6955-11-19

Ramezani T, karameh z T, Karimi Z (2019) Exploring spiritual needs and its relation with anxiety and depression in the elderly patients with chronic diseases. Health Spiritual Med Ethics 6:10–16

Rassouli M, Sajjadi M (2014) Palliative care in the Islamic Republic of Iran. In: Silberman M (ed) Palliative care to the cancer patient: The Middle East as a model for emerging countries. Nova Scientific Publisher, New York

Rassouli M, Sajjadi M (2016) Palliative care in Iran: moving toward the development of palliative care for cancer. Am J Hosp Palliat Care 33:240–244

Rassouli M, Shirinabadi Farahani A, Khanali Mojen L (2019) Palliative care research in Iran: a review of current status. In: Silbermann M (ed) Palliative care: the role and importance of research in promoting palliative care practice. Nova Scientific Publisher, New York

Sajjadi M, Rassouli M, Abbaszadeh A, Brant J, Majd HA (2016) Lived experiences of 'illness uncertainty' of Iranian cancer patients: a phenomenological hermeneutic study. Cancer Nurs 39(4):E1–E9. https://doi.org/10.1097/NCC.0000000000000282

Sandor M, Sierpina V, Vanderpool H, Owen S (2006) Spirituality and clinical care: exploring developmental changes in nursing and medical students. Explore (NY) 2:37–42

Sharma RK, Astroko AB, Texeria K (2012) The spiritual needs assessment for patients (SNAP): development and validation of a comprehensive instrument to assess unmet spiritual need. J Pain Symptom Manage 44:44–51

Shirinabadi Farahani A, Rassouli M, Yaghmaie F, Alavi Majd H (2016) Hope, the foundation of spiritual health in adolescents: a qualitative study. Iranian Red Crescent Medical J 18:1–7

Shirinabadi Farahani A, Rassouli M, Salmani N, Mojen L, Sajjadi M, Heidarzadeh M, Masoudifar Z, Khademi F (2019a) Evaluation of health-care providers' perception of spiritual care and the obstacles to its implementation. Asia Pac J Oncol Nurs 6:122–129

Shirinabadi Farahani A, Salmani N, Al Sadat K, Khoshnazar T, Karami M, Hatamipour KH, Yazdani S, Pourazarhagh P, Rassouli M (2019b) The perspective of cancer patients on the use of complementary medicine. Int J Cancer Manag 12(2):e89916

Taheri-Kharameh Z, Moeini B (2017) Validation of the Persian version of the spiritual needs questionnaire. Eur J Public Health 27(3):471. https://doi.org/10.1093/eurpub/ckx186.200

Torabi F, Rassouli M, Nourian M, Borumandnia N, Shirinabadi Farahani A, Nikseresht F (2018) The effect of spiritual care on adolescents coping with cancer. Holist Nurs Pract 32:149–159

Yousefi H, Abedi HA (2011) Spiritual care in hospitalized patients. Iran J Nurs Midwifery Res 16:125–132

Zand S, Rafiei M (2016) Patients' religious care: a neglected need in medical education. J Med Educ Dev 8:50–58

Zhao Y, Wang Y, Yao X, Jiang L, Hou M, Zhao Q (2019) Reliability and validity of the Chinese version of spiritual needs questionnaire with 27 items (SpNQ-Ch-27) in cancer patients. Int J Nurs Sci 6:141–147

Zibad HA, Foroughan M, Shahboulaghi FM, Rafiey H, Rassouli M (2017) Perception of spiritual health: a qualitative content analysis in Iranian older adults. Educ Gerontol 43:21–32

CHAPTER 13

Development of Spiritual Needs during Chemotherapy of Breast Cancer Patients

Arndt Büssing, Pia Marie Hartmann, Yvonne Beerenbrock, and Daniela Rodrigues Recchia

Background

Breast cancer is the most common cancer type in women and the second leading worldwide. Its multimodal treatment involves surgery (increasingly breast-conserving approaches, but also mastectomy in several cases), adjuvant and neoadjuvant chemotherapy, radiotherapy, endocrine therapy and targeting agents (McDonald et al. 2016; Wörmann 2017). Good

A. Büssing (✉)
Professorship Quality of Life, Spirituality and Coping, Faculty of Health, Witten/Herdecke University, Herdecke, Germany

IUNCTUS—Competence Center for Christian Spirituality, Philosophical-Theological University of Münster, Münster, Germany
e-mail: Arndt.buessing@uni-wh.de

P. M. Hartmann • Y. Beerenbrock • D. R. Recchia
Professorship Quality of Life, Spirituality and Coping, Faculty of Health, Witten/Herdecke University, Witten, Germany
e-mail: pia.hartmann@gmx.at; Yvonne.Beerenbrock@uni-wh.de; Daniela.RodriguesRecchia@uni-wh.de

A. Büssing (ed.), *Spiritual Needs in Research and Practice*,
https://doi.org/10.1007/978-3-030-70139-0_13

prognosis of women with breast cancer is increasing during the last decades, particularly those in early stages.

During the course of their antitumor treatment, patients' physical and mental health, their hopes and expectations, and maybe also their spiritual needs may change, depending on the phase of their treatment. One can expect that prior to their treatment patients are in fear of the side effects of chemotherapy and whether the tumor will respond to the intended treatment. Indeed, Schneider et al. (2016) approved that the time before chemotherapy was the "most anxiety-provoking". Moreover, patients' self-efficacy expectation during chemotherapy is usually low (Akin and Kas Guner 2019), but may increase when anxiety decreases (Papadopoulou et al. 2017). During the phase of chemotherapy patients have a more realistic view than before of how the chemotherapy affects their physical and mental health and whether or not the tumor is responding. Several women experience side effects of chemotherapy such as nausea and vomiting despite the use of antiemetic treatment (Fernández-Ortega et al. 2012), pain, loss of weight, fatigue/tiredness and loss of hair—and thus their quality of life decreases—and often a loss of their abilities to perform daily-life activities (Kayl and Meyers 2006; Niklasson et al. 2017). After chemotherapy, patients recover from the treatment and their quality of life and life satisfaction increase again (Lötzke et al. 2016).

How patients' spiritual needs are related to these different phases, whether or not they change at all during the treatment, is so far unclear. Therefore, we started a longitudinal study enrolling patients with breast cancer from Germany. Here we refer to findings from an interim analysis. Within the sample of 87 patients treated for breast cancer (79% with chemotherapy, 17% with antihormonal therapy, 4% other or unclear), 84 persons were women, one was a man and two did not state their gender. Patients' mean age was 53 ± 10 (34–79) years. Of these, 60% had a Christian affiliation, 11% other religious affiliations and 29% had none; however, 48% regarded themselves as neither religious nor spiritual (R-S-), 37% as religious (R+) and 16% as spiritual but not religious (R-S+).

Development of Life Satisfaction and Intention to Escape from the Situation during Antitumor Treatment

As shown in Table 13.1, patients' general life satisfaction, as measured with the 10-item Brief Multidimensional Life Satisfaction Scales (BMLSS-10) addressing intrinsic (myself, overall life), social (friendships, family life), external (work, where I live), perspective (financial situation, future prospects) and health (health situation, abilities to cope with daily life affairs) dimensions (Büssing et al. 2009) was quite high prior to their antitumor treatment. Patients were very satisfied with the support by the hospital team and their partners, as measured with the BMLSS Support module (Büssing et al. 2017), and they had low intentions to escape from their illness or life situation, as measured with the 3-item Escape scale (Büssing et al. 2006). During the antitumor treatment patients' life satisfaction significantly decreased, while the satisfaction with team support marginally decreased, and their escape intentions remained stable. Three months after the end of the antitumor treatment, patients' life satisfaction was higher than prior to the treatment, but not significantly, and their intention to escape from the situation was much lower than before; their satisfaction with team support was stably high.

With respect to health-related life satisfaction parameters, satisfaction with the health situation (item G1 of the BMLSS) and satisfaction with treatment success (item G2) increased both during therapy and after treatment when they were the highest (Table 13.1). Satisfaction with abilities to cope with daily-life activities (item G3) and satisfaction with vitality/fitness (item G4) decreased during treatment and increased again three months after the end of the antitumor treatment.

Development of Spiritual Needs during Antitumor Treatment

Prior to their therapy (T0), *Religious* needs and *Existential* needs scored rather low, while *Inner Peace* needs and *Giving/Generativity* needs were of stronger relevance. For the intensity of these needs, the underlying spiritual–religious self-perception was of relevance, as religious and spiritual persons scored high on *Religious* needs (R+S+: 1.81 ± 0.86) compared to religious but not spiritual ones (R+S-: 0.81 ± 0.83) or nonreligious but spiritual persons (R-S+: 0.56 ± 0.66), while nonreligious and non-spiritual persons scored the lowest (R-S-: 0.18 ± 0.33); these differences are significant ($F = 24.1$, $p < 0.0001$). *Existential* needs scored the highest in R+S+ (1.26 ± 0.99), followed by R-S+ (0.83 ± 0.87), while R+S- (0.49 ± 0.54) and R-S- (0.45 ± 0.54) scored similarly low; these differences are significant too ($F = 4.0$, $p = 0.010$). *Inner Peace* needs scored highest in spiritual persons (R+S+: 1.98 ± 0.70; R-S+: 2.00 ± 0.90) compared to non-spiritual ones (R+S-: 1.37 ± 0.83; R-S-: 1.33 ± 0.69); these differences are also significant ($F = 4.3$, $p = 0.007$). For *Giving/Generativity*

Table 13.1 Quality-of- life indicators and spiritual needs within the course of treatment

	T0 *(prior to therapy)*	**T1** *(3 months after start of therapy)*	**T2** *(5 months after start of therapy)*	**T3** *(3 months after end of therapy)*	*p values (Friedman; n = 30)*	*p values (Wilcoxon)*[a]
Included number	$n = 83$	$n = 58$	$n = 45$	$n = 33$		
Quality-of-life indicators						
Life satisfaction (BMLSS-10) [0–100]	73.60 ± 15.30	69.80 ± 16.52	67.94 ± 17.74	77.15 ± 19.33	0.014	T0:T1 $p = 0.003$ T0:T2 $p = 0.005$ T2:T3 $p = 0.010$
Satisfaction with health situation (G1 of BMLSS) [0–6]	2.60 ± 1.73	2.66 ± 1.66	2.84 ± 1.60	3.70 ± 1.49	<0.0001	T0:T2 $p = 0.025$ T0:T3 $p = 0.001$ T2:T3 $p = 0.006$
Satisfaction with current treatment success (G2 of BMLSS) [0–6]	4.36 ± 1.24	4.44 ± 1.24	4.51 ± 1.08	5.21 ± 0.74	0.002	T0:T2 $p = 0.009$ T0:T3 $p = 0.001$ T2:T3 $p = 0.002$
Satisfaction with abilities to cope with daily life activities (G3 of BMLSS) [0–6]	4.39 ± 1.32	4.07 ± 1.38	3.76 ± 1.48	4.39 ± 1.27	n.s.	T2:T3 $p = 0.030$
Satisfaction with vitality/fitness (G4 of BMLSS) [0–6]	3.53 ± 1.59	3.24 ± 1.57	3.04 ± 1.81	3.28 ± 1.44	n.s.	/

Support satisfaction (BMLSS support) [0–100]	84.84 ± 13.48	79.13 ± 18.58	80.01 ± 19.85	81.37 ± 22.37	n.s.	T0:T1 $p = 0.029$
Escape from illness (ECAPE) [0–100]	33.33 ± 24.97	28.12 ± 24.27	32.78 ± 25.77	22.47 ± 22.10	n.s.	T2:TK $p = 0.035$
Spiritual needs						
Religious needs [0–3]	0.64 ± 0.82	0.61 ± 0.76	0.59 ± 0.70	0.49 ± 0.66	n.s.	/
Existential needs [0–3]	0.66 ± 0.82	0.70 ± 0.85	0.62 ± 0.69	0.45 ± 0.59	n.s.	/
Inner Peace needs [0–3]	1.56 ± 0.80	1.59 ± 0.96	1.42 ± 0.65	1.22 ± 0.97	0.034	T0:TK $p = 0.040$
Giving/Generativity needs [0–3]	1.10 ± 0.81	1.11 ± 0.80	1.06 ± 0.71	0.93 ± 0.83	n.s.	/
SpNQ-20 index [0–3]	0.92 ± 0.65	0.92 ± 0.66	0.86 ± 0.61	0.71 ± 0.60	n.s.	T0:TK $p = 0.013$

[a]only significant differences are depicted; values in square brackets are expected ranges

needs there were no significant differences with respect to the spiritual–religious self-categorization (R+S+ 1.31 ± 1.10; R+S-: 0.67 ± 0.62; R-S+: 1.21 ± 0.86; R-S-: 1.13 ± 0.72; $F = 1.9$, n.s.).

Among the *Religious* needs, the need to pray for one self (N20: 0.99 ± 1.18) was most relevant and among the *Existential* needs, particularly the need to dissolve/clarify open aspects of life (N5: 1.02 ± 1.25). Among the *Inner Peace* needs, talking with others about fears and worries (N2: 2.06 ± 0.98) was of strong importance, while among the *Giving/Generativity* needs it was the need to be assured that life was meaningful and of value (N27: 1.64 ± 1.26). The additional item N36, which addresses the need to have hope again, scored high (1.65 ± 1.36), while being connected with the family scored the highest (2.53 ± 0.82).

Patients had the option to state further unmet needs. Among these at T0 were the following: to just take care of me; need for pity; to continue to live as before; need for places of pilgrimage; to be able to see and accept myself as a creature of God in his image and parable; to surrender, let go, be given; seeking silence; to convert unrest into relaxation; sorting unclarified processes and tidying up; to put on makeup and put on nice clothes; go to the hairdresser to shorten hair (to prepare for chemotherapy); get good advice from medical doctors.

Within the time of antitumor therapy (T1 and T2), all spiritual needs remained stable and decreased after antitumor therapy had ended (T3). This decrease was significant for patients' *Inner Peace* needs, particularly comparing the posttreatment needs (T3) with the pretreatment needs (T0), while for *Religious* needs this decrease was only a statistically remarkable trend (T3 versus T0).

With respect to chemotherapy or other treatment regimes, in this interim analysis there were no significant differences in patients' unmet spiritual needs (data not shown).

Correlations between Spiritual Needs, Life Satisfaction and Escape from Illness during the Course of Treatment

Prior to treatment (T0), in this interim analysis the spiritual needs were not significantly related to patients' life satisfaction or their intention to escape from the situation. There was a trend toward weak association between *Existential* needs and low life satisfaction ($r = -0.21$, $p = 0.061$), while all other needs did not show relevant associations. Then in the first phases of treatment (T1), *Existential* needs were moderately related to low life satisfaction (r = -0.42, p = 0.02) and to the intention to escape from the situation (r = 0.39, p = 0.003). At the end of the treatment (T2), *Existential* needs were moderately related to escape (r = 0.48, p = 0.001). Three months after treatment ended, *Existential* needs were still moderately related to low life satisfaction (r = -0.36, p = 0.038) and to escape from illness (r = 0.35, p = 0.049). However, *Existential* needs were also moderately negatively related to satisfaction with team support (r = -0.46, p = 0.008).

Detailed analyses at T1 revealed that among the different dimensions of life satisfaction, *Existential* needs were particularly related to low satisfaction with the abilities to cope with daily-life activities (r = -0.40, p = 0.002), reduced vitality and fitness (r = -0.44, p = 0.001), low satisfaction with oneself (r = -0.43, p = 0.001) and life in general (r = -0.35, p = 0.009). Reduced vitality and fitness at T1 were moderately related to *Inner Peace* needs (r = -0.36, p = 0.007) as well. Interestingly, within the last phases of treatment, these moderate correlations became insignificant and irrelevant. However, three months after the treatment ended (T3) there were still relevant associations between *Existential* needs and reduced satisfaction with family life (r = -0.43, p = 0.012), life in general (r = -0.39, p = 0.028) and financial situation (r = -0.35, p = 0.044), while the associations with health-related satisfaction became irrelevant.

Which specific *Existential* needs were related with the respective satisfaction dimensions? At the start of the treatment (T1), low satisfaction with the abilities to cope with daily life activities, life in general, financial situation, workplace and with oneself were all moderately inversely related to the items N12 (talking with someone about the possibility of life after death) and N17 (being forgiven), while reduced vitality and fitness were moderately inversely related to items N16 (to forgive someone) and N17 (being forgiven). Three months after treatment (T3), satisfaction with workplace, life in general and also with oneself were moderately inversely related to N16 (to forgive someone).

Conclusions

Preliminary findings from this interim analysis showed that the principle pattern of spiritual needs prior to antitumor therapy is similar compared to that in other tumor patients from Germany (Büssing et al. 2010; Höcker et al. 2014; Haußmann et al. 2017), even when they are treated in palliative care units (Büssing et al. 2020). During antitumor therapy these needs remained unchanged, and decreased three months after the active treatment had ended, indicating that the reasons for the respective needs had either vanished or had become less relevant. So far, it seems that particularly *Existential* needs are related to low life satisfaction and patients' depressive intention to escape from their situation. A further important variable which may explain patients' intensity of unmet needs is their spiritual–religious self-assessment. Those who regarded themselves as R+S+ had significantly higher needs compared to the other groups, while R-S- had usually the lowest spiritual needs. The R+S+ patients are probably more open to recognizing and valuing their spiritual needs than their R-S- counterparts. These skeptic R-S- persons have unmet spiritual needs too, particularly *Inner Peace* needs and *Giving/Generativity* needs. The reason why *Existential* needs are lower in R-S- patients, too, remains unclear.

Thus, it is important to take a short spiritual history in terms of an anamnestic interview to differentiate the underlying spiritual attitudes of patients prior to and during the treatment as their attitudes may influence how strongly they perceive unmet spiritual needs. As their life satisfaction decreases during antitumor treatment and as it is inversely related with patients' *Existential* needs, they may require further support. Dissatisfaction with the health situation and also with life in general and its perspective (work and financial situation) may be associated with specific existential needs that could be addressed by a multi-professional team (i.e. social worker, psychotherapist, physiotherapists, nurses, medical doctors).

References

Akin S, Kas Guner C (2019) Investigation of the relationship among fatigue, self-efficacy and quality of life during chemotherapy in patients with breast, lung or gastrointestinal cancer. Eur J Cancer Care 28:e12898. https://doi.org/10.1111/ecc.12898

Büssing A, Keller N, Michalsen A, Moebus S, Dobos G, Ostermann T, Matthiessen P (2006) Spirituality and adaptive coping styles in German patients with chronic diseases in a CAM health care setting. J Complement Integr Med 3:4. https://doi.org/10.2202/1553-3840.1049

Büssing A, Fischer J, Haller A, Heusser P, Ostermann T, Matthiessen PF (2009) Validation of the brief multidimensional life satisfaction scale in patients with chronic diseases. European Journal of Medicine Research 14:171–177

Büssing A, Balzat HJ, Heusser P (2010) Spiritual needs of patients with chronic pain diseases and cancer – validation of the spiritual needs questionnaire. Eur J Med Res 15:266–273

Büssing A, Wassermann U, Hvidt NC, Längler A, Thiel M (2017) Spiritual needs of mothers with sick new born or premature infants. Woman and Birth 31:e89–e98

Büssing A, Baumann K, Rentschler J, Becker G (2020) Spirituelle Bedürfnisse von Tumorpatienten verändern sich während der palliativmedizinischen Betreuung kaum. Deutsche Zeitschrift für Onkologie Online first. https://doi.org/10.1055/a-1135-3566

Fernández-Ortega P, Caloto MT, Chirveches E, Marquilles R, Francisco JS, Quesada A, Suárez C, Zorrilla I, Gómez J, Zabaleta P, Nocea G, Llombart-Cussac A (2012) Chemotherapy-induced nausea and vomiting in clinical practice: impact on patients' quality of life. Support Care Cancer 20(12):3141–3148

Haußmann A, Schäffeler N, Hautzinger M, Weyel B, Eigentler T, Zipfel S, Teufel M (2017) Religiöse/spirituelle Bedürfnisse und psychosoziale Belastung von Patienten mit malignem Melanom. Psychother Psych Med 67:413–419

Höcker A, Krüll A, Koch U, Mehnert A (2014) Exploring spiritual needs and their associated factors in an urban sample of early and advanced cancer patients. Eur J Cancer Care 23:786–794

Kayl AE, Meyers CA (2006) Side-effects of chemotherapy and quality of life in ovarian and breast cancer patients. Curr Opin Obstet Gynecol 18(1):24–28

Lötzke D, Wiedemann F, Recchia DR, Ostermann T, Sattler D, Ettl J, Kiechle M, Büssing A (2016) Iyengar-yoga compared to exercise as a therapeutic intervention during (neo)adjuvant therapy in women with stage I-III breast cancer: health-related quality of life, mindfulness, spirituality, life satisfaction and cancer-related fatigue. Evidence-based complementary and alternative medicine 2016. Article ID 5931816. https://doi.org/10.1155/2016/5931816

McDonald ES, Clark AS, Tchou J, Zhang P, Freedman GM (2016) Clinical diagnosis and Management of Breast Cancer. J Nucl Med 57(Suppl 1):9S–16S

Niklasson A, Paty J, Rydén A (2017) Talking about breast cancer: which symptoms and treatment side effects are important to patients with advanced disease? Patient 10:719–727

Papadopoulou C, Kotronoulas G, Schneider A, Miller MI, McBride J, Polly Z, Bettles S, Whitehouse A, McCann L, Kearney N, Maguire R (2017) Patient-reported self-efficacy, anxiety, and health-related quality of life during chemotherapy: results from a longitudinal study. Oncol Nurs Forum 44:127–136

Schneider A, Kotronoulas G, Papadopoulou C, McCann L, Miller M, McBride J, Polly Z, Bettles S, Whitehouse A, Kearney N, Maguire R (2016) Trajectories and predictors of state and trait anxiety in patients receiving chemotherapy for breast and colorectal cancer: results from a longitudinal study. Eur J Oncol Nurs 24:1–7. https://doi.org/10.1016/j.ejon.2016.07.001

Wörmann B (2017) Breast cancer: basics, screening, diagnostics and treatment. Grundlagen, Früherkennung, Diagnostik und Therapie. Med Monatsschr Pharm 40:55–64

CHAPTER 14

Psychosocial, Existential and Spiritual Needs of Persons with Cystic Fibrosis

Jörg Große-Onnebrink and Arndt Büssing

Background

Cystic fibrosis (CF) occurs in 1/3500 births and thus is the most common autosomal recessive disease in Caucasians (Mehta et al. 2010). CF is caused by mutations on chromosome 7 in the region which encodes for the cystic fibrosis transmembrane conductance regulator (CFTR) protein, which, in short, is a chloride channel and maintains low viscosity in secretions such as the bronchial epithelium, biliary ducts, pancreatic ducts and so forth. Decreased function of CFTR results in the different disease manifestations. The disease is mainly characterized by poor weight gain and

J. Große-Onnebrink (✉)
Department of General Pediatrics, Pediatric Respiratory Medicine Unit, University Hospital Münster, Münster, Germany
e-mail: joerg.grosse-onnebrink@ukmuenster.de

A. Büssing
Professorship Quality of Life, Spirituality and Coping, Faculty of Health, Witten/Herdecke University, Herdecke, Germany

IUNCTUS—Competence Center for Christian Spirituality, Philosophical-Theological University of Münster, Münster, Germany
e-mail: Arndt.buessing@uni-wh.de

A. Büssing (ed.), *Spiritual Needs in Research and Practice*,
https://doi.org/10.1007/978-3-030-70139-0_14

frequent respiratory infection in childhood, while later in life bronchiectasis, as well as infertility, hepatobiliary disease, diabetes mellitus and many other conditions may decrease patients' quality of life. The respiratory disease of CF mainly accounts for the disease burden and is the most important causal factor for reduced life expectancy. The CF lung disease is characterized by highly viscous secretions of the bronchial epithelium, which results in decreased airway clearance, repetitive pulmonary infections and a high inflammatory state. Later, formation of bronchiectasis and ongoing pulmonary destruction are frequently seen. Patients with CF with end-stage lung disease suffer from frequent hospitalizations for intravenous antibiotic treatment courses, supplementary oxygen insufflation, mechanical ventilation, need for additional high caloric intake via gastral feeding tubes and severely decreased physical fitness. Lung transplantation serves as a treatment option in end-stage lung disease and results in 50% survival of patients 6–7 years after lung transplantation (International Society for Heart and Lung Transplantation n.d.).

Spirituality and religion have been studied in relation to health for a considerable period of time, and numerous reviews have been published (Koenig et al. 2015; Hill and Pargament 2003). Many studies have linked various dimensions of faith, including religiosity (Berman et al. 2004; Cotton et al. 2006, 2010), worship attendance (Chida et al. 2009), and spiritual coping with different health outcomes, both physical (Pargament et al. 2001) and mental (Pargament et al. 2004). In general, spirituality and religion have been understood as a resource to cope with disease.

Grossoehme et al. (2016) examined 11–19 year old children and adolescents with CF and found that their treatment adherence was related to their spirituality and lower spiritual strife/worries; this treatment adherence in turn was the predictor of airway clearance adherence, which is therapeutically important. A qualitative study by that working group addressed whether people who were diagnosed with CF in adulthood use their spirituality to cope better with the disease and disease management. It turned out that spirituality was actually helpful to find meaning and to "deal cooperatively" with God and the pulmonologist (Grossoehme et al. 2012). An early qualitative study by Pendleton et al. (2002) found a variety of religious/spiritual coping strategies in 5–12 year old children with CF that were almost always associated with favorable adaptive health behaviors.

Spirituality is generally seen as a resource to find meaning in life, and support and hope by praying to a helping source. Prayer is indeed often intensified in times of need and illness, and can thus be inversely associated with health (Ladd and Spilka 2013), while it is also of relevance independently to a person's health situation (Büssing 2017).

So far there are not many studies on the impact of spirituality on patients with CF, and there are no studies on their spiritual needs. Therefore, a study among persons with CF (adolescents and young adults) was performed to assess which spiritual needs were of relevance to them and how these are triggered. Due to the limited life expectancy we hypothesized that questions regarding end-of-life scenarios are more urgent and prominent for patients with CF. We further hypothesized that spiritual needs are thus relevant to CF patients and that disease progress is associated with an increase in specific spiritual needs. If this is the case, we might be able to address specific spiritual consulting services for CF patients.

Description of Enrolled Patients

Patients with CF were recruited from four specialized hospitals in West Germany. All were informed about the purpose of the respective study, were assured of confidentiality and were asked to provide informed consent. For adolescents, their parents provided informed consent. Ethical approval for the study was obtained by the Institutional Review Board (IRB) of Witten/Herdecke University and from IRBs of the involved hospitals. Patients were asked for basic sociodemographic data and further for clinical details (i.e. lung function parameters—forced expiratory Volume in one second % predicted [FEV1 %pred], days of antibiotic treatment in hospital, frequency of infection of lower airways with the opportunistic pathogen *Pseudomonas aeruginosa*, nebulization with antibiotics, long-term oxygen treatment, usage of noninvasive ventilation, being on waitlist for lung transplantation or already having received lung transplantation). Here, the Spiritual Needs Questionnaire (SpNQ) in its adapted adolescent version (see Chap. 8) was applied which uses an additional relational item (N38: That there is someone who is always at your side) and two affirmative items (N43: That your situation improves for the better; N44: To have someone who assures that your situation will improve for the better).

The sample consisted of 115 persons (48% women and 52% men) with a mean age of 30.4 ± 13.1 years; 17% were adolescents. The majority was nominally Christian; however, only 42% regarded themselves as "believers". Nevertheless, 20% stated that their belief in God played a major role in their life, 21% were undecided and 59% rejected this statement. In line with this finding, 17% are praying often/very often, 35% seldom and 54%

never. Patients' life satisfaction was in the upper range (BMLSS [0–100]: 71.6 ± 15.0) and their symptom score in the lower third (VAS [0–100]: 35.7 ± 23.2). Their FEV1 %pred was 56.1 ± 32.8 [0–135]. Of these, 10% of persons with CF had already received a lung transplantation, and 3% were on the waitlist. Most did not need long-term oxygen supplementation (82%), and 7% required noninvasive ventilator support.

Spiritual Needs of Persons with Cystic Fibrosis

Within this group the strongest needs were relational needs (Table 14.1), particularly the needs that "there is someone who is always at your side" (N38), to be assured by someone "that your situation improves for the better" (N43), "to turn to someone in a loving attitude" (N13) and also needs for "inner peace" (N8) and the intention to "plunge into beauty of nature" (N6). With respect to the factors, *Attention/Positive Affirmation* needs and *Inner Peace* needs scored highest, followed by *Existential* needs, while *Religious* needs scored much lower. Women had significantly higher *Attention/Positive Affirmation* needs than men ($F = 5.4$, $p = 0.021$), while *Inner Peace* needs were significantly higher in the older age group ($F = 6.2$, $p = 0.001$). Being a believer was associated with higher *Religious* needs ($F = 28.9$, $p < 0.0001$), while lacking this faith was associated with lower *Existential* needs ($F = 3.3$, $p = 0.042$) (data not shown).

With respect to the clinical situation, respirator usage (which was required by eight persons) was associated with higher *Attention/Positive Affirmation* needs ($F = 11.5$, $p = 0.001$) and *Inner Peace* needs ($F = 6.2$, $p = 0.015$), while there were no relevant differences with respect to oxygen application (which was necessary in 20 persons), except a trend towards higher *Attention/Positive Affirmation* needs in the user group ($F = 3.5$, $p = 0.065$). Being on the waitlist for lung transplantation ($n = 3$) resulted in significantly higher *Religious/Praying* needs ($F = 15.5$, $p < 0.0001$) and *Existential/Giving* needs ($F = 10.8$, $p = 0.001$), while they did not significantly differ for those after lung transplantation ($n = 11$) and those without with respect to the needs scores ($F < 2.7$, n.s.) (data not shown).

Correlation analyses between spiritual needs and health related indicators (life satisfaction, symptom score, antibiotics in hospital, lung function) and self-efficacy expectation revealed weak to moderate associations. Life satisfaction (BMLSS) was moderately inversely related to *Attention/Positive Affirmation* needs ($r = -0.45$) and *Existential/Giving* needs

Table 14.1 Spiritual needs scores (0–3) in the sample

Scale and items	*M ± SD*
Religious/Praying needs	**0.51 ± 0.78**
N18 To pray with someone	0.28 ± 0.66
N19 That someone prays for you	0.49 ± 0.89
N20 To pray for yourself	0.61 ± 0.97
N23 To turn to a higher presence (i.e. god, Allah, angels, saints)	0.67 ± 1.02
Existential/Giving needs	**1.04 ± 1.09**
N11 To talk with someone about the question of meaning in life	0.61 ± 0.90
N13 To turn to someone in a loving attitude	1.57 ± 1.08
N15 To give solace to someone	1.08 ± 1.08
N25 To be assured that your life is meaningful and of value	0.87 ± 1.07
Need for attention / positive affirmation	**1.60 ± 0. 49**
N2 To talk with someone about your fears and worries	1.50 ± 1.09
N38 That there is someone who is always at your side	1.89 ± 1.18
N43 That your situation improves for the better	1.73 ± 1.16
N44 To have someone who assures that your situation will improve for the better	1.26 ± 1.19
Inner Peace Needs	**1.39 ± 0.97**
N6 To plunge into beauty of nature	1.47 ± 1.21
N7 To dwell at a place of quietness and peace	1.14 ± 1.23
N8 To find inner peace	1.54 ± 1.18
Additional items	
N4 To reflect back on your life	1.00 ± 1.00
N5 To dissolve / clarify open aspects of your life	0.87 ± 0.99
N10 To find meaning in illness and/or suffering	0.59 ± 0.95
N16 To forgive someone from a distinct period of your life	0.73 ± 0.97
N25 To feel connected with family	1.11 ± 1.07

(r = -0.31) and weakly with *Inner Peace* needs (r = -0.24), but not with *Religious/Praying* needs (r = -0.06). Symptom scores were weakly positively associated with *Inner Peace* needs (r = 0.27), *Attention/Positive Affirmation* needs (r = 0.26) and *Existential/Giving* needs (r = 0.22), but not with *Religious/Praying* needs (r = 0.02). Days for antibiotics in hospital were weakly related only to *Religious/Praying* needs (r = 0.26), while lung function scores were weakly related to *Inner Peace* needs only (r = -0.25). Patients' self-efficacy expectation (GSS) was weakly negatively related to *Attention/Positive Affirmation* needs (r = -0.27) and *Inner Peace* needs (r = -0.23).

Because there were several significant influencing variables which may predict the intensity of patients' spiritual needs, stepwise regression analyses with the variables gender, age, praying (as an indicator of religiosity) and the clinical indicators were performed.

- *Religious/Praying* needs were predicted primarily by praying (54% of explained variance) with further contribution of days in hospital for antibiotic therapy (adding 3%) and low self-efficacy expectation (adding 2%). These variables explain together 59% of variance.
- *Existential/Giving* needs were predicted by reduced life satisfaction and praying with low predictive power ($R^2 = 0.15$).
- *Attention/Positive Affirmation* needs were predicted best by reduced life satisfaction (which explains 21% explained variance), and further by respirator usage (adding 7% of explained variance) and praying (adding further 4%). These three variables together explain 32% of variance.
- *Inner Peace* needs were predicted with low power ($R^2 = 0.15$) by higher age and reduced lung function.

In none of these models were patients' symptom score or gender and age among the significant predictors.

Discussion of Findings

The strongest needs among patients with CF were those for attention and positive affirmation which is comprehensible in case of a progressive and "incurable" disease. That these patients also have higher *Inner Peace* needs which were weakly related to respirator usage and reduced lung function is comprehensible, too. *Religious* needs were of lowest relevance, which could be explained by the low age of the patients, as in Germany, interest in religious issues is very low among younger persons. This contrasts with findings from the USA. Population-based studies indicate that 63% of German participants believe in God, while 44% state that God is important in their life and only 12% attend religious service at least once (www.europeanvaluesstudy.eu). In the USA, 83% believe in God absolutely or fairly certainly, 77% find religion very important or somewhat important in their lives and 36% attend religious services at least once a week (Pew Research Center n.d.). Within these studies, the number of older persons is high, and thus low religious interest of younger persons is masked. These differences suggest different religious attitudes and different grades of secularism within these populations, which also applies to different European countries (www.europeanvaluesstudy.eu).

The younger group of patients with cystic fibrosis has a differential pattern of spiritual needs. Aspects of organized religiosity (i.e. praying with others) were of lower interest compared to non-organized private prayers. However, this seems to be a general trend and can be found in other groups of patients, too. Among German patients with cancer, trust in higher sources or search for meaningful support was more important than for patients with chronic pain diseases (Büssing et al. 2007). Possibly, for patients with recently diagnosed life-threatening disease, the need to address existential issues is more acute, while patients with chronic diseases like CF have a different focus. To them concrete persons who are available and are there for relieving talk about their fears and worries and who give hope, are obviously more relevant.

It might be that the activity of disease is crucial for the intensity of spiritual needs; during the progression of lung disease in patients with CF, they may strongly change. While in patients with CF disease burden during the first years of life is relatively low and medical treatment is mainly characterized by nutritional care and antibiotic treatment during infective pulmonary exacerbations, later, the disease burden increases and is characterized by an increase in frequency of pulmonary exacerbations and need for hospitalization. Furthermore, shortness of breath with dependency on technical equipment (oxygen supplementation, respirator) develops and, if lung transplantation becomes an option, fear of dying and end-of-life scenarios become more relevant to patients. This might raise the intensity of spiritual needs. In fact, there was a positive association between specific spiritual needs with age, lung function and respirator usage on the one hand, and very strong needs in those few who are on the waitlist for lung transplantation (i.e. end-stage lung disease) on the other, while the intensity of spiritual needs was similar to the others when transplantation was done.

Conclusions

Obviously, in patients who are confronted with end of life, special spiritual needs come to the fore. The aspect that specific disease stages are associated with specific spiritual needs is highly relevant to CF care, because specific spiritual care may be offered to selected patients, respective to their clinical situation.

The following practical consequences may result from these findings: the anamnesis in patients with CF should address spiritual issues as it already contains questions on psychological well-being, relationship status and physical signs and symptoms. Especially in patients with advanced lung disease or during phases with disease deterioration, spiritual needs can change in pattern and degree. Herein possible spiritual needs should be addressed in patients. Furthermore, spiritual offers should respect the different needs in secularized communities. While denominational spiritual care is regularly implemented in hospital organization structure, non-confessional offers of spirituality are widely lacking—structural development is useful and necessary here. Positive affirmation and attention are important to several patients: visitor regulations should enable personal contacts between patients and relatives/friends. If face-to-face contacts are limited, provision of electronically aided communication devices (e.g. for video calls) and internet access may help patients to stay in touch with friends and relatives.

Taken together, spiritual needs with different characteristics are relevant to patients with CF and might change during disease progression. A comprehensive medical approach should recognize spiritual needs and offer appropriate options to patients.

Acknowledgements We are grateful to all who have helped to enroll the patients, particularly Charlotte Roche, who worked on this project as a part of her thesis, Florian Stehling, Sutharsan Sivagurunathan and Michaela Schiller from the collaborating university hospitals in Essen and Homburg/Saar and all patients who have filled the questionnaire.

References

Berman E, Merz JF, Rudnick M, Snyder RW, Rogers KK, Johnson JLD, Mosenkis A, Israni A, Wolpe PR, Lipschutz JH (2004) Religiosity in a hemodialysis population and its relationship to satisfaction with medical care, satisfaction with life, and adherence. Am J Kidney Dis 44(3):488–497

Büssing A (2017) Empirische Zugänge zum Beten im Horizont von Krankheit und Gesundheit. In: Peng-Keller S (ed) Gebet als Resonanzereignis. Annäherungen im Horizont von Spiritual Care. Vandenhoeck & Ruprecht, Göttingen, pp 151–181

Büssing A, Ostermann T, Koenig HG (2007) Relevance of religion and spirituality in German patients with chronic diseases. Int J Psychiatry Med 37(1):39–57. https://doi.org/10.2190/60W7-1661-2623-6042

Chida Y, Steptoe A, Powell LH (2009) Religiosity/spirituality and mortality. A systematic quantitative review. Psychother Psychosom 78(2):81–90

Cotton S, Puchalski CM, Sherman SN, Mrus JM, Peterman AH, Feinberg J, Pargament KI, Justice AC, Leonard AC, Tsevat J (2006) Spirituality and religion in patients with HIV/AIDS. J Gen Intern Med 21(Suppl 5):S5–S13. https://doi.org/10.1111/j.1525-1497.2006.00642.x

Cotton S, McGrady ME, Rosenthal SL (2010) Measurement of religiosity/spirituality in adolescent health outcomes research: trends and recommendations. J Relig Health 49(4):414–444

Grossoehme DH, Ragsdale JR, Cotton S, Meyers MA, Clancy JP, Seid M, Joseph PM (2012) Using spirituality after an adult CF diagnosis: cognitive reframing and adherence motivation. J Health Care Chaplain 18(3–4):110–120

Grossoehme DH, Szczesniak RD, Mrug S, Dimitriou SM, Marshall A, McPhail GL (2016 Oct) Adolescents' spirituality and cystic fibrosis airway clearance treatment adherence: examining mediators. J Pediatr Psychol 41(9):1022–1032

Hill PC, Pargament KI (2003) Advances in the conceptualization and measurement of religion and spirituality. Implications for physical and mental health research. Am Psychol 58(1):64–74

International Society for Heart and Lung Transplantation (n.d.) International Thoracic Organ Transplant (TTX) Registry Quarterly Data Reports. https://ishltregistries.org/registries/quarterlydatareport.asp. Accessed 28 Aug 2020

Koenig HG, King DE, Carson VB (2015) Handbook of religion and health, 2nd edn. Oxford University Press, Oxford

Ladd KL, Spilka B (2013) Prayer: a review of the empirical literature. In: Pargament KI (ed) APA handbook of psychology, religion, and spirituality. American Psychological Association, Chapter 16, pp 1–18

Mehta G, Macek M Jr, Mehta A, European Registry Working G (2010) Cystic fibrosis across Europe: EuroCareCF analysis of demographic data from 35 countries. J Cyst Fibros 9(Suppl 2):S5–S21

Pargament KI, Koenig HG, Tarakeshwar N, Hahn J (2001) Religious struggle as a predictor of mortality among medically ill elderly patients: a 2-year longitudinal study. Arch Intern Med 161(15):1881–1885

Pargament KI, Koenig HG, Tarakeshwar N, Hahn J (2004) Religious coping methods as predictors of psychological, physical and spiritual outcomes among medically ill elderly patients: a two-year longitudinal study. J Health Psychol 9(6):713–730. https://doi.org/10.1177/1359105304045366

Pendleton SM, Cavalli KS, Pargament KI, Nasr SZ (2002) Religious/spiritual coping in childhood cystic fibrosis: a qualitative study. Pediatrics 109(1):E8. https://doi.org/10.1542/peds.109.1.e8

Pew Research Center (n.d.) Religion and Public life. https://www.pewforum.org/religious-landscape-study/belief-in-god. Accessed 28 Aug 2020

CHAPTER 15

Spiritual Needs of HIV-Infected Persons from Brazil

Tânia Cristina de Oliveira Valente and Ana Paula Rodrigues Cavalcanti

Background

The diagnosis of Acquired Immunodeficiency Syndrome (AIDS) is marked by a set of feelings, attitudes, and practices that reveal the difficulty of giving a new meaning to life and suffering (Espírito Santo et al. 2003). However, the evolution of scientific knowledge about this disease caused by an infection with the Human Immunodeficiency Virus (HIV) has increased the survival of people living with HIV/AIDS (PLWHA), giving the disease a recurring character (Poorolajal et al. 2016).

Among the coping strategies, religiosity/spirituality (R/S) can represent an element of support for the weaknesses exposed by the disease

T. C. de Oliveira Valente (✉)
Interdisciplinary Medical Anthropologic Studies and Research Laboratory, Rio de Janeiro State Federal University, Rio de Janeiro, Brazil

A. P. R. Cavalcanti
Religious Sciences Department, Federal University of Paraíba, João Pessoa, Brazil

A. Büssing (ed.), *Spiritual Needs in Research and Practice*,
https://doi.org/10.1007/978-3-030-70139-0_15

(Caixeta et al. 2012), improving the quality of life of the PLWHA as proposed by the World Health Organization (WHO 2003) which included this indicator when proposing the WHOQOL-HIV.

Despite this, these individuals can be affected by guilt, fear, anxiety, depression, suicidal ideation, among other reactions associated with the disease's stigma (Chambers et al. 2015). Spiritual needs (SpN) can be a source of support and resilience to address threats to PLWHA's physical and mental health (Arrey et al. 2016).

Since the biopsychosocial model proposed by Engel (1977), several elements have been added to the study of the health–disease relationship, to expand its understanding, previously restricted to its purely biological aspects. Sulmasy (2002) was a pioneer in adding the spiritual dimension to this structure, but his focus was on patients in palliative care. In 2010, Büssing and Koenig (2010) discussed the application of the biopsychosocial–spiritual model to the care of patients with chronic diseases and emphasized the multidimensional character of spirituality, and identified and discriminated four major (interconnected) dimensions of SpN: social needs, associated with the need for connection (love, belonging, communication with close people); emotional needs, associated with the need for peace (inner peace, hope, balance, ability to forgive, fear of relapse); existential needs, associated with the need to have a meaning/objective (meaning in life, assign a role in life); and religious needs, associated with transcendence (spiritual resources, relationship with God, the sacred, prayers).

Based on this model and considering that the importance of R/S for PLWHA is still questioned (Doolittle et al. 2018), the recent review by Valente et al. (2020) identified 59 different designations related to the SpN in PLWHA in several dimensions of this construct.

Regarding the religious needs the following were mentioned: individual prayer, religious readings, support from religious groups, intercessory prayers, belonging to religious communities or spiritual support, visits by spiritual leaders, religious songs, religious TV programs, religious purification, water, drinks or medicines prepared by religious persons, religious rituals involving herbal baths and animal sacrifice, attendance at religious services, religious experiences, veneration of ancestral spirits, the intervention of pastors of other religious or traditional healers, and religious behavior. Other topics that often referred to the faith dimension were previous beliefs, spiritual connection, belief in biblical promises of healing, belief in divine or spiritual healing, belief in ancestral spirits, belief in God's forgiveness, belief in karma, divine intervention, belief in a supreme deity, belief in spiritual reconciliation with illness, belief in promises to obtain a cure, practices such as curing possession by demonic spirits, curing spells, spiritual passes, spiritual practices, practices that lead to the return of power or energy lost when falls ill, divination practices or clairvoyance, as well as the ingestion of miracle medicines.

The emotional needs listed were needs to repair, feelings of abandonment, forgiveness, forgiveness for offending deities, as well as needs for feelings of peace.

Regarding social needs the authors cited social support needs, needs of affective relationships, relations with the family, social support of religious groups, spiritual support, participation in cultural activities that give meaning to the disease and counseling received from health professionals.

Less frequently cited, the existential needs were reflected through the meaning of life, disease and death, life goals, acceptance of the disease, spiritual matters, and reflections that give rise to a positive outlook on life.

Given the relevance shown by Valente's review about SpN as a factor that can step directly or indirectly into the results of health care, several research instruments have been proposed for the investigation of these needs. One of these instruments is the Spiritual Needs Questionnaire (SpNQ) (Büssing et al. 2010, 2018). This questionnaire, initially written in German, translated and validated in other languages, explores four aspects related to SpN: Religious needs, Inner Peace needs, Existential needs, and Giving/Generativity needs; avoiding the exclusive use of religious terminology and also applying to agnostic or atheistic patients, and focusing on a holistic health perspective. Previous studies in patients with other chronic pathologies have shown different results using the SpNQ (Büssing et al. 2013a, 2016). Among cancer patients, in a secular society, the needs for *Giving/Generativity* and for *Inner Peace* were considered more relevant (Büssing et al. 2013a), as well as among patients with fibromyalgia (Offenbaecher et al. 2013) and patients with chronic disease from China (Büssing et al. 2013b) and Poland (Büssing et al. 2015).

To study and culturally adapt the SpNQ for use on adults with chronic states/diseases in Brazil, two studies were conducted among two samples of patients with PLWHA using previous SpNQ versions (Büssing et al. 2013b, 2016) which will be discussed as examples of what these patients value while facing the adversities imposed by the disease and their SpN. At present, the 20-item version of SpNQ (SpNQ-20) is considered definitive (Büssing et al. 2018).

Specificities of the HIV Patient Regarding Spirituality

Regarding the usage of spirituality as a resource, AIDS cannot be considered as any other chronic illness. Because of its social stigma, it is not always regarded as legitimate to seek spiritual help to obtain a cure (or miracle) for this. Some people have the prejudice that the sick person somehow 'deserved' to be infected by 'divine punishment' against any deviation from the moral rules defended by some religious authorities (Pinho et al. 2017).

In this sense, PLWHA are seen by some persons as scapegoats, an HIV/AIDS as material proof of 'divine wrath' against 'perversions' and various sins committed in disobedience to the rules. Thus, these patients start to wear a label of 'perversion,' of moral indignity, who would deserve to hate themselves, for being guilty of their illness, and being detested by everyone. It is a reverberation of what in the Modern Age is consolidated as a social prejudice against "the plague"—considered by the clergy as demons installed within society (Delumeau 1989). In the nineteenth century, a hygienist science brought the notion of 'filth' and its consequence, the notion of who was 'filthy': the stigmatized social types or "fallen faithful and impossible return." It is not uncommon for PLWHA waiting in the outpatient care waiting room (especially when they come to the first consultations) to be 'in disguise,' hiding themselves behind sunglasses, caps, and large coats, in fear of being recognized and blamed.

Based on the (idealistic) idea that religion consolidates the integration of people into the community (Koenig 2004), safeguards society and spirituality, focuses on individual reflection, as well as on the examination of conscience and divine judgment, PLWHA may experience an exclusion from the religious institution. It can affect the moments of socialization of that faith, due to social prejudices, but not from the internalized spiritual experience acquired by the methods of the religious institution and others, throughout life.

For Boff (2009), "the drama of the current human being is to have lost spirituality and his ability to live a feeling of connection. What is opposed to spirituality is not irreligion or atheism, but the inability to connect and reconnect with all things."

Two Brazilian Studies About SpN in PLWHA

To understand SpN among Brazilian PLWHA in Rio de Janeiro, we relied on the existing dataset used for transcultural adaptation to the Portuguese version of SpNQ (Valente TC de et al. 2018) that included 200 PLWHA, randomly selected among patients followed up at the AIDS Outpatient Clinic of the Rio de Janeiro State Federal University Medical School Hospital, Brazil. This hospital is accredited as a National AIDS Reference Center by the Brazilian Ministry of Health, and is the largest clinic with this specialty in Rio de Janeiro State. In Paraíba State, 157 PLWHA assisted in the outpatient clinic of the Infectious Diseases Hospital Complex Dr. Clementino Fraga (CHCF) were studied. CHCF is a reference for the treatment of contagious infectious diseases in the State of Paraíba, with emphasis on the care of people with tuberculosis, Hansen's disease, and HIV/AIDS (Silva 2020).

Among the patients from Rio de Janeiro and João Pessoa, 57% and 49% were of male gender, and 57% and 54% were 30–49 years old, respectively. Regarding the level of education, most of them had incomplete high school education and high school education, respectively. Most preferred not to state their religion (42% in Rio de Janeiro and 69% in João Pessoa). For people who had declared their religion, the most cited were Kardecist Spiritism in Rio de Janeiro and Catholic in João Pessoa, both with non-organizational practice.

Regarding SpNQ domains and items, differences between the samples from Rio de Janeiro and João Pessoa are presented in Table 15.1. SpNQ Scores are show in Table 15.2.

The spiritual needs scores were significantly higher in the João Pessoa PLWHA, who are predominantly Catholics, than in the Rio de Janeiro PLWHA, where the religious diversity is greater (Table 15.2).

The *Religious* needs domain showed more significance to PLWHA in Paraíba than in Rio de Janeiro. It is interesting to note the difference between "turn to a higher presence" (N23) and "pray for yourself" (N20), because both were not considered as relevant in Rio. "Participate in a religious ceremony" (N21) was remarkably crucial to Paraíba, but not for Rio respondents. Prayer presented far-reaching importance to Paraíba, which is confirmed by local history and traditions. This distinction is also met in "Read religious/spiritual books" (N22). To have a pastor or priest caring for the respondent (N3) was far more critical in Paraíba, which was

Table 15.1 SpNQ domains and items responses among PLWHA from Rio de Janeiro and João Pessoa samples of PLWHA

Domains and Items		*No (%)*		*YES*					
				Somewhat (%)		*Strong (%)*		*Very Strong (%)*	
		RJ	*PB*	*RJ*	*PB*	*RJ*	*PB*	*RJ*	*PB*
1—RELIGIOUS NEEDS									
N21	Participate in a religious ceremony (e.g. service)	46.00	27.74	19.00	23.23	29.50	16.77	**5.50**	**32.26**
N23	Turn to a higher presence (e.g. God, Allah)	**27.00**	**8.39**	22.00	20.00	39.50	34.19	11.50	37.42
N19	Someone prays for you	34.00	21.15	30.50	22.44	29.00	28.21	**6.50**	**28.21**
N20	Pray for yourself	**40.00**	**5.84**	31.50	33.77	23.50	32.47	**5.00**	**27.92**
N18	Pray with someone	57.00	24.36	27.00	28.85	13.50	24.36	**2.50**	**22.44**
N03	Someone of your religious community (e.g. pastor) cares for you	71.50	50.64	19.00	22.44	9.00	14.74	**0.50**	**12.80**
N22	Read religious/spiritual books	60.00	40.00	22.50	21.33	12.00	16.67	**5.50**	**22.00**
2—EXISTENTIAL NEEDS									
N10	Find meaning in illness and/or suffering	59.50	33.12	25.50	23.38	10.50	25.32	4.50	18.18
N11	Talk about the question of meaning in life	31.00	32.43	37.00	26.35	26.00	27.70	6.00	13.51
N13	Turn to someone in a loving attitude	18.00	17.20	51.00	21.02	26.50	28.66	**4.50**	**33.12**
N12	Talk about the possibility of life after death	54.00	58.33	26.00	12.18	11.00	14.10	9.00	15.38
N02	Talk with others about your fears and worries	**34.00**	**0.00**	32.50	37.50	31.00	15.91	**2.50**	**46.59**
N17	Be forgiven	37.50	22.73	25.00	22.08	30.00	24.03	**7.50**	**31.17**

(*continued*)

Table 15.1 (continued)

Domains and Items		*No (%)*		*YES*					
				Somewhat (%)		*Strong (%)*		*Very Strong (%)*	
		RJ	*PB*	*RJ*	*PB*	*RJ*	*PB*	*RJ*	*PB*
N14	Give away something from yourself	30.50	30.14	45.00	28.08	20.50	21.92	**4.00**	**19.86**
N15	To solace someone	32.00	17.33	33.00	27.33	29.00	24.00	**6.00**	**31.33**
N16	To forgive someone from a distinct period of your life	40.00	17.83	31.00	21.66	23.50	30.57	**5.50**	**29.94**
N05	To solve the "open aspects" of your life	18.50	42.76	41.50	13.16	33.00	30.92	7.00	13.16
3—INNER PEACE NEEDS									
N07	Dwell in a place of quietness and peace	4.00	3.95	**31.50**	**6.58**	47.50	15.79	**17.00**	**73.68**
N08	Find inner peace	4.50	5.96	**27.00**	**5.30**	46.50	14.57	**22.00**	**74.17**
N06	Plunge into beauty of nature	7.00	2.58	**37.00**	**9.03**	42.50	16.77	**13.50**	**71.61**
N04	Reflect on your previous life	33.00	29.03	40.00	30.32	22.00	20.65	**5.00**	**20.00**
N24	Am I complete and safe?	3.50	9.15	19.50	30.07	54.00	33.99	23.00	**26.80**
4—SOCIAL and GENERATIVITY NEEDS									
N30	Receive more support from your family	19.50	17.31	**56.00**	**17.95**	21.00	26.28	**3.50**	**38.46**
N25	Feel connected with your family	17.00	12.26	**57.00**	**21.94**	21.50	29.03	**4.50**	**36.77**
N26	To transmit your own life experiences to others	29.00	14.94	46.00	24.68	21.00	30.52	**4.00**	**29.87**
N27	To be assured that your life was meaningful and of value	**14.50**	**4.55**	31.00	11.04	47.50	29.22	**7.00**	**55.19**
N28	Be inserted again in your family concerns	71.50	16.77	21.00	15.48	**5.50**	**30.97**	**2.00**	**36.77**

Abbreviations: RJ—Rio de Janeiro (Rio de Janeiro State), PB—João Pessoa (Paraíba State)

Table 15.2 SpNQ Scores among Brazillian Rio de Janeiro and João Pessoa samples of PLWHA

		Religious Needs	*Existential Needs*	*Inner Peace Needs*	*Giving/ Generativity Needs*	*SpNQ-20 Mean Scores*
Sample from…						
João Pessoa (n = 157)	Mean	1.54	1.31	2.45	1.93	1.72
	SD	0.57	0.54	0.50	0.51	0.39
Rio de Janeiro (n = 200)	Mean	0.97	0.95	1.57	1.23	1.11
	SD	0.67	0.62	0.64	0.56	0.53
All persons (n = 357)	Mean	1.22	1.11	1.95	1.54	1.38
	SD	0.69	0.61	0.73	0.64	0.57
F-value		69.84	32.33	202.42	147.66	145.03
p-value		<0.001	<0.001	<0.001	<0.001	<0.001

a social indicator in this place and was considered a positive aspect to live under collective norms.

The *Existential* needs domain basically showed relevant differences between those who perceived it as a "very strong" need: Paraíba was markedly higher. Forgiveness and prayer showed their value for Paraíba's sample, too.

Inner Peace needs, in turn, almost opposed Rio de Janeiro to Paraíba; the latter showed noticeably higher scores. As the opposite side of the "social coin," Paraíba is far more prejudiced against gays, lesbians, and, therefore, PLWHA. These patients know well how importantly this dimension represents them.

Social and Generativity needs, as well, were more robust for Paraíba's respondents—except concerning receiving more support from the family and the feeling of connection with the family, where both samples agree on the importance of these situations. However, PLWHA from Paraíba again presented a more acute pattern. Family ties are actively cultivated on this State, and to dismiss them could be a threat, socially reproachable, and hard to bear keeping good mental health.

The differences between these samples point to psychosocial and religious/spiritual characteristics as to how people deal with AIDS in Northeast Brazil, where social justice is insecure, ubiquitous, and harmful. The awareness of this discrimination and isolation in moments of collective experience of faith and religion—mass, worship, contact—with a priest or pastor proved to be relevant, as did support from the religious community, and the consequent greater importance given to spiritual growth "within yourself," out of the view of society. It is a paradox that religions embrace all "who are suffering and burdened"—but not the LGBT people, or PLWHA (as far as considering the reactions against these groups goes, especially among those who pick Old Testimony versicles to condemn LGBT and justify the suffering of PLWHA as a deserved curse) (Bluthenthal et al. 2012; Pereira and Monteiro 2015; Reyes-Estrada et al. 2018).

da Silva (2019) demonstrated a strong need for João Pessoa's PLWHA to feel supported by the family, and thereby achieve inner peace. As a second priority, these individuals differentiated the social side from the religious experience (approaching what Allport and Ross (1967) argued to be "extrinsic religiosity") from the inner side, the spiritual dimension (which would, in contrast, be the "intrinsic religiosity" defined by Allport).

The strength found in what the PLWHA in Silva's study differentiated as "spirituality" can be seen both as a coping strategy and as a characteristic of the human condition (da Silva 2019). These are aspects of human life that once again proved to be donors of resilience, meaning, and animus to continue living after the diagnosis, facing the necessary and lifelong therapy against the virus, and experiencing the anguish of the predominant emotional state in the first moment of coping with the disease.

These findings are remarkably diverse from those of Rio de Janeiro, a cosmopolitan city where social constraints are less harmful to PLWHA. Despite this, these Brazilian studies pointed out that for these patients, family support is not replaceable, and this lack worsens the quality of life of these patients. The family can provide the support that the rest of society denies or diminishes, complementing the inner strength achieved by spirituality in coping with chronic illness.

Although the religious profile of Brazil is undergoing a significant transformation, with an increase in religious plurality, some regions such as the Northeast, where João Pessoa is located, still have a predominant Catholic profile (approximately 75% of the population is Catholic, 9% are neo-Pentecostal evangelicals, 5% evangelicals, and 0.7% spiritualists). In the Southeast, where Rio de Janeiro is located, there is greater diversity (64%, the population is Catholic, 13% neo-Pentecostal evangelicals, 8% evangelicals, and 3% spiritualists).

Despite this, these percentages are not reflected in religious practices in the surveyed PLWHA, where 58% in Rio de Janeiro and only 10% in João Pessoa stated that they had religious organizational practices.

Practical Implications

The relationship between spirituality and mental and physical health has been explored in scientific literature, emphasizing the role of religion and spirituality in the practice of health care, as a way for human beings to find meaning in the disease they are suffering from to stay alive (Lucchetti et al. 2011; Manning et al. 2019; Demir 2019; Rudaz et al. 2019).

The encouragement of religious practices and spirituality, previously denied by the biomedical model, is increasingly present in the approach to patients with chronic diseases.

It is necessary to consider the cultural differences that concern the beliefs and practices of PLWHA and the vital importance of this to their spiritual needs. The health professional must also have in view to meet this demand to contribute to better acceptance of the disease, adherence to treatment, reduction of depressive conditions, and subsequent improvement in the quality of life of these patients (Kremer and Ironson 2009; Ironson et al. 2016).

Conclusion

These comparisons testify that SpNQ is a practical tool to evaluate the spiritual needs of culturally different backgrounds. Its items may be arranged differentially, depending on the illness but also the sample size, country, and cultural characteristics. Besides, between these Brazilian samples, an application of the Item Response Theory was conducted afterward, to verify if the questionnaire items showed satisfactory discrimination and variability of difficulty. SpNQ passed this test, showing appropriate psychometric qualities to discriminate between respondents as to the probability of marking one answer and not another, in the same item, showing whether or not the questionnaire was biased toward a pattern of response desired by the researcher, confirming once more the good psychometric quality of SpNQ for screening of SpN in the PLWHA.

References

Allport GW, Ross JM (1967) Personal religious orientation and prejudice. J Pers Soc Psychol 5(4):432–443

Arrey AE, Bilsen J, Lacor P, Deschepper R (2016) Spirituality / religiosity: a cultural and psychological resource among migrant women from sub-Saharan Africa with HIV / AIDS in Belgium. PLoS One 11(7)

Bluthenthal RN, Palar K, Mendel P, Kanouse DE, Corbin DE, Derose KP (2012) Attitudes and beliefs related to HIV/AIDS in urban religious congregations: barriers and opportunities for HIV-related interventions. Soc Sci Med 74(10):1520–1527

Boff L (2009) Jung e o mundo espiritual. Caxias do Sul, Correio Rio-Grandense

Büssing A, Koenig HG (2010) Spiritual needs of patients with chronic diseases. Religions 1:18–27. https://doi.org/10.3390/rel1010018

Büssing A, Balzat HJ, Heusser P (2010) Spiritual needs of patients with chronic pain diseases and cancer – validation of the spiritual needs questionnaire. Eur J Med Res 15:266–273

Büssing A, Janko A, Baumann K, Hvidt NC, Kopf A (2013a) Spiritual needs among patients with chronic pain diseases and cancer living in a secular society. Pain Med 14:1362–1373. https://doi.org/10.1111/pme.12198

Büssing A, Zhai X, Peng W, Ling C (2013b) Psychosocial and spiritual needs of patients with chronic diseases: validation of the Chinese version of the spiritual needs questionnaire. Journal of Integrative Medicine 11:106–115. https://doi.org/10.3736/jintegrmed2013020

Büssing A, Pilchowska I, Surzykiewicz J (2015) Spiritual needs of polish patients with chronic diseases. J Relig Health 54:1524–1540

Büssing A, Recchia DR, Koenig H, Baumann K, Frick E (2018) Factor structure of the spiritual needs questionnaire (SpNQ) in persons with chronic diseases, elderly and healthy individuals. Religions 9:13. https://doi.org/10.3390/rel9010013

Büssing A, Tânia Cristina de OV, Ana Paula RC, Anderson LCT Jr., Daniela RR (2016)

Caixeta CR, Nascimento LC, Pedro IC d S, Rocha SMM (2012) Spiritual support for people living with HIV/aids: a Brazilian explorative, descriptive study. Nurs Health Sci 14(4):514–519. https://doi.org/10.1111/j.1442-2018.2012.00705.x

da Silva CAO, Cavalcanti APR, Lima KS, Cavalcanti CAM, de Valente TCO, Büssing A (2020) Spiritual needs questionnaire (SpNQ): validity evidence among HIV+ patients in Northeast Brazil. Religions 11(5):234. https://doi.org/10.3390/rel11050234

Chambers LA, Rueda S, Baker DN, Wilson MG, Deutsch R, Raeifar E, Rourke SB, The Stigma Review Team (2015) Stigma, HIV and health: a qualitative synthesis. BMC Public Health 3(15):848. https://doi.org/10.1186/s12889-015-2197-0

Delumeau J (1989) História do medo no ocidente: 1300–1800, uma cidade sitiada.Companhia das Letras, São Paulo

Demir E (2019) The evolution of spirituality, religion and health publications: yesterday, today and tomorrow. (2019). Journal of Religion & Health 58:1–13. https://doi.org/10.1007/s10943-018-00739-w

Doolittle BR, Justice AC, Fiellin DA (2018) Religion, spirituality, and HIV clinical outcomes: a systematic review of the literature. AIDS Behav 22:1792–1801. https://doi.org/10.1007/s10461-016-1651-z

Engel GL (1977) The need for a new medical model: a challenge for biomedicine. Science 196(4286):129–136. https://doi.org/10.1126/science.847460

Espirito Santo CC, Gomes AMT, de Oliveira DC, Marques SCI (2003) Adesão ao Tratamento Antirretroviral e à Espiritualidade de pessoas com HIV/aids: Estudo de Representações Sociais. Rev Enfem UERJ 21(4)458–463. Available at: https://www.e-publicacoes.uerj.br/index.php/enfermagemuerj/article/view/10005

Ironson G, Kremer H, Lucette A (2016) Relationship between spiritual coping and survival in patients with HIV. J Gen Intern Med 31(9):1068–1076. https://doi.org/10.1007/s11606-016-3668-4

Koenig HG (2004) Religion, spirituality, and medicine: research findings and implications for clinical practice. South Med J 97:1194–2000. https://doi.org/10.1097/01.SMJ.0000146489.21837.CE

Kremer H, Ironson G (2009) Everything changed: spiritual transformation in people with HIV. The International Journal of Psychiatry in Medicine 39(3):243–262. https://doi.org/10.2190/PM.39.3.c

Lucchetti G, Lucchetti ALG, Koenig H (2011) Impact of spirituality/religiosity on mortality: comparison with other health interventions. Journal of Science and Healing 7(4):234–238. https://doi.org/10.1016/j.explore.2011.04.005

Manning L, Ferris M, Rosario CN, Prues M, Bouchard L (2019) Spiritual resilience: understanding the protection and promotion of well-being in the later life. J Relig Spiritual Aging 31:168–186. https://doi.org/10.1080/15528030.2018.1532859

Offenbaecher MN, Kohls LL, Toussaint C, Sigl C, Winkelmann A, Hieblinger R, Walthe A, Büssing A (2013) Spiritual Needs in Patients Suffering from Fibromyalgia Evidence-Based Complementary and Alternative Medicine Article ID:178547. https://doi.org/10.1155/2013/178547

Pereira CR, Monteiro SS (2015) A criminalização da transmissão do HIV no Brasil: avanços, retrocessos e lacunas. Physis Revista de Saúde Coletiva 25(4):1185–1205. https://doi.org/10.1590/S0103-73312015000400008

Pinho CM, Dâmaso BFR, Gomes ET, Trajano M de FC, Andrade MS, Valença MP (2017) Religious and spiritual coping in people living with HIV/aids. Rev Bras Enferm 70:392–399. https://doi.org/10.1590/0034-7167-2015-0170

Poorolajal J, Hooshmand E, Mahjub H, Jenabi E (2016) Survival rate of AIDS disease and mortality in HIV-infected patients: a meta-analysis. Public Health 139:3–12. https://doi.org/10.1016/j.puhe.2016.05.004

Reyes-Estrada M, Varas-Díaz N, Parker R (2018) Religion and HIV-related stigma among nurses who work with people living with HIV/AIDS in Puerto Rico. Journal of the International Asociation of providers of AIDS Care – JIAPAC. https://doi.org/10.1177/2325958218773365

Rudaz M, Ledermann T, Grzywacz JG (2019) The influence of daily spiritual experiences and gender on subjective well-being over time in cancer survivors. Arch Psychol Relig. https://doi.org/10.1177/0084672419839800

Silva CAO da (2019) AIDS e religiosidade: influências intersubjetivas aos acometidos pela epidemia. Thesis (Master in Religious Studies) – Universidade Federal da Paraíba, João Pessoa. Available from: https://repositorio.ufpb.br/jspui/handle/tede/4212?locale=pt_BR

Silva CAO da, Cavalcanti APR, Lima KS, Cavalcanti CAM, Valente TC de O, Büssing A (2020) Spiritual Needs Questionnaire (SpNQ): Validity Evidence among HIV+ Patients in Northeast Brazil. Religions 11(5):234. https://doi.org/10.3390/rel11050234

Sulmasy DP (2002) A biopsychosocial-spiritual model for care of patients at the end of life. Gerontologist 42:24–33. https://doi.org/10.1177/1359105307074251

de Valente TCO, Silva LM, Cavalcanti APR (2020) Spiritual needs of people living with HIV/AIDS: a systematic review of literature. AIDS CARE (submitted)

de Valente TCO, Cavalcanti APR, Büssing A, da Costa Júnior CP, Motta RN (2018) Transcultural adaptation and psychometric properties of Portuguese version of the spiritual needs questionnaire (SpNQ) among HIV positive patients in Brazil. Religions 9(4):135. https://doi.org/10.3390/rel9040135

World Health Organization. WHOQOL HIV Group (2003) Initial steps to developing the World Health Organization's quality of life instrument (WHOQOL) module for international assessment in HIV/AIDS. AIDS Care 15:347–357. https://doi.org/10.1080/0954012031000105405

CHAPTER 16

Spiritual Needs in People with Mild to Moderate Dementia

Wilson Correia de Abreu, Margarida Abreu, and Arndt Büssing

Background

Dementia is a clinical condition that has become a concern for many countries, particularly for those who are facing progressive aging of the population. The number of people currently living with dementia is estimated as 47.7 million and is expected to reach 75.63 million by 2030 and 135.46 million by 2050 (WHO 2015).

The Diagnostic and Statistical Manual of Mental Disorders V (American Psychiatric Association 2013) characterizes dementia as a major

W. C. de Abreu (✉) • M. Abreu
Porto School of Nursing, Porto, Portugal CINTESIS (Center for Health Technology and Services Research), University of Porto, Porto, Portugal
e-mail: wjabreu@esenf.pt; mabreu@esenf.pt

A. Büssing
Professorship Quality of Life, Spirituality and Coping, Faculty of Health, Witten/Herdecke University, Herdecke, Germany

IUNCTUS—Competence Center for Christian Spirituality, Philosophical-Theological University of Münster, Münster, Germany
e-mail: Arndt.buessing@uni-wh.de

A. Büssing (ed.), *Spiritual Needs in Research and Practice*,
https://doi.org/10.1007/978-3-030-70139-0_16

neurocognitive disorder. The syndrome is characterized by a significant cognitive decline, while multiple other functions can be disturbed, including thinking, executive function, orientation, comprehension, learning capacity, language, complex attention, perception, social cognition and judgment. Dementia is a clinical syndrome characterized by progressive acquired global impairments of cognitive skills and ability to function independently (Sheeman 2012).

The clinic shows that dementia is common in acute medical inpatients over the age of 70 years and is associated with severe acute physical illness, comorbidity situations and longer hospital stays. The progressive loss of cognitive and functional abilities has repercussions on self-care and activities of daily living, which puts enormous pressure on family caregivers (Muders et al. 2015; Abreu et al. 2019).

The incidence and prevalence of dementia are strongly age- and culture-dependent (Sheeman 2012). There are cultural patterns that shape social representations and strategies of care. By age 60, the major burdens of disability and death arise from age-related losses in hearing, seeing and moving, and noncommunicable diseases, including heart disease, stroke, chronic respiratory disorders, cancer and dementia (WHO 2015). Comorbidities are common in people with dementia (Crowther 2015).

The growth rate of dementia prevalence calls for new interventions, involving social and political decision-makers (Burla et al. 2014). Studies show incremented expenditures by health and social institutions, and a growing need for support from family caregivers. There is, however, a consensus on the need to provide more humane and better quality care to people with dementia and avoid unnecessary hospitalizations (Abreu et al. 2019).

The care provided to people with dementia is often fragmented and many may die as a result of unrecognized and untreated symptoms and needs, experiencing considerable suffering (Jones et al. 2016). Care based on health-care needs is crucial to provide adequate care (Abreu et al. 2019). The assessment must be comprehensive and include not only physical, but also social and psychological functioning, including emotions and spirituality domains (Miranda-Castillo et al. 2010; Schölzel-Dorenbos et al. 2010). The evaluation of these needs facilitates the provision of non-medicated interventions, of a sensory nature, that promote comfort and preserve the person's dignity. Some dimensions are frequently underestimated, for example past life experiences, cultural background, preferences, spirituality and identities (Holmerová et al. 2016). Evidence which was available clearly pointed to a need for a positive approach to practice that embraces physical, psychological, social, spiritual and existential needs (Tolson et al. 2017).

The spiritual needs, which are the core of this study, are clearly overlooked in relation to others. Health professionals do not develop skills in their professional training to deal with spirituality and provide spiritually competent care. Often, the health systems themselves are not prepared to make and save an assessment of peoples' needs in terms of spirituality, which marginalizes those needs in a consistent anamnesis. Conducting a comprehensive health-care needs assessment can prevent fragmented care and considerable suffering in people living with dementia.

Sullivan (1993) defined spirituality as an individual and unique characteristic that links the "I" to the universe and to others, whether or not it may include a belief in a God. Puchalski et al. (2014) described spirituality as a way to find meaning and purpose in life, connecting the interior with the sacred. Koenig et al. (2012) stated that spirituality is distinct from humanism, values, morals and mental health, due to its connection with what is sacred, transcendent, inferring that religion involves beliefs, practices and rituals related to the transcendent, where there may be a God or a divine entity. Spirituality is defined as a dynamic and intrinsic aspect of humanity through which persons seek ultimate meaning, purpose and transcendence, and experience relationship to self, family, others, community, society, nature and the significant or sacred, expressed through beliefs, values, traditions and practices (Puchalski et al. 2014).

People can seek spirituality as a way of dealing with illnesses, minimizing suffering, dealing with deficits or even maintaining hope for a cure. Spirituality, as studies in the area of palliative care show, can be relevant to promote comfort in terminal situations (Meredith et al. 2012). These spiritual needs or wishes can be interpreted as the intention to (re)connect with the environment/nature, with others and with one's own life; the intention to "pass own life experiences to others," to "give away something" and to "solace someone" can also be seen in this light (Erichsen and Büssing 2013). Spirituality helps to give meaning to patients' personal life, history and reality (Balboni et al. 2013), and can be an important strategy for dealing with difficult situations and even reducing suffering and pain (Penderell and Brazil 2010).

A broad definition assumes spirituality as all attempts to find meaning, purpose and hope in relation to the sacred or significant (which may have a secular, religious, philosophical, humanist or personal dimension), and the related spiritual practices have commitment to values, beliefs, practices or philosophies which may have an effect on patients' cognition, emotion and behavior (Büssing et al. 2014). Büssing (2015) added that although spirituality is often used as a divergent dimension of religiosity, spirituality can be found through religious engagement, but also independent from specific religion through an individual experience of the Divine, and/or through a connection to other people, the environment and the sacred (Büssing 2015).

The Spiritual Needs Questionnaire (SpNQ) has been widely used in diverse cultural contexts and in very different health situations. In this chapter, we aim to summarize the results of a study that assessed spiritual needs in a sample of people with dementia in Portugal, using for data collection the Portuguese version of SpNQ (Portugal) that was used on people with mild and moderate dementia.

Methodological Background of the Study

These results, obtained using the SpNQ, are part of an umbrella project related to people from mild to advanced dementia. The project was positively evaluated by the ESEP Committee of Ethics and the use of the instruments was also authorized by the institutions where the data were collected. All the participants of the study were already evaluated clinically and were diagnosed with mild to advanced dementia.

The study was conducted within different sites in Portugal (Continent and Islands). Participants, who filled the questionnaire themselves, were recruited from two tertiary hospitals and the community using a convenience sampling. On both sites, data were collected by researchers with experience in dealing with patients with chronic diseases. The researchers described the study to participants and clarified sentences that were unclear. Participants with high levels of anxiety or depression, or users with severe cognitive impairment that did not allow understanding of the questions were not interviewed (exclusion criteria). Although the umbrella project included people with mild to advanced dementia, in this evaluation we will only use data referring to people with mild to moderate dementia.

The sample comprised 176 people formally diagnosed with mild or moderate dementia. Among them, 50% were men and 50% women, their mean age was 77.4 ± 10.5 (59–97) years. The majority of the sample was married (39%) and most had completed primary school (69%).

Participants were mainly retired (by age) (63%), professed a religion (73%), were Christian Catholic (89%) or had other religious affiliations (2%) or no religious affiliation (9%), and were diagnosed with either mild dementia (51%) or moderate dementia (49%).

Main Results of the Study

For this study the Portuguese version of the SPNQ with 27 items was used to assess patients' spiritual needs. This version shows good psychometric properties (Cronbach's alpha = 0.91). It differentiates among five factors: *Religious* needs (Cronbach's alpha = 0.71), *Existential* needs (Cronbach's alpha = 0.66), *Inner Peace* needs (Cronbach's alpha = 0.75), *Giving/Generativity* needs (Cronbach's alpha = 0.66) and *Forgiveness* needs (Cronbach's alpha = 0.75). Internal consistency was assessed using Cronbach's alpha for the entire instrument (Cronbach's alpha = 0.83). Usually, reliability coefficients higher than 0.7 are deemed adequate. However, in two subscales the values were slightly lower (*Existential* and *Giving/Generativity*).

The mean scores of these factors were high: *Religious* needs 1.19 ± 0.73, *Existential* needs 1.07 ± 0.75, *Inner Peace* needs 1.41 ± 0.70, *Giving/Generativity* needs 1.39 ± 0.67 and *Forgiveness* needs 1.33 ± 0.99. The mean values of the subscales varied between 1.07 and 1.41. The mean of the values for the 27-item instrument (SpNQ-27) were 1.36 ± 0.57.

As the questionnaire could be used as a 20-item research instrument (SpNQ-20) which was tested on persons with chronic diseases, we calculated also the averages of the subscales and the Cronbach's alpha to study the internal consistency of the subscale values. The results obtained were as follows: *Religious* needs (Cronbach's alpha = 0.71; 1.19 ± 0.62), *Existential* needs (Cronbach's alpha = 0.79; 0.95 ± 0.77), *Inner Peace* needs (Cronbach's alpha = 0.70; 1.43 ± 0.74) and *Giving/Generativity* needs (Cronbach's alpha = 0.74; 1.39 ± 0.80). The mean of the values for the entire instrument (SpnQ-20) was 1.25 ± 0.56. Internal consistency was also assessed using Cronbach's alpha for the 20-item instrument (0.87), and was better compared to the 27-item version; here, none of the factors had an alpha < 0.70.

An Analysis of variance (ANOVA) test was applied to compare the scores of each dimension (SpNQ-27) according to the two groups (two levels of dementia—mild or moderate). The results obtained were as follows: *Religious* needs ($Z = 9.57$; $p = 0.002$), *Existential* needs ($Z = 68.40$;

$p < 0.001$), *Inner Peace* needs ($Z = 73.68$; $p < 0.001$), *Giving/Generativity* needs ($Z = 61.31$; $p < 0.001$) and *Forgiveness* needs ($Z = 39.49$; $p < 0.001$). A main effect of the level of dementia in the way people feel (verbalize) their needs in each scale was found (the highest values of the subscales were found in the group of people with mild dementia—the difference was significant, as shown in Fig. 16.1). The results achieved in all statistical tests show that in all subscales differences are significant at the 95% confidence level ($p < 0.01$).

The linear correlations among the SpNQ subscales were also calculated, using the Pearson correlation coefficient *r*. The purpose was to evaluate whether there would be a linear relationship between those values of the subscales. Basically, we wanted to know if variations in one subscale would make similar variations occur in others. There were several strong correlations between the values of the subscales, particularly between *Inner Peace* needs and *Existential* needs (Table 16.1).

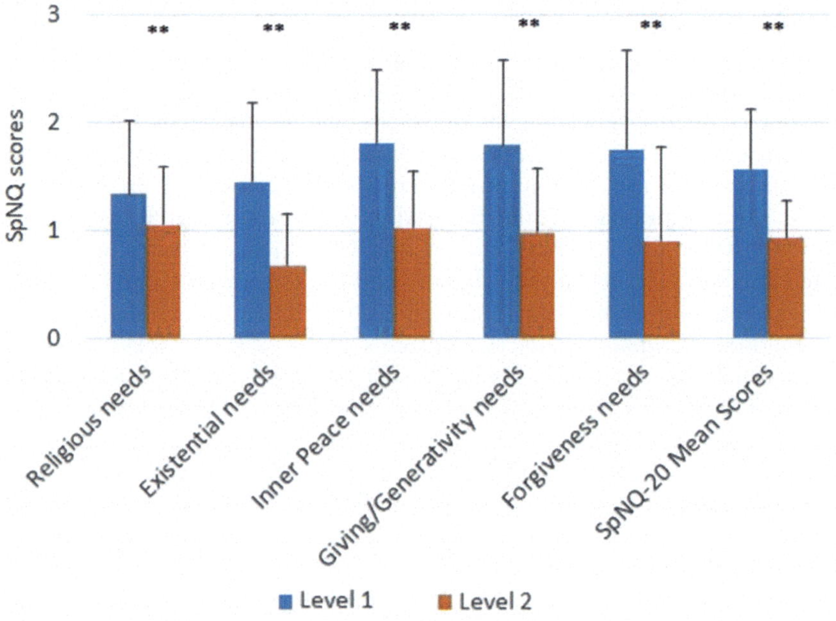

Fig. 16.1 Spiritual needs in people with mild (level 1) or moderate (level 2) dementia. (** $p < 0.001$; $p = 0.002$ (ANOVA))

Table 16.1 Correlations (r) between the subscales of the Portuguese version of the SpNQ

	Religious needs	*Existential needs*	*Inner peace needs*	*Giving/ generativity needs*	*Forgiveness needs*
Religious needs	1				
Existential needs	0.290**	1			
Inner peace needs	0.349**	**0.713****	1		
Giving/ Generativity needs	0.214**	**0.687****	**0.648****	1	
Forgiveness needs	0.296**	**0.658****	**0.601****	**0.538****	1

**$p < 0.0001$ (Pearson); strong correlations were highlighted (bold)

What We Emphasize in the Study

In this study, with a sample comprising 176 people formally diagnosed with mild or moderate dementia, we found that the sociodemographic characteristics are in line with others found in similar studies. It should be noted that this is a population in the North of Portugal, where people (together with those living in Galicia, Spain) are deeply Catholic, a reality that conditions habits, beliefs, lifestyles and even behaviors in disease situations.

In the last years, societies have paid more attention to people with dementia and their caregivers. Traditional care models, based only on the management of the therapeutic regimen and management of symptoms and signs, have given rise to holistic care perspectives, with a view of respecting the dignity of people and alternative interventions to medications. More attention is given to comfort, quality of life and the well-being of the person, using sensory interventions. Interventions related to spirituality have still been poorly systematized and introduced in care models, but they cannot be forgotten in holistic models (Weathers et al. 2017). The provision of holistic care is recognized and promotes best practices in caring for people with chronic diseases (Egan et al. 2013); it involves assessing and caring bearing in mind physical, emotional and spiritual needs (Koenig 2012).

To identify patients' spiritual needs, we used the SpNQ (Büssing et al. 2010, 2018), which has been shown to be adequate for understanding spiritual needs in people with chronic illness and with different religions. When analyzing the results of the averages of the subscale values, it appears that these are slightly lower than those found in old people living in residential/nursing homes (Erichsen and Büssing 2013).

Let us note some questions that are part of the subscales *Religious*, *Existential*, *Inner Peace*, *Giving/Generativity* and *Forgiveness* needs. Given the memory decline and sometimes psychological distress present in dementia situations, it is understood that people not only express less interest, but also consider less relevance of the item in the context of their health situation. Very often, people forget the names of family members, lose functional skills, forget to eat their meals and fail to give importance to their habits. Although unconsciously, most of the time, the absence of this contact with the world and with people causes disturbance and even some depersonalization. Participants find it difficult to value issues such as "To pray for yourself" (*Religious* needs), "To reflect back on your life" (*Existential* needs), "To dwell in a place of quietness and peace" (*Inner Peace* needs), "To pass own life experiences to others" (*Giving/Generativity* needs) and "To forgive someone from a distinct period of your life" (*Forgiveness* needs). These, among other issues, arouse concern, suffering and sometimes conflicting feelings in people with dementia. They forget where they were happy. In the Church, they feel shame for not being able to follow the prayers. If they sometimes assume these difficulties, at other times they manifest flight and denial behaviors, which alleviate their suffering. So objectively, in situations of advanced dementia, the mediation of family members can be decisive.

After calculating the correlations between the subscales, we can state that there are strong intercorrelations. We can conclude, in this population, that the different variations in the spiritual needs in each subscale accompany the variations in the others, which allows us to accept that it is a consistent instrument to assess the spiritual needs of people with dementia, moreover reinforced with a Cronbach's alpha value of 0.83 for the global instrument.

What Should Be Done to Support These Patients' Needs

Chronic illness is defined as a long-term illness with no expectations of a cure. These diseases have unpredictable episodes and uncertainty regarding progress, with signs and symptoms that can be manifested slowly over time, or intermittently or with progressive disabilities that can lead to death. Dementia, as a chronic syndrome, has specific characteristics, for example in matters of needs of palliative care (Tolson et al. 2017).

A person with a chronic illness feels his or her quality of life affected and experiences distress symptomatology and identity disturbances. Often, people with chronic illness manifest feelings of guilt, loss, sadness, anxiety, decreased self-esteem, loss of function and problems with communication with family and friends (Büssing and Koenig 2010). In people with dementia, these aspects can be amplified because the person feels that memory is affected, is afraid of the response of family members and can spend years in palliative situations ("extended palliative phase").

People with mild dementia show higher values in different subscales, but this does not mean that as the cognitive decline progresses, people have fewer spiritual needs—they just cannot verbalize them adequately. This result is important for more humane and dignified assistance.

After 20 years in contact with people with dementia, we had the opportunity to deepen interventions of a cognitive nature (cognitive stimulation), with the purpose of delaying cognitive decline and promoting quality of life. We concluded, throughout this time, that interventions of a spiritual nature have a strong potential for cognitive stimulation. In the last decades, literature has demonstrated the important role of religiosity and spirituality in the physical and mental health of patients (Koenig et al. 2012). It is shown that there are positive correlations between spiritual well-being and the quality of life of some patients with chronic diseases (Lucchetti et al. 2013). However, there are no studies that demonstrate that interventions of a spiritual nature can provide episodes of memory recovery (even if very short), during which the person can recover contact with the environment, remember the name of family members and recognize loved ones in photographs. However, there are reports that persons with dementia singing religious songs they were used to sing in their youth can remember all lyrics while singing - but cannot remember when they are asked for. Furthermore, spiritual interventions can provide health professionals with moments to learn about users' preferences, a process that is relevant for humanistic assistance that respects the dignity of the person.

Implications for Practice

In the national health systems, terms and expressions related to spiritual dimensions (needs, distress, well-being, suffering) are not yet properly consolidated and included in the data classification systems.

Schultz et al. (2017) concluded that spiritual distress is not enough to identify spiritual suffering. For Davison and Jhangri (2010), patients with chronic diseases with unmet spiritual needs had more difficulty in psychological adaptation to the disease. Büssing et al. (2010) infer that for many patients confronted with chronic diseases, spirituality/religiosity is a relevant resource to cope; both chronic illness and life-threatening diseases confront patients with the question of meaning and purpose in life. Moreover, dimensions related to spirituality can interfere with quality of life, well-being, acceptance of resources for disease management, obtaining inner peace to mobilize forces to face suffering, and help from a supernatural being to live with the disease or wait for death. How to formulate specific diagnoses related to spiritual dimensions in the documentation systems that are everywhere?

Professionals reveal the need to accept the relationship between health outcomes and religiosity, but they do not understand or recognize the multidimensional nature of this relationship (Wilt et al. 2019). Patients suffering from chronic or life-threatening diseases often report unmet needs, which are mostly not addressed or recognized by health professionals (Büssing and Koenig 2010; Balboni et al. 2010; Daly et al. 2016). The curricula of health professionals must include more information on this whole theme.

Increasingly, health services work with "paper-free" registration systems, which means that data relating to assessment, data design and intervention either exist in taxonomies or are simply overlooked. Work on spiritual needs, spiritual well-being, spiritual suffering, spiritual comfort or spiritual distress implies work of ontologies, systematization, education and transfer to documentation systems.

Conclusion

In Ancient Egypt, physicians invested in clinical observation, diagnosis and treatment, producing knowledge that was later deepened by Greek medicine. Medical practice accepted that patients' spirituality and a strong belief in healing may play a large part in the effectiveness of the treatment (Aboelsoud 2010). Spirituality as part of the therapeutic regimen was considered relevant to the management of signs and symptoms and to the adherence to treatment, key points for obtaining better medical outcomes. In today's societies, the secularization of states, whose logic is accepted, has led to less attention to spirituality and religiosity. Even models of holistic intervention or cultural competence fail to explain and systematize spirituality in the context of health care.

The Spiritual Needs Questionnaire (SpNQ) was designed to explore peoples' spiritual needs and can be used in both secular and religious societies by avoiding exclusive religious terminology. After its application to people with mild or moderate dementia, we conclude that it can be used in this population for clinical and research purposes. More problematic would be its application in patients with advanced dementia. Our suggestion is to build a linguistically adapted and shortened specific version for patients with advanced or severe dementia. In the case of people with advanced dementia, with severe cognitive impairment, it could be filled out by family caregivers, bearing in mind the history of the person with dementia. Competent assessment of spiritual needs in people with dementia allows more humane assistance and respect for the dignity of people in such a precarious clinical situation.

References

Aboelsoud N (2010) Herbal medicine in ancient Egypt. J Med Plant Res 4:082–086. https://doi.org/10.5897/JMPR09.013

Abreu W, Tolson D, Jackson GA, Staines H, Costa N (2019) The relationship between frailty, functional dependence, and healthcare needs among community-dwelling people with moderate to severe dementia. Health Soc Care Community 11:3–18. https://doi.org/10.1111/hsc.12678

American Psychiatric Association (2013) Diagnostic and statistical manual of mental disorders, 5th edn. American Psychiatric Association, Arlington

Balboni TA, Paulk ME, Balboni MJ, Phelps AC, Loggers ET, Wright AA, Block SD, Lewis EF, Peteet JR, Prigerson HG (2010) Provision of spiritual care to patients with advanced cancer: associations with medical care and quality of life near death. J Clin Oncol 28:445–452

Balboni MJ, Sullivan A, Amobi A, Phelps AC, Gorman DP, Zollfrank A, Balboni TA (2013) Why is spiritual care infrequent at the end of life? Spiritual care perceptions among patients, nurses, and physicians and the role of training. J Clin Oncol 31(4):461–467. https://doi.org/10.1200/JCO.2012.44.6443

Burla C, Rego G, Nunes R (2014) Alzheimer, dementia and the living will: a proposal. MED HEALTH CARE PHIL 17:389–395. https://doi.org/10.1007/s11019-014-9559-8

Büssing A (2015) Spirituality/religiosity as a resource for coping in soldiers: a summary report. Medical Acupuncture 27:360–366

Büssing A, Koenig HG (2010) Spiritual needs of patients with chronic diseases. Religions 1(1):18–27

Büssing A, Recchia DR, Koenig H, Baumann K, Frick E (2018) Factor structure of the Spiritual Needs Questionnaire (SpNQ) in persons with chronic diseases, elderly and healthy individuals. Religions 9(1):13. https://doi.org/10.3390/rel9010013

Büssing A, Balzat HJ, Heusser P (2010) Spiritual needs of patients with chronic pain diseases and cancer—validation of the Spiritual Needs Questionnaire. Eur J Med Res 15:266–273

Büssing A, Baumann K, Hvidt NC, Koenig HG, Puchalski CM, Swinton J (2014) Spirituality and health. Evid Based Complement Alternat Med:682817. https://doi.org/10.1155/2014/682817

Crowther G (2015) Palliative care in dementia. Radcliffe Publishing, London

Daly L, Fahey-McCarthy E, Timmins F (2016) The experience of spirituality from the perspective of people living with dementia: a systematic review and meta-synthesis. Dementia 18(2):448–470. https://doi.org/10.1177/1471301216680425

Davison S, Jhangri G (2010) Existential and supportive care needs among patients with chronic kidney disease. J Pain Symptom Manag 40(6):838–843. https://doi.org/10.1016/j.jpainsymman.2010.03.015

Egan R, McKechnie R, Jobson J, Herbison P, Richards R (2013) Perspectives on psychosocial and spiritual cancer support services in New Zealand. J Psychosoc Oncol 31:659–674

Erichsen N, Büssing A (2013) Spiritual needs of elderly living in residential/nursing homes. Evid Based Complement Alternat Med. https://doi.org/10.1155/2013/913247

Holmerová I, Waugh A, MacRae R, Veprková R, Sandvide A, Hanson E, Jackson G, Watchmen K, Tolson D (2016). Best practice statement. Project: dementia Palliare: interprofessional experiential learning solutions: equipping the quali!ed dementia workforce to champion evidence informed improvement to advanced dementia care and family caring project. EU, Erasmus Plus, Palliare Project

Jones L, Candy B, Davis S, Elliott M, Gola A, Harrington J, Kupeli N, Lord K, Moore K, Scott S, Vickerstaff V, Omar RZ, King M, Leavey G, Nazareth I, Sampson EL (2016) Development of a model for integrated care at the end of life in advanced dementia: a whole systems UK-wide approach. Palliat Med 30:279–295

Koenig H (2012) Religion, spirituality, and health: the research and clinical implications. International Scholarly Research Network. https://doi.org/10.5402/2012/278730

Koenig H, King D, Carson V (2012) Handbook of religion and health, 2nd edn. Oxford University Press, New York

Lucchetti G, Oliveira L, Koenig HG, Leite JR, Lucchetti A (2013) Medical students, spirituality and religiosity-results from the multicenter study SBRAME. BMC Med Educ 13:162. https://bmcmededuc.biomedcentral.com/articles/10.1186/1472-6920-13-162

Meredith P, Murray J, Wilson T, Mitchell G, Hutch R (2012) Can spirituality be taught to health care professionals? J Relig Health 51:879–889. https://doi.org/10.1007/s10943-010-9399-7

Miranda-Castillo C, Woods B, Galboda K, Oomman S, Olojugba C, Orrell M (2010) Unmet needs, quality of life and support networks of people with dementia living at home. Health Qual Life Outcomes 8:132. https://doi.org/10.1186/1477-7525-8-132

Muders P, Zahrt-Omar C, Bussmann S, Haberstroh J, Weber M (2015) Support for families of patients dying with dementia: a qualitative analysis of bereaved family members' experiences and suggestions. Palliat Support Care 13:435–442. https://doi.org/10.1017/S1478951513001107

Penderell A, Brazil K (2010) The spirit of palliative practice: a qualitative inquiry into the spiritual journey of palliative care physicians. Palliat Support Care 8(4):415–420. https://doi.org/10.1017/S1478951510000271

Puchalski C, Blatt B, Kogan M, Butler A (2014) Spirituality and health: the development of afield. Acad Med 89(1):10–16

Schölzel-Dorenbos C, Meeuwsen E, Rikkert M (2010) Integrating unmet needs into dementia health-related quality of life research and care: introduction of the hierarchy model of needs in dementia. Aging Ment Health 14:113–119. https://doi.org/10.1080/13607860903046495

Schultz M, Meged-Book T, Mashiach T, Bar-Sela G (2017) Distinguishing between spiritual distress, general distress, spiritual well-being, and spiritual pain among cancer patients during oncology treatment. J Pain Symptom Manag 54(1):66–73. https://doi.org/10.1016/j.jpainsymman.2017.03.018

Sheeman B (2012) Assessment scales in dementia. Ther Adv Neurol Disord 5(6):349–358. https://doi.org/10.1177/1756285612455733

Sullivan, W. P. (1993). "It helps me to be a whole person": The role of spirituality among the mentally challenged. Psychosocial Rehabilitation Journal, 16(3), 125–134. https://doi.org/10.1037/h0095669

Tolson D, Holmerova I, Macrae R, Waugh A, Hvalič-Touzery S, Abreu W, Lillo-Crespo M, Merta A, Hanson E (2017) Improving advanced dementia care: an interprofessional Palliare learning framework. J Am Med Dir Assoc 18:561–563. https://doi.org/10.1016/j.jamda.2017.03.014

Weathers E, Weathers G, McCarthy G, Coffey A (2017) Concept analysis of spirituality: an evolutionary approach. Nurs Forum 51(2):79–96. https://doi.org/10.1111/nuf.12128

Wilt JA, Pargament KI, Exline JJ, Barrera TL, Teng EJ (2019) Spiritual transformation among veterans in response to a religious/spiritual struggle. Psychol Relig Spiritual 11(3):266–277. https://doi.org/10.1037/rel0000208

World Health Organization (2015) The epidemiology and impact of dementia current state and future trends. World Health Organization, Geneva

CHAPTER 17

Spiritual Needs in Psychiatry and Psychotherapy

Klaus Baumann, Eunmi Lee, and Franz Reiser

What about Spiritual Needs in the Context of Psychiatry and Psychotherapy?

Contemporary medicine cherishes a patient-centered approach which integrates biopsychosocial aspects of patients' health and disorders into the therapeutic process. Concerning patients' spiritual (and religious) needs, this seems less controversial in other realms of clinical practice than in psychiatry and psychotherapy, for many historical, epistemological, and practical reasons. In recent years several position papers of relevant psychiatric associations have pled for the respectful attention and explicit integration of patients' spiritualities and religiosities into the treatment process (APA 2006; RCPsych 2009, 2013, 2014; Utsch et al. 2016; WPA 2017; Reiser 2018, 95–105). The need for such recommendations indicates two things implicitly: first, that such attention and integration cannot be taken

K. Baumann (✉) • E. Lee • F. Reiser
Caritas Science and Christian Social Work, Faculty of Theology,
Albert-Ludwigs University, Freiburg, Germany
e-mail: klaus.baumann@theol.uni-freiburg.de; eunmi.lee@theol.uni-freiburg.de;
franz.reiser@theol.uni-freiburg.de

A. Büssing (ed.), *Spiritual Needs in Research and Practice*,
https://doi.org/10.1007/978-3-030-70139-0_17

for granted (Cook et al. 2009; Huguelet and Koenig 2009), and second, that it is not an easy task (Aten and Leach 2009; Pargament 2007) given the basically secular and methodologically atheistic professional training and settings of clinical practice. Actually, there is a deeply rooted double ambivalence in the history of psychiatry and psychotherapies toward patients' religious beliefs and spiritual needs due to their individual dynamic interactions with the clinical syndromes to be dealt with in therapy (Baumann 2012). First, are religious beliefs pathological themselves? Second, to what degree are they resources or rather obstacles in the patients' situation of depression or mood disorder, anxiety disorder, personality disorder, or psychosis? Do they favor treatment and healing or do they resist and worsen the clinical process?

These questions for discernment need to be addressed in order to realize true patient-centered psychiatry and psychotherapy. In order to address them in a professionally appropriate manner, psychiatrists and psychotherapists need to become familiar with their patients' religious/spiritual needs on the one hand, and to know their *own* needs, attitudes, and behaviors in this regard on the other hand.

In the German-speaking context, there is a dearth of empirical studies which tackle these or related questions (Hofmann & Walach 2011), especially in inpatient clinical settings (Unterrainer 2010).

Starting with a pilot study at Freiburg University Hospital and extending it to a Germany-wide survey first of psychiatric staff (and regional survey in South Korea, later on), followed by a survey among patients at Freiburg University Hospital, we tried to empirically contribute to the following questions in the context of inpatient psychiatry and psychotherapy:

- How important are patients' spiritual needs for psychiatric staff, and how spiritual do they consider themselves?
- How important are spiritual needs for inpatients in psychiatry and psychotherapy?
- How do patients feel treated with regard to their spiritual needs by staff, and how does staff say they treat patients with regard to their spiritual needs?

You Need to Ask Both Patients and Staff

Hence, two main studies were conducted in order to shed more light onto these questions: a survey with staff in psychiatry and psychotherapy and a survey among psychiatric inpatients.

The Survey with Staff (Lee 2014)

A nationwide study was conducted in German university hospitals and confessional clinics within the same cities (Lee and Baumann 2013; Lee et al. 2014; Lee 2014; Lee et al. 2015). In total 53 clinics were asked to participate, of which 21 took part in the survey with paper-based questionnaires. Respondents were staff who directly worked with patients, such as psychiatrists, psychotherapists, nurses or social workers.

The main instrument was a revised version of Religion and Spirituality in Medicine: Physicians' Perspectives (RSMPP) by Farr Curlin (Curlin et al. 2007; Kørup et al. 2019). In addition, we used the Duke University Religion Index (DUREL), which measures extrinsic as well as intrinsic religiosity (Koenig and Büssing 2010). Both instruments were used in valid German versions for the first time.

The Survey with Patients (Reiser 2018)

In the department of psychiatry and psychotherapy at the Freiburg University Hospital, an open, prospective, explorative and cross-sectional survey was conducted over the course of 18 months (June 2010–December 2011). All new inpatients (except the acute locked ward) consecutively received a paper-based questionnaire. Participation was completely voluntary, without any incentives.

The study was registered by the WHO Universal Trial Number (UTN) U1111–1115-0735, for which the University Ethic Committee had given approval in January 2010 (Nr. 7/10). For this study the SpNQ in a previous version 1.2 (Büssing et al. 2010) was utilized, which contains 19 items in four scales (Table 17.1): *Religious needs* (six items), *Inner Peace needs* (five items), *Existential needs* (Reflection/Meaning) (five items) and *Actively Giving/Generativity needs* (three items). In addition, patients were asked in the beginning how they wished their spiritual and religious needs should be dealt with during their inpatient stay and by whom

Table 17.1 Spiritual needs of 248 patients from clinical survey at University Hospital, Department of Psychiatry and Psychotherapy, Freiburg, Germany

Factors and items (SpNQ Version 1.2)	*Mean (SD)*
Religious needs (Cronbach's alpha = 0.88)	**0.75 (0.83)**
N20 pray for yourself	0.95 (1.12)
N21 participate in a religious ceremony (i.e. service)	0.58 (0.95)
N23 turn to a higher presence (i.e. god, Allah, angels)	1.07 (1.20)
N18 pray with someone	0.52 (0.93)
N19 that someone prays for you	0.79 (1.15)
N22 read religious/spiritual books	0.62 (0.91)
Existentialistic needs (Cronbach's alpha = 0.66)	**1.32 (0.77)**
N4 reflect on your previous life	1.60 (1.20)
N11 talk with someone about the question of meaning in life	1.17 (1.20)
N5 dissolve open aspects of your life	1.91 (1.15)
N10 find meaning in illness and/or suffering	1.31 (1.27)
N12 talk with someone about the possibility of life after death	0.60 (1.04)
Actively giving/generative needs (Cronbach's alpha = 0.70)	**1.54 (0.91)**
N15 provide solace to someone	1.45 (1.12)
N14 give away something from yourself	1.20 (1.22)
N13 turn to someone in a loving attitude	1.98 (1.09)
Inner peace needs (Cronbach's alpha = 0.62)	**2.04 (0.67)**
N6 plunge into beauty of nature	1.68 (1.13)
N7 dwell at a place of quietness and peace	1.97 (1.17)
N2 talk with others about my fears and worries	2.24 (0.89)
N8 find inner peace	2.43 (0.96)
N1 higher devotion by others	1.90 (1.14)
Additional items	
N24 being complete and safe	2.56 (0.88)
N17 be forgiven	1.34 (1.30)
N16 forgive someone from a distinct period of your life	1.11 (1.22)

[a]Responses to these need-items were given as yes/no, the latter then scored on a scale with 1 (somewhat), 2 (strong) and 3 (very strong). "No" was scored as zero.

preferably. When leaving, they were asked again how these expectations were met and by whom.

And What Was Their Answer?

In the first survey with staff in psychiatry and psychotherapy (Lee 2014), within five months (October 2010–February 2011) 404 of 1654 questionnaires were returned, of which 401 questionnaires were complete enough for statistical analysis (response rate: 24.4%). Most of the respondents were nurses and psychiatrists (respectively 42% and 32%). Two-thirds were women.

In these inpatient settings, German psychiatric professionals not rarely experienced religious/spiritual issues being presented by their patients: More than half of the respondents reported that their patients sometimes bring up religious/spiritual topics to talk about, for example God, meditation, or the Bible; 18% experienced this quite often. Furthermore, psychiatric staff reported both positive and negative influences of their patients' religiosity/spirituality. For instance, they observed that religiosity/spirituality helps psychiatric patients to cope with their mental health problems or gives them hopeful and stable emotional conditions. Psychiatrists stated this most among all the staff groups, while nurses were those who most saw negative influences.

Mental health professionals generally consider it appropriate to cover religious/spiritual issues with patients, especially if this is restricted to verbal exchange rather than doing any religious/spiritual practices together. For example, about 75% of respondents found that questions or discussions about religious/spiritual issues are appropriate for the professional therapeutic process. Not surprisingly, almost all respondents declared that they listen carefully and empathetically when patients want to talk about religious/spiritual issues. About 67% of respondents said they encourage their patients in religious/spiritual beliefs and practices, and they consider such issues as part of their professional responsibilities.

As to their own religious or spiritual stances, the majority of staff denied talking about their own beliefs or experiences with patients (38% rather not, 34% definitely not) or even to practice religious/spiritual exercises together, for example prayer (26% rather not, 55% definitely not).

Why would it be hard or wrong to integrate religious/spiritual issues into therapeutic processes? Almost half of the respondents mentioned *professional neutrality* (46%). Other frequently ticked reasons were *insufficient time*, *lack of knowledge* and *not their responsibility* (respectively 33%, 27% and 24%). In additional free texts, respondents deemed talking about religious or spiritual issues to be too private and intimate for them to be professional and neutral.

Therefore, Then, How Religious or Spiritual Do Psychiatric Staff Consider Themselves?

First of all, more than 75% declared having a religious affiliation. About 60% characterized themselves as a "believing person". In this regard, there was no significant difference between nurses and psychiatrists (respectively 66% and 56%). According to DUREL, the mean intrinsic religiosity of psychiatric staff was somewhat moderate with M = 7.01 (on a scale from 3 to 12). About 55% replied that religious beliefs influence their whole approach to life. About 42% answered that they try to carry their religion into other areas of their lives and also experienced God's presence. There was no significant correlation between the staff's intrinsic religiosity (DUREL) and their experience of how often their patients bring up religious and/or spiritual issues (one-tailed correlation: $r = 0.07$). Their intrinsic religiosity and their appraisal of the influences of patients' religious/spiritual issues on therapeutic outcome, however, showed significant correlations (moderate with questions about positive influences, $r = 0.41$, $p < 0.001$; negligible with questions about negative influences, $r = -0.14$, $p = 0.006$). In other words, the more spiritual psychiatric staff were, the more positively they rated the influence of patients' religion-related issues for the therapeutic process.

With these self-reports of the staff, it will be interesting to check how they are perceived by the patients. How open do psychiatric patients feel their staff are toward their religious/spiritual issues and their readiness to address them, if needed?

Before addressing these questions, we need to ask another question.

How Important Are Spiritual Needs for Inpatients? How Much Do They Desire That Their Needs Are Dealt with in Therapeutic Settings of Psychiatry and Psychotherapy?

The second survey (Reiser 2018) offers the following answers. Within 18 months, 248 patients participated *at admission* (60% women; mean age 39.6 ± 13.4 years), with a response rate of 23.3%; their primary diagnoses were 7% Psychotic Disorders, 11% Alcohol Addiction, 42% Depressive Disorders, 5% Bipolar Disorders, 14% Obsessive-Compulsive Disorders, 11% Borderline-Personality Disorder, 11% others. The distribution of sex, age, education and diagnoses was similar to the general patient population of the clinic. Concerning their religious orientation, they reported 77% Christian (Catholics/Protestants equally), 9% other, 15% none. Their self-rating as religious and/or spiritual was 17% religious and spiritual, 23% religious but not spiritual, 14% spiritual but not religious, 46% neither religious nor spiritual. These distributions of religious orientation and of self-rating are similar to the regional general population (Reiser 2018, 175–184).

The SpNQ 1.2 in this specific sample (4 scales,[1] about 60% explained variance) shows a good reliability for the first scale, and acceptable moderate reliability for the rest: *Religious needs* (Cronbach's alpha = 0.88), *Inner Peace needs* (Cronbach's alpha = 0.62), *Existentialistic needs* (Reflection/Meaning) (Cronbach's alpha = 0.66), *Actively Giving/Generativity needs* (Cronbach's alpha = 0.70). In detail, the mean values of the scales and items can be found in Table 17.1.

Inner Peace needs got the highest scores (2.04 ± 0.67), followed by *Actively Giving/Generativity needs* (1.54 ± 0.91), *Existentialistic needs* (1.32 ± 0.77) and *Religious Needs* (0.75 ± 0.83). The acutely stressed patients at the beginning of their stay in psychiatry seemed to need relief and human support most of all (N8: find inner peace 2.43 ± 0.96; N2: talk with others about my fears and worries 2.24 ± 0.89). Caring for others

[1] Analyzing the factor structure of the SpNQ 1.2 in our sample (principle components analysis; Varimax rotation with Kaiser normalization), we got *five* factors: The factor *Inner Peace needs* turned out to be divided into a more interpersonal factor (N1 and N2 with loadings of 0.85 and 0.76 respectively in the rotated component matrix) and a more general factor (N6, N7 and N8 with loadings of 0.78, 0.72 and 0.58 in the rotated component matrix). In order to maintain comparability with other studies, we kept these two aspects within one scale.

and being a "giving" person seems nonetheless important (e.g. N13: turn to someone in a loving attitude 1.98 ± 1.09). The need for meaning and reflection is frequent (e.g. N5 dissolve open aspects of your life 1.91 ± 1.15). Although *Religious needs* seem to be less frequent, selected items show high relevance: the need to turn to a higher presence (N23) is "strong" for 19% and "very strong" for 19% of patients; the need to pray for yourself (N20) is "strong" for 20% and "very strong" for 13%.

The scales of SpNQ 1.2 did not show any significant differences for sex, family status, education or diagnosis (ANOVA). Only in *Religious Needs* we found a difference between age groups (ANOVA, $F_{4.243} = 3.6$; $p = 0.008$): The oldest group over 60 years (1.3±0.9) scoring significantly higher (Tukey-HSD) than the two youngest groups 18–39 years (0.6±0.8). The self-rating group "neither spiritual nor religious" reported the lowest mean scores in all four of the spiritual needs scales (not only for *Religious needs*).

The additional *forgiveness* items are not part of the four scales in SpNQ Version 1.2, but they give important clinical hints to spiritual realities and worries of patients: The need "to forgive someone from a distinct period of your life" (N16) was "strong" for 20% and "very strong" for 20% of patients; the need "to be forgiven" (N17) was strong for 17% and even very strong for 30% (both items without significant differences in ANOVA regarding diagnoses, $N = 248$).

Inpatients' spiritual needs were significantly correlated ($p < 0.001$) with spirituality as a resource to cope in the scales of the SpREUK-15 (Büssing 2010). In our sample, patients' *Search for access to spirituality* was strongly associated with *Religious needs* (Pearson $r = 0.67$), moderately with *Existential needs* ($r = 0.38$) and weakly with *Inner Peace needs* ($r = 0.29$) and *Giving/Generativity needs* ($r = 0.28$). Their (religious) *Trust in higher Guidance/Source* was strongly related with *Religious needs* ($r = 0.67$), moderately with *Existential needs* ($r = 0.30$) and weakly with *Giving/Generativity needs* ($r = 0.26$) and *Inner Peace* needs ($r = 0.22$). *Reflection/Positive Interpretation of Disease* was moderately related with *Existential needs* ($r = 38$), *Inner Peace* needs ($r = 0.34$), *Religious needs* ($r = 0.33$) and *Giving/Generativity needs* ($r = 0.31$).

The scales of the SpNQ 1.2 in our sample showed only minimal correlations with measures of life satisfaction (BMLSS) and depression (BDI-2) and therefore seem to be independent. The only exception is a weak correlation of *Inner Peace needs* with a Visual Analog Scale of distress ($r = 0.23$; $p < 0.001$).

How Satisfied Were Patients at the End of Their Inpatient Treatment with the Way Their Spiritual Needs Were Met by Staff/Physicians/Nurses?

The samples at admission (n = 243) and on discharge (n = 228) were not identical; there was an overlap of participants with n = 121 ("matches"). At entry (n = 243), 26% of inpatients considered it at least "important" (16%, and "very important" 10%) that staff address their faith or spirituality, while 18% did not want this at all; 43% considered it as less important, while 13% "did not know". Overall, patients wanted psychotherapists (35%), chaplains (33%), physicians (19%) or nurses (16%) to address this (several options could be chosen).

On discharge (n = 218), 45% were satisfied with what was offered regarding their faith or spirituality during their stay, 7% were rather not or not at all satisfied, while 48% did not know, usually commenting that they had no expectations in this regard. Staff who actually addressed aspects of faith or spirituality (several options) were nurses (21%), chaplains (20%), psychotherapists (18%) and physicians (16%). The differences between expectations at entry and realities on discharge concerning the staff groups' behavior became even more acute among the sample of "matches" which were possible for 121 patients: a stronger role of nurses was confirmed (expectation: 17% vs 19% corresponding behavior), while the negative gap for psychotherapists (40% vs 16%), chaplains (33% vs 18%) and physicians (17% vs 11%) tended to increase further (Reiser 2018, 215–216, 231–232, 239).

How Do the Answers of Patients and Staff Fit Together: And What Do They Tell Us about Spiritual Needs in Psychiatry and Psychotherapy

These results provide answers to the following study questions:

- How important are patients' spiritual needs for psychiatric staff, and how spiritual do they consider themselves?

Psychiatric staff reported that they were open to religion- and spirituality-related issues and, in keeping with professional standards, that they are open and empathetic when their patients bring such issues to bear into the clinical process or therapeutic communication. With a majority reporting some religious affiliation, on average, there is a slightly moderate intrinsic religiosity (DUREL) among psychiatric staff. The more religious or spiritual staff report to be themselves, the more positively they experience and estimate the positive effects of religiosity and spirituality on their patients for the therapeutic outcome, while there is no such difference among staff regarding negative effects.

- How important are spiritual needs for inpatients in psychiatry and psychotherapy?

In our survey, inpatients mirrored the distribution of religious affiliations and orientations in the general regional population. Taking into account the situation of distress and crisis at entry, two response groups are especially remarkable: about a quarter of patients considered it important and very important that their religious and spiritual needs are taken care of in the clinical setting, too, while 18% were very outspoken in their desire that this should not happen at all. Among the spiritual needs of the SpNQ, *Inner Peace Needs* were most salient at entry, and explicitly *Religious Needs* the least salient. Among these latter, strong and very strong needs of the patients to turn to a higher presence (38%) and to pray on one's own (33%) qualified as remarkable exceptions. In addition, needs for reconciliation showed up to be important, too. There were no significant differences among the patient groups with regard to diagnoses, age and sex (except for age with regard to *Religious Needs*). The spiritual needs of the inpatients also appeared to be variables independent of life satisfaction (BMLSS) and depression (BDI-2). In other words, spiritual needs do not depend on diagnosis (pathology) or life satisfaction or depression in this sample: They are present even in moments or processes of acute crisis (usually given at entry). More or less, 'spiritually needy' inpatients do not differ significantly among each other with regard to diagnosis, life satisfaction and depression. A patient-centered approach ought to be mindful of these needs as relevant dimensions of any human person. Individual spiritual practices and, for example, personal prayer as a relationship with the divine are important for many patients, more than mindfulness meditation or participating in religious ceremonies. Chaplains as well as psychiatric staff may encourage these individual spiritual practices in a sensitive way.

- How do patients feel treated with regard to their spiritual needs by staff, and how do staff say they treat patients with regard to their spiritual needs?

On leaving, 45% of the patients were satisfied with the way the staff dealt with religious or spiritual issues. This satisfaction may include those who hoped that their spiritual needs would be taken care of, as well as those who did not want this realm to be touched at all, and finally also patients who did not consider this an important topic. Another 48% were satisfied enough because they had no expectations in this regard. It was only 7% who were explicitly unsatisfied with what was offered regarding faith or spirituality during their stay. Presumably, these patients may have had high expectations though we cannot exclude the fact that some patients felt confronted inappropriately with religious or spiritual topics. Apart from a considerably high general satisfaction, the resulting picture seems inconclusive, which may also be due to the general character of the survey questions. A more detailed picture is provided by the results of who took care of the inpatients' religious/spiritual needs and issues. Although the samples at entry and on discharge were not identical and could be matched only in more than 50% of cases, the results are sobering: It was only the nurses who met or exceeded the expectations that they would take care of their spiritual needs, while physicians, other therapists and even chaplains did not live up to their patients' expectations. These results strongly put into question the self-report of psychiatric professionals of being open to, and taking care of, their patients' religious and spiritual needs in treatment, except to some extent for the nurses who were reported to do more than initially expected by the patients.

While one could object that our survey among patients took place almost ten years ago, unmet spiritual needs of mental health patients were also found in other surveys, such as a recent study in the Netherlands (van Nieuw Amerongen-Meeuse et al. 2020). In other words, professional attention to, and integration of, patients' spiritual needs into the treatment settings cannot be taken for granted yet. The Code of Ethics of the Royal College of Psychiatrists (2014, no. 1.3) in contrast claims that "Psychiatrists strive to work collaboratively with patients, respecting the patient's views, beliefs and priorities". At any rate, however, there was no indication in both of our surveys that psychiatric staff considered religious beliefs as indicators of pathology or mental health problems. This is in keeping with Code of Ethics norm 7.3 "Psychiatrists shall not diagnose or treat a person as mentally ill on the basis of that person's political, religious, ideological, moral or philosophical beliefs".

How Can Staff Respond Appropriately to Patients' Religious and Spiritual Needs?

Addressing spiritual needs professionally has to respect therapeutic boundaries (Poole et al. 2019). Then, surely, the necessary therapeutic skills and knowledge are requested (Juckel et al. 2018; Koenig et al. 2020; Mönter et al. 2020; Utsch et al. 2018). Our study with psychiatric staff reported that less than 30% had participated in training programs with religion- or spirituality-related topics. In particular, professionals working in confessional clinics had got significantly more chances to do so than staff in (secular) university clinics (39% vs. 21%; $p < 0.001$). Of all respondents 74% declared themselves ready to take part in such programs. Such programs are what the WPA (2017, no. 2) calls for: "An understanding of religion and spirituality and their relationship to the diagnosis, etiology and treatment of psychiatric disorders should be considered as essential components of both psychiatric training and continuing professional development."

Verhagen (2009, 209; cf. Verhagen et al. 2010; RCPsych 2014, no. 9; Reiser 2018) is more explicit about a curriculum aiming at knowledge, skill and attitude competences:

> With regard to training and education, a curriculum should offer sufficient opportunity for teaching trainees to address the existential, religious and spiritual needs of our patients, including: *Knowledge*: basic knowledge of major belief systems; knowledge about the developmental, experiential, and mental health; consequences of religious experiences. *Skills*: improvement of skills; improvement of diagnostic skills with respect to people having all kinds of religious backgrounds; therapeutic skills. *Attitudes*: systematic reflection on the professional's own belief system (atheism included) and the influence of it on their functioning; analysis of transference and counter-transference issues; empathy.

Unconscious transference and counter-transference issues and biases were given evidence in our survey with professionals. While there was no difference in the negative impacts of patients' religiosity/spirituality in the eyes of psychiatric staff, the difference was significant with regard to positive effects: When psychiatric professionals report higher scores of intrinsic religiosity (DUREL), they acknowledge positive effects of patients' religiosity/spirituality more frequently than colleagues with lower scores do (Lee and Baumann 2013). These results underline the need for more or less religiously minded psychiatric staff "to be sensitive to their own biases and beliefs, how these might influence their practice and to ensure that the patient's best interests are paramount" (RCPsych 2014, 1.4). This certainly needs appropriate training programs, coaching, supervision and didactic therapies. It is not an impossible "neutrality" that is called for but professionality, self-reflection and openness toward the patients' religious and spiritual needs (Lee and Baumann 2013, 2019a; RCPsych 2014, 3.1). In addition to (reflected) clinical intuitions and empathy, such professional formation is the necessary condition for discerning to which degree religious and spiritual needs are resources or rather obstacles in a patient's situation of depression or mood disorder, anxiety disorder, personality disorder or psychosis. How much do they serve a progressive function for healing and treatment or rather a regressive one as part of the pathological process in this particular patient? These questions can only be answered in a patient-centered treatment approach in combination with appropriate training.

The combination of both of our surveys has enabled us to answer the three main study questions of this paper and to formulate consequences for professional training.

We Are Aware of Several Limitations of our Present Endeavor, a Few of Which Are the Following

In spite of our significant and valid results which the DGPPN position-paper (Utsch et al. 2016) called for, they compared the results of a nation-wide study of psychiatric staff with results obtained from inpatients of one university site. There is need for more studies, especially involving inpatients, in order to improve the comparative and representative character of such surveys.

In addition, our surveys have been performed in Germany. Similar studies in different countries are needed. Depending on cultural backgrounds, for example histories, traditions and ethnicities, patients' religious and spiritual needs are different and are also regarded differently. For example, in Korea, one of the multicultural Asian countries, religious/spiritual issues in psychiatric settings seem to be less familiar and welcome than in Germany (Lee and Baumann 2019a, b). According to our regional survey, Korean psychiatric staff commonly consider religious/spiritual needs and practices as an insalubrious influence or even part of a missionary, proselytizing activity. As a result, staffs usually try to keep them strictly apart from clinical settings, no matter what kind of meaning these issues have for patients or how acutely patients want to talk about them.

Finally, we used different questionnaires and tools in the main two of our reported and compared surveys in this paper. The early version of SpNQ we used in the patients' survey proved its usefulness convincingly. Büssing has continued the further development of this tool, based on plenty of research, for the operationalization of spiritual needs, including so-called secular spiritual needs. Similar topics to the ones operationalized by the SpNQ can be found in a qualitative systematic review by Milner et al. (2020) with 594 participants in 38 qualitative studies from 15 countries which found six core themes: *Meaning-making*, *Identity*, *Service-provision*, *Talk about it*, *Interaction with symptoms* and *Coping*. These results of *qualitative* research converge with our *quantitative* results, thereby adding to the validity of the SpNQ and, at the same time, indicating further aspects of patients' spiritual needs, while other aspects are missing which have been empirically validated in the SpNQ (e.g. Generative Altruism). In addition to empirical research, both qualitative and quantitative, patient-centered approaches also call for conceptual reflection on what is meant by spiritual needs and their implications for treatment and doing justice to the patients and their best interests (Pargament 2007; Aten and Leach 2009; Reiser 2018).

Conclusions

Mental health professionals are faced with patients' spiritual or religious needs, even though these needs may seem to be weaker or more silent than other needs. This does not mean that these patient needs are negligible. According to our survey with the SpNQ among psychiatric inpatients, they affirmed spiritual needs which deserve attention. These needs indicate mental aspects in need of support and clarification and could be important resources to be encouraged for recovery and in their own rights as part of the patients' personalities.

Psychiatric staff report their own openness to welcome their patients' spiritual and religious needs as part of the clinical treatment situation and their readiness for training to do so appropriately. Though these results call for more representativeness and for intercultural studies, they indicate the need for curricula which integrate the manifold religious and spiritual realities of both patients and staff, in accordance with the useful guidelines of psychiatric associations.

Acknowledgments We sincerely thank all respondents who participated in our studies, and to Dr. Anne Zahn for her strong support, especially for the patients' survey, and Professor Dr. Ulrich Voderholzer and Professor Dr. Mathias Berger who encouraged and facilitated both surveys. All stated studies were funded by resources of the department of Caritas Science and Christian Social Work at Freiburg University. In part, the writing of papers was supported by the National Research Foundation of Korea Grant funded by the Korean Government [2016S1A3A2924944].

References

APA (2006) American Psychiatric Association, committee on religion, spirituality and psychiatry: resource document on religious/spiritual commitments and psychiatric practice, Arlington. http://www.psychiatry.org/File%20Library/Psychiatrists/Directories/Library-and-Archive/resource_documents/rd2006_Religion.pdf. Accessed 21 August 2020

Aten JD, Leach MM (eds) (2009) Spirituality and the therapeutic process. A comprehensive resource from intake to termination. American Psychological Association, Washington DC

Baumann K (2012) Remarks on religions and psychiatry/psychotherapies. In: Hefti R, Bee J (eds) Spiritualität und Gesundheit. Spirituality and Health. Ausgewählte Beiträge im Spannungsfeld zwischen Forschung und Praxis. Selected Contributions on Conflicting Priorities in Research and Practice. Peter Lang, Bern, pp 99–118

Büssing A (2010) Spirituality as a resource to rely on in chronic illness: the SpREUK Questionnaire. Religions 1:9–17

Büssing A, Balzat HJ, Heusser P (2010) Spiritual needs of patients with chronic pain diseases and cancer—validation of the spiritual needs questionnaire. Eur J Med Res 15:266–273

Cook C, Powell A, Sims A (eds) (2009) Spirituality and psychiatry. RCPsych Publications, London

Curlin FA, Lawrence RE, Odell S, Chin MH, Lantos JD, Koenig HG, Meador KG (2007) Religion, spirituality, and medicine: psychiatrists' and other physicians' differing observations, interpretations, and clinical approaches. Am J Psychiatr 164:1825–1831

Hofmann L, Walach H (2011) Spirituality and religiosity in psychotherapy—a representative survey among German psychotherapists. Psychother Res 21(2):179–192. https://doi.org/10.1080/10503307.2010.536595

Huguelet P, Koenig HG (eds) (2009) Religion and spirituality in psychiatry. Cambridge University Press, New York

Juckel G, Hoffmann K, Walach H (eds) (2018) Spiritualität in Psychiatrie und Psychotherapie. Pabst Science, Lengerich

Koenig HG, Büssing A (2010) The Duke university religion index (DUREL): a five-item measure for use in epidemiological studies. Religions 1(1):78–85. https://doi.org/10.3390/rel1010078

Koenig HG, Peteet JR, VanderWeele TJ (2020) Religion and psychiatry: clinical applications. BJPsych Advances. https://doi.org/10.1192/bja.2020.11

Kørup AK, Søndergaard J, Lucchetti G, Ramakrishnan P, Baumann K, Lee E, Frick E, Büssing A, Alyousefi NA, Karimah A, Schouten E, Wermuth I, Hvidt NC (2019) Religious values of physicians affect their clinical practice. A meta-analysis of individual participant data from 7 countries. Medicine 98:38(e17265). https://doi.org/10.1097/MD.0000000000017265

Lee E (2014) Religiosität bzw. Spiritualität in Psychiatrie und Psychotherapie. Ihre Bedeutung für psychiatrisches Wirken aus der Sicht des psychiatrischen Personals anhand einer bundesweiten Personalbefragung. Echter, Würzburg

Lee E, Baumann K (2013) German psychiatrists observation and interpretation of religiosity/spirituality. Evid Based Complement Alternat Med:280168. https://doi.org/10.1155/2013/280168

Lee E, Baumann K (2019a) How Korean psychiatric staff deal with religious and spiritual issues of patients: what is professional? Religions 10:544. https://doi.org/10.3390/rel10100544

Lee E, Baumann K (2019b) Religiosity and spirituality: is it an appropriate issue in psychiatry and psychotherapy?—Comparative studies of Germany and South Korea. Open J Soc Sci 7:300–310. https://doi.org/10.4236/jss.2019.73025

Lee E, Zahn A, Baumann K (2014) Religiosity/spirituality and mental health: psychiatric staff's attitudes and behaviors. Open J Soc Sci 2:7–13. https://doi.org/10.4236/jss.2014.211002

Lee E, Zahn A, Baumann K (2015) How do psychiatric staffs approach religiosity/spirituality in clinical practice? Differing perceptions among psychiatric staff members and clinical chaplains. Religions 6:930–947. https://doi.org/10.3390/rel6030930

Milner K, Crawford P, Edgley A, Hare-Duke L, Slade M (2020) The experiences of spirituality among adults with mental health difficulties: a qualitative systematic review. Epidemiol Psychiatr Sci 29:e34. https://doi.org/10.1017/S2045796019000234

Mönter N, Heinz A, Utsch M (eds) (2020) Religionssensible Psychotherapie und Psychiatrie. Kohlhammer, Stuttgart

Pargament KI (2007) Spiritually integrated psychotherapy. Understanding and addressing the sacred. The Guilford Press, New York

Poole R, Cook CCH, Higgo R (2019) Psychiatrists, spirituality and religion. BJ Psych 214:181–182. https://doi.org/10.1192/bjp.2018.241

RCPsych (2009) Good psychiatric practice. 3rd ed. Royal College of Psychiatrists London (College Report, CR154). https://www.rcpsych.ac.uk/docs/default-source/improving-care/better-mh-policy/college-reports/college-report-cr154.pdf?sfvrsn=e196928b_2. Accessed 21 August 2020

RCPsych (2013) Recommendations for psychiatrists on spirituality and religion. Royal College of Psychiatrists London (Position Statements, PS03/2013). http://www.rcpsych.ac.uk/pdf/PS03_2013.pdf. Accessed 21 August 2020

RCPsych (2014) Good psychiatric practice. Code of Ethics. Royal College of Psychiatrists London (College Report, CR186). https://www.rcpsych.ac.uk/docs/default-source/improving-care/better-mh-policy/college-reports/college-report-cr186.pdf?sfvrsn=15f49e84_2. Accessed 21 August 2020

Reiser F (2018) Menschen mehr gerecht werden. Zur Religiosität bzw. Spiritualität von Patientinnen und Patienten in Psychiatrie und Psychotherapie. Echter, Würzburg

Unterrainer H-F (2010) Seelenfinsternis? Struktur und Inhalt der Gottesbeziehung im klinisch-psychiatrischen Feld. Waxmann, Münster

Utsch M, Anderssen-Reuster U, Frick E, Gross W, Murken S, Schouler-Ocak M, Stotz-Ingenlath G (2016) Empfehlungen zum Umgang mit Religiosität und Spiritualität in Psychiatrie und Psychotherapie. Position paper of the DGPPN (Deutsche Gesellschaft für Psychiatrie, Psychotherapie und Nervenheilkunde). http://www.dgppn.de/presse/stellungnahmen/stellungnahmen-2016/religiositaet.html. Accessed 21 August 2020

Utsch M, Bonelli R, Pfeifer S (2018) Psychotherapie und Spiritualität, 2nd edn. Springer, Heidelberg

van Nieuw Amerongen-Meeuse JC, Schaap-Jonker H, Westerbroek G, Anbeek C, Braam AW (2020) Conversations and beyond: religious/spiritual care needs among clinical mental health patients in the Netherlands. J Nerv Ment Dis 208:524–532. https://doi.org/10.1097/NMD.0000000000001150

Verhagen PJ (2009) Religion, spirituality and psychiatry. Reflections and directions for thorough action. In: Christodoulou GN, Jorge M, Mezzich JE (eds) Advances in psychiatry, vol 3. BETA, Athen, pp 201–211

Verhagen PJ, van Praag HM, López-Ibor JJ, Cox J, Moussaoui D (eds) (2010) Religion and psychiatry. Beyond boundaries (World Psychiatric Association Book 32). John Wiley & Sons, Chichester

WPA (2017) Position statement on spirituality and religion in psychiatry. World Psychiatric Association Section on Religion, Spirituality and Psychiatry. https://www.wpanet.org/position-statements. Accessed 21 August 2020

CHAPTER 18

Spiritual Needs of Tumor Patients During Their Stay at a Palliative Care Unit

Arndt Büssing, Klaus Baumann, Jochen Rentschler, and Gerhild Becker

Background

Most health care providers are well aware that several of their patients consider the question of what constitutes their lives, what specifically gives their life orientation, meaning, and hold, what can and must still be clarified and resolved, and which resources they have to instill them with support and hope. Also in secular societies, for many people their faith and spirituality is an important resource. However, this resource is in most cases only theoretically acknowledged by health care providers and only rarely actively supported, because an important argument against it is that there is no additional time during their routine care, that specific knowledge is lacking, and that the pastoral care practiced by the church(es) is

A. Büssing (✉)
Professorship Quality of Life, Spirituality and Coping, Faculty of Health, Witten/Herdecke University, Herdecke, Germany

IUNCTUS—Competence Center for Christian Spirituality, Philosophical-Theological University of Münster, Münster, Germany
e-mail: Arndt.buessing@uni-wh.de

A. Büssing (ed.), *Spiritual Needs in Research and Practice*,
https://doi.org/10.1007/978-3-030-70139-0_18

"responsible" for this task. Moreover, some physicians would point to "value neutrality" as an argument against addressing spiritual concerns. All these arguments might be true in specific situations, as it is well known that health care providers are working mostly "at their limits." However, many patients want to talk to their doctor about their spiritual needs, not necessarily with a pastor (Büssing et al. 2009a) or want their doctor to be informed about their spiritual concerns (Frick et al. 2006).

Balboni et al.'s study among North American cancer patients clearly revealed that most of them do not feel adequately supported by the medical system, and about half of them not by a religious community (Balboni et al. 2007). Also in more secular Germany, chronically ill and tumor patients have circumscribed spiritual needs (Büssing et al. 2011, 2013; Höcker et al. 2014; Haußmann et al. 2017). However, their support is barely anchored in the clinical setting. An exception is palliative care, where the subject area of spirituality should be considered. Actually, the WHO definition of palliative care is very clear: Palliative care "prevents and relieves suffering through the early identification, correct assessment and treatment of pain and other problems, whether physical, psychosocial or spiritual." (World Health Organization 2018). These spiritual "problems" could be the domain of spiritual care (Boothe and Frick 2017), which is not identical to pastoral care, and addresses the multi-professional responsibility for the spiritual dimension of being human in care (Frick 2009).

K. Baumann
Caritas Science and Christian Social Work, Faculty of Theology,
Albert-Ludwigs University, Freiburg, Germany
e-mail: klaus.baumann@theol.uni-freiburg.de

J. Rentschler
Department Hematology/Oncology/Palliative Medicine, Ortenau Clinic,
Offenburg-Kehl, Germany
e-mail: Jochen.Rentschler@ortenau-klinikum.de

G. Becker
Chair of Palliative Care, Department of Palliative Care, Medical Center – University of Freiburg, Faculty of Medicine, University of Freiburg, Freiburg im Breisgau, Germany

Medical Center – University of Freiburg, Faculty of Medicine,
University of Freiburg, Freiburg im Breisgau, Germany
e-mail: gerhild.becker@uniklinik-freiburg.de

To address this adequately, it is important first to analyze what specific spiritual needs patients in a palliative situation have, and whether or not these needs change during their stay. Are patients at a palliative care unit (PCU) satisfied with the support of their spiritual needs?

Findings from Patients with Cancer at a PCU

In a sample of patients from South-West Germany (n = 118; 97% with cancer, mean age 63 ± 11 [35–84] years; 74% with a Christian background, 2% other, and 25% without a religious affiliation), their needs for *Inner Peace* (1.58 ± 0.89) and *Giving/Generativity* (a concern for giving, being useful to, and guiding the next generation or others in general) (1.49 ± 0.93) were the strongest, while *Religious* needs (0.95 ± 0.92) and *Existential* needs (0.79 ± 0.85) were expressed less strongly (Büssing et al. 2020). The SpNQ-20 mean scores within this sample was 1.12 ± 0.71. There were no gender-related differences in the intensity of these needs. Their spiritual well-being as measured with the FACIT-Sp (Peterman et al. 2002; Bredle et al. 2011) was particularly pronounced in terms of the Meaning dimension, weaker for the Peace dimension and least for the Faith dimension (Büssing et al. 2020). Here, there were significant gender-related differences in both the Meaning and the Peace dimension, with men having higher well-being scores.

The analysis of patients' needs at two time points during their stay at the PCU was quite difficult, because several were dying more rapidly than expected or were leaving the PCU earlier than expected. Most were treated for 2–3 weeks at the PCU (82%) and 9% for 4–6 weeks. The study group was thus able to analyze data of 62 resp. 58 patients at the beginning and at end of their stay. These were in 60% women and in 40% mean, with a mean age of 64 ± 11 [37–84] years.

Interestingly, there were neither significant changes of their spiritual needs scores (Fig. 18.1) nor of their spiritual well-being (Büssing et al. 2020). During this period, the patients experienced a significant increase in their perceived health status (VAS: 33.05 ± 17.63 versus 42.06 ± 16.35; $p < 0.0001$), which, however, can still be seen as reduced. Moderate multidimensional life satisfaction scores (BMLSS) remained unchanged, as did high satisfaction with support received by the hospital team, which was rated as very good (Büssing et al. 2020).

Within the limited period of 2–3 weeks there were no significant changes in both patients' spiritual needs and their spiritual well-being. It

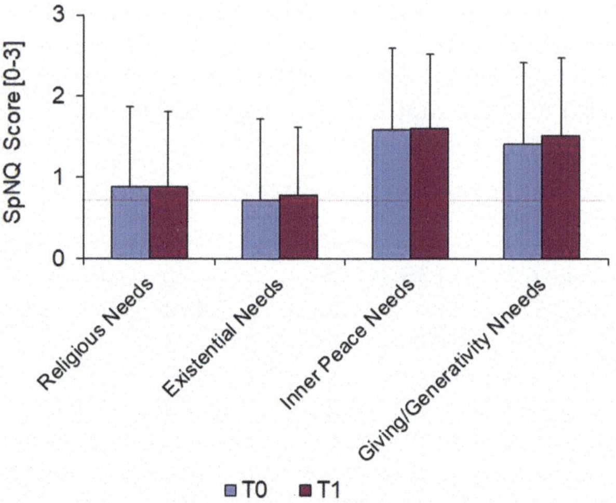

Fig. 18.1 Spiritual needs of patients at the start (t1) and end (t2) of their PCU stay

was not to be expected that the reduced life satisfaction would change significantly, but it was noticeable that patients' support satisfaction was very high and could, therefore, hardly be increased. In both palliative care institutions where these patients have been recruited, however, there was no one with an explicit training for spiritual care; it is thus unclear whether the findings would have been different when a whole PCU team would have had some spiritual care training.

The dimension of *Inner Peace* was striking, as its relevance (as recorded by means of two survey instruments) was very high. This calls for the health care system to provide adequate support for it. The SpNQ (Büssing et al., 2010, 2018) addresses this topic with items such as needs to talk to someone about fears and worries, needs to stay at a place of quietness and peace, to be able to "immerge" into the beauty of nature in order to find inner peace, etc. This topic was operationalized in the FACIT-Sp (Bredle et al. 2011) as well-being—that is, in terms of living in peace with oneself, finding solace in oneself, feelings of inner harmony, but also troubles to find inner peace. Persons from the field of psychotherapy and pastoral care would therefore be considered as contact persons for these topics, but also other professions that would assume a responsibility here (art therapists, health care professionals, etc.). It is interesting, however, that the need to talk to someone about a (possible) life after death was only small (12% had a great need here, 12% a medium, 7% a small, and 69% with no need at all).

The topic of *Giving/Generativity*, which would go beyond one's own life, was also strongly pronounced by the PCU patients. This is about the needs to tell from the own life and to pass on the acquired life experiences, but also to comfort someone else (and thus to be able to step out of the passive role of the "treated" person), and to have the certainty that one's own life has been and is meaningful and valuable. Here, the aim is to build on one's own life story so that it can be carried on and taken up by the next generation. This value of life could be confirmed through persons who are willing to listen and to address the generative concerns of patients—and this would facilitate (at least a bit) to let go fears and concerns because their life was approved as "worth it."

Even when it is true that the time resources of health care providers are limited, this does not argue against the fact that patients need spiritual care support, too, and that the structural and organizational framework conditions should be improved as well as individual solutions. Further education and training in the field of spiritual care are an essential prerequisite for this. With the help of the Spiritual Care Competence Questionnaire (SCCQ), the corresponding skills and the readiness of the team for this topic can also be mapped (Frick et al. 2019), so that specific competences could be promoted.

A further relevant insight from these findings is that the pattern of spiritual needs as described here in palliative care patients is identical to that of tumor patients in earlier stages (Büssing et al. 2011, 2013; Höcker et al. 2014; Haußmann et al. 2017). This is important because the consideration of spiritual needs in palliative care is fundamentally sought, while the support of these is still given little attention to in the early stages of cancer. Especially in the social–spatial environment, that is, in the time span between the hospital (at the time of diagnosis and first treatment) and the palliative care unit or hospice, many questions would arise for support, particularly who is available as a contact person? Pastoral care providers are trained for this, but not always available.

Working with the SpNQ as a Tool in Palliative Medicine

After reading the items for the first time, patients often stated that some of the questions were very close to them. After a short time, many put the questionnaire aside to target it at a time when they felt psychologically and physically stable enough for it. Again and again, patients perceived some of these questions first as an imposition and an additional burden, but then they noticed that it was ultimately good for them to face these issues. Especially when collecting the questionnaires, that is, about 48 h after delivery, there were many in-depth discussions with the nursing staff or the doctors about points that had particularly touched and concerned the patients. It is important to note that the conversation initiative always started with the patient. Ideally, the only thing the doctors or nurses communicated in this regard was that there was no time pressure to stand in the way of a conversation. In many cases, the relevant topics could be deepened with clinic pastors or external clergy, our psycho-oncologist, and music therapist.

In our interdisciplinary anamnestic interviews, we routinely integrate a spiritual anamnesis (CSI-MEMO modified according to Harold G. Koenig). However, this does not usually lead to an in-depth exchange about spiritual needs and satisfaction as triggered by the Spiritual Needs questionnaire. This may be due to the setting and timing. Feedback from one of the enrolled centers was that the regular use of the questionnaire has noticeably increased both the quantity and the quality of the Spiritual Care provision on the ICU.

Ways to React Toward the Addressed Spiritual Needs

There are different ways to deal with the responses. First of all, readiness for conversations is important. Addressing spiritual needs of patients is a core component of comprehensive cancer and palliative care (WHO Definition 2007; Sinclair et al. 2012). National Cancer Networks in the United States and Germany recommend routine screening and assessment of spiritual issues (National Comprehensive Cancer Network 2011; Gahr et al. 2020).

The dimension of *Inner Peace* needs can be met through creative, often small, but individually tailored actions. For example, to put up a photo/picture that means a lot to the patient. It often depicts children, grandchildren or friends, and often also memories of important experiences such as climbing a mountain or a big motorcycle tour. Music therapy is also very important. One may play music that suits the patient. Especially in patients in an advanced phase of dying, a significant calming down can often be observed through sensitive music therapy. The breath becomes steadier and calmer, muscle spasms loosen, facial features relax. Another action like facilitating saying goodbye to loved places, for example, by medically assisted transports to the patient's apartment or garden for a few hours is also of outstanding importance.

The dimension of *Generativity* is quite complex. Nearly every specialist in the palliative team (doctors, nurses, physiotherapy, nutritional therapy, psycho-oncology, music therapy) immerses himself or herself into different areas of the patient's biography during the repeated encounters. The patient "controls" who is given insight, where, and how. The repeated encounters create relationships and make them grow over time. The professionals listen, ask questions, and reflect what has been said in their own experience, and thus the patient can experience himself or herself as both a giver and a gift recipient. With almost every farewell of a patient when he or she is discharged home, to the nursing home, or to the hospice, the ICU team explicitly tells him/her that it was a pleasure and a privilege to be able to look after him/her and that he/she enriched us with his/her presence and communication.

Conclusions

The use of the SpNQ as part of a research project to which patients voluntarily gave their consent, transformed spiritual care from a more or less random possibility to a structured, regular offer. It increased the team's awareness of spiritual needs and provided a good framework and stimulus for patients to make personalized, specific remarks and requests. While addressing patients' spiritual needs has been endorsed by health care organizations and clinical guidelines, there is little guidance on what constitutes spiritual care and how physicians and nurses might meet these needs as good practice. The use of instruments such as the SpNQ may help to integrate spiritual care in routine bedside clinical care as part of holistic patient care.

Acknowledgments We are grateful to all patients who have filled the questionnaire.

References

Balboni TA, Vanderwerker LC, Block SD, Paulk ME, Lathan CS, Peteet JR, Prigerson HG (2007) Religiousness and spiritual support among advanced cancer patients and associations with end-of-life treatment preferences and quality of life. J Clin Oncol 25:555–560

Boothe B, Frick E (2017) Spiritual care. Über das Leben und das Sterben. Orell Füssli Verlag, Zürich

Bredle JM, Salsman JM, Debb SM, Arnold BJ, Cella D (2011) Spiritual well-being as a component of health-related quality of life: the functional assessment of chronic illness therapy—spiritual well-being scale (FACIT-Sp). Religions 2:77–94

Büssing A, Michalsen A, Balzat HJ, Grünther RA, Ostermann T, Neugebauer EAM, Matthiessen PF (2009a) Are spirituality and religiosity resources for patients with chronic pain conditions? Pain Med 1:327–339

Büssing A, Balzat HJ, Heusser P (2010) Spiritual needs of patients with chronic pain diseases and cancer – validation of the spiritual needs questionnaire. Eur J Med Res 15:266–273

Büssing A, Lux EA, Janko A, Kopf A (2011) Psychosoziale und spirituelle Bedürfnisse bei Patienten mit chronischen Schmerz- und Krebserkrankungen. Deutsche Zeitschrift für Onkologie 41:39–73

Büssing A, Janko A, Baumann K, Hvidt NC, Kopf A (2013) Spiritual needs among patients with chronic pain diseases and cancer living in a secular society. Pain Med 14:1362–1373

Büssing A, Recchia DR, Koenig H, Baumann K, Frick E (2018) Factor structure of the spiritual needs questionnaire (SpNQ) in persons with chronic diseases, elderly and healthy individuals. Religions 9:13. https://doi.org/10.3390/rel9010013

Büssing A, Baumann K, Rentschler J, Becker G (2020) Spirituelle Bedürfnisse von Tumorpatienten verändern sich während der palliativmedizinischen Betreuung kaum. Deutsche Zeitschrift für Onkologie. Online first: https://doi.org/10.1055/a-1135-3566

Frick E (2009) Spiritual care – ein neues Fachgebiet der Medizin. Zeitschrift für medizinische Ethik 55:145–155

Frick E, Riedner C, Fegg MJ, Hauf S, Borasio GD (2006) A clinical interview assessing cancer patients' spiritual needs and preferences. Eur J Cancer Care 15:238–243

Frick E, Theiss M, Recchia DR, Büssing A (2019) Validierung einer deutschsprachigen Skala zur Messung von Spiritual Care Kompetenzen. Spiritual Care 8:193–207

Gahr S, Lödel S, Berendt J, Thomas M, Ostgathe C (2020) Implementation of best practice recommendations for palliative care in German comprehensive cancer centers. Oncologist 25:e259–e265

Haußmann A, Schäffeler N, Hautzinger M, Weyel B, Eigentler T, Zipfel S, Teufel M (2017) Religiöse/spirituelle Bedürfnisse und psychosoziale Belastung von Patienten mit malignem Melanom. Psychother Psych Med 67:413–419

Höcker A, Krüll A, Koch U, Mehnert A (2014) Exploring spiritual needs and their associated factors in an urban sample of early and advanced cancer patients. Eur J Cancer Care 23:786–794

National Comprehensive Cancer Network (2011) NCCN clinical practice guidelines in oncology: paliative care. (Version 2.2011) National Comprehensive Cancer Network. https://www.nccn.org/professionals/physician_gls/pdf/palliative.pdf. Accessed 7 July 2020

Peterman AH, Fitchett G, Brady MJ, Hernandez L, Cella D (2002) Measuring spiritual well-being in people with cancer: the functional assessment of chronic illness therapy – spiritual well-being scale (FACIT-Sp). Ann Behav Med 24:49–58

Sinclair S, Bouchal SR, Chochinov HM, Hagen N (2012) Spiritual care: how to do it. BMJ Support Palliat Care 2:319–327

Word Health Organization (2007) Definition of palliative care. https://www.who.int/cancer/palliative/definition/en. Accessed 7 July 2020

World Health Organization (2018) Palliative care. https://www.who.int/newsroom/fact-sheets/detail/palliative-care. Accessed 7 July 2020

PART IV

Findings in Different Populations: Persons with Special Needs in Difficult Situations

CHAPTER 19

Spiritual Needs of Patients in the Emergency Room

Charlotte Wapler, Christoph Dodt, Arndt Büssing, Andreas Beivers, Kristin Härtl, and Eckhard Frick

Background

Over the last years, the number of patients treated in emergency rooms in Germany has grown continuously (Eiff et al. 2016). Due to various factors like an increasing number of old and multimorbid patients or structural difficulties and restrictions in the health care system, the emergency department has become an important key point in patient care (Weyrich et al. 2012). This is a critical development because emergency rooms often present very stressful and precarious surroundings for the patients. They in an exceptional physical situation and are also exposed to a new environment with intense medical examinations and numerous unusual sensory

C. Wapler • E. Frick (✉)
Research Unit Spiritual Care, Clinic and Policlinic for Psychosomatic Medicine and Psychotherapy, Klinikum rechts der Isar, Technical University of Munich, Munich, Germany
e-mail: eckhard.frick@tum.de

C. Dodt
Clinic for Emergency Medicine, Clinic Bogenhausen, Munich, Germany
e-mail: Christoph.Dodt@muenchen-klinik.de

A. Büssing (ed.), *Spiritual Needs in Research and Practice*,
https://doi.org/10.1007/978-3-030-70139-0_19

impressions (Fleischmann 2016). Other difficulties are the uncertainty of the outcome, the sensation of pain, or the feeling of being left alone. Altogether, coping with all this can be very challenging and therefore trigger spiritual distress (Wensley et al. 2017).

A Taiwanese study surveyed boarded patients in the emergency department who were waiting for a bed for more than 8 h. During this time, the patients were not only burdened by the physical effects of their illness, but also by the anxiety caused by the long waiting time, the possibility of dying, and the sense of passivity and helplessness. Therefore, emergency care should not only respect the medical and physical needs, but also involve attention to the individual's spiritual concerns like discomfort and emotional challenges (Han et al. 2017).

In order to do so, it is important to first recognize the patients' spiritual needs and concerns and, second, find the willingness and time to address them. Often there is a mismatch between the perception of patients' spiritual needs by medical staff and the expression of those needs by the patients. This could be shown in an American study surveying EMTs (emergency medical technicians) and paramedics' reports regarding their patients' needs. Most EMTs/paramedics reported to rarely or occasionally have the impression that the patients have spiritual needs or concerns. While 55% of the patients stated that they would have wanted to discuss spiritual issues with them, 78% of the EMTs/paramedics have never or rarely discussed spiritual concerns with their patients (Jang et al. 2004). This may lead to the conclusion that emergency patients have a tendency not to voice their spiritual needs. A similar reluctance could be found in patients with end-stage heart failure or lung cancer, because they did not want to bother the busy health professionals with those issues. At the same time, those who had the opportunity to address their concerns often were relieved and felt valued. Consequently, it is of importance to actively

A. Büssing
Professorship Quality of Life, Spirituality and Coping, Faculty of Health, Witten/Herdecke University, Herdecke, Germany

IUNCTUS—Competence Center for Christian Spirituality, Philosophical-Theological University of Münster, Münster, Germany
e-mail: Arndt.buessing@uni-wh.de

A. Beivers • K. Härtl
Hochschule Fresenius, Munich, Germany
e-mail: beivers@hs-fresenius.de; kristin.haertl@hs-fresenius.de

provide a possibility for the patient to voice spiritual distress (Murray et al. 2004). Since it is known that meeting spiritual needs of patients has many beneficial effects both on spiritual and physical health (Balboni et al. 2007, 2011; Edwards et al. 2010), it seems important to identify unmet spiritual needs as early as possible over the course of the illness to be able to react appropriately (Gordon et al. 2018).

In German hospitals, it is a frequent practice to register patients' religion, while usually there is no other religious/spiritual assessment. However, the informative value of the religious affiliation is only limited in an ever more secular society and provides little insight into the role of religion or spirituality in the individual's everyday life (Glenister and Prewer 2017). According to our knowledge, the present study is the first one in German-speaking countries to assess spiritual needs of patients in the emergency room (Frick et al. 2020). It focuses on the following research questions:

1. Is it possible to assess spiritual needs of patients in the emergency room?
2. What kind of spiritual needs can be found?
3. Do sociodemographic characteristics like age, gender, or religious affiliation influence the expression of spiritual needs in emergency room patients?
4. Do clinical parameters like affected organ system, Emergency Severity Index, the experience of pain, etc. influence the expression of spiritual needs in emergency room patients?

To address these questions, we enrolled patients during a 4-week time period coming to the emergency room of a municipal hospital (Frick et al. 2020). They gave informed consent to the collection of sociodemographic and medical data and responded to the SpNQ in its SpNQ-20 version. Field notes were made in order to document any particularities like special reactions to the questionnaire or extraordinary situations in the emergency room (Frick et al. 2020).

Patients in the Emergency Room

Of the 479 patients approached, 383 were willing to take part in the study (80% response rate). The gender (52% women, 48% men) and age distribution was well balanced; the average age was 58 ± 21 years. Among them, 69% were Christian, 6% Muslim, 2% had other and 23% no religious affiliation. Patients were treated by the departments of internal medicine

(29%), general medicine (29%), and surgery or urology (41%). The organ systems the main diagnosis referred to were in most cases the cardiovascular and nerve systems (15% each) and the musculoskeletal system (28%); 66% of the surveyed patients experienced physical pain. The average length of the hospital stay was 4 ± 6 days, ranging from 0 to 57 days; 51% were in-patients, while 49% got an ambulant treatment.

The Emergency Severity Index (ESI), a tool that is used to evaluate the urgency of the patients' treatment (Grossmann et al. 2009), was 2 for 22% of the patients, indicating an urgent, possibly life-threatening situation, 3 for 57%, and 4 or 5 for 19%. The ESI scores of 3, 4, and 5 differ in the number of resources that are expected to be necessary for diagnostics and treatment, with 3 being the most resource-consuming one. The Charlson Comorbidity Index (CCI) served to assess the severity of a patient's health status and the connected prospective mortality (Charlson et al. 1987). It encloses 17 conditions of illness that are weighed by severity: The higher the CCI, the larger is the mortality risk. The average CCI was 1.1 ± 1.7 ranging from 0 to 13 points.

Compared to a reference sample of patients (n = 694) treated in the emergency room in the same period one year prior to the spiritual needs assessment study, there were no significant differences with respect to age, gender, ESI score, and treatment conditions (data not shown). Therefore, the sample can be regarded as representative for the hospital's emergency patients (Frick et al. 2020).

Several times it was documented in the field notes that patients had a great need to talk. Sometimes answering the questionnaire facilitated that patients started a conversation about their current situation, important life topics, or experiences. It was noted that after those conversations, some of the patients were grateful for the empathic attention.

Patients' Spiritual Needs and Their Relation to Sociodemographic and Clinical Parameters

In the sample of patients in the emergency room, *Inner Peace* needs and *Giving/Generativity* needs were of stronger importance than *Religious* or *Existential* needs (Table 19.1). Only 2% of the patients stated not having any *Giving/Generativity* needs and only 4% not having any *Inner Peace* needs, while no *Existential* needs were expressed by 23% and no *Religious* ones by 33%. The most significant needs (considered either strong or very

Table 19.1 Expression of spiritual needs in patients in the emergency room[a]

Item ID and topic	*Agreement score [Mean ± SD]*
Number	379
Religious needs score	**0.73 ± 0.84**
N18 pray with someone	0.49 ± 0.97
N19 someone prays for you	0.65 ± 1.06
N20 pray for yourself	1.08 ± 1.24
N21 participate at a religious ceremony (i.e., Sunday service)	0.84 ± 1.09
N22 read religious/spiritual books	0.48 ± 0.93
N23 turn to a higher presence (i.e., God, Allah)	0.85 ± 1.15
Existential needs score	**0.67 ± 0.61**
N5 dissolve/clarify open aspects of your life	0.69 ± 1.07
N10 find meaning in illness and/or suffering	0.39 ± 0.81
N11 talk with someone about the question of meaning in life	0.73 ± 1.05
N12 talk with someone about the possibility of life after death	0.73 ± 1.05
N16 forgive someone from a distinct period of your life	0.69 ± 1.06
N17 be forgiven	0.78 ± 1.09
Inner Peace needs score	**1.49 ± 0.74**
N2 talk with others about your fears and worries	0.94 ± 1.14
N6 plunge into beauty of nature	2.31 ± 1.03
N7 dwell at a place of quietness and peace	1.48 ± 1.24
N8 find inner peace	1.21 ± 1.20
Giving/Generativity needs score	**1.59 ± 0.73**
N14 give away something of yourself	1.56 ± 1.19
N15 give solace to someone	1.52 ± 1.19
N26 pass own life experiences to others	1.73 ± 1.10
N27 be assured that your life was meaningful and of value	1.55 ± 1.21
SpNQ-20 mean score	**1.04 ± 0.54**

[a]data from Frick et al. (2020)

strong) were to plunge into beauty of nature (N6: 82%), to pass on their own life experience to others (N26: 63%), to be assured that life was meaningful and of value (N27: 59%), to give away something of yourself (N14: 56%), to give solace to someone (N15: 55%), and to dwell at a place of quietness and peace (N7: 54%) (Frick et al. 2020).

Women had significantly higher scores for *Religious*, *Existential* and *Inner Peace* needs than men and therefore also higher SpNQ-20 Scores (Frick et al. 2020). For the age groups, there was a significant difference for *Inner Peace* needs ($F = 2.25$; $p = 0.049$) and a trend for *Religious* needs ($F = 2.21$; $p = 0.065$); both were expressed the least by the younger patients (<30 years of age). The older ones (>70 years of age) had the strongest *Religious* needs, while the group of 51–60-year-old patients had the strongest *Inner Peace* needs. Patients with religious affiliations expressed more *Religious* needs ($F = 42.0$, $p < 0.0001$) and *Giving/Generativity* needs ($F = 4.5$, $p = 0.036$) than those without a religious affiliation. Among the religious patients, *Religious* needs of Muslim patients ($n = 24$) were stronger than that of Christians ($n = 261$) (1.34 ± 1.10 vs. 0.85 ± 0.83) (Frick et al. 2020).

The expression of spiritual needs did not depend on the Emergency Severity Index or on the duration of stay in the hospital (Frick et al. 2020). Whether patients were perceiving pain or not, whether the illness was caused in a traumatic or nontraumatic way, whether they were treated as an in-patient or ambulant, and whether the condition of illness was acute or chronic—none of these parameters had any significant effect on the spiritual needs score. Also, the organ system the main diagnosis referred to and the comorbidity index did not have any statistically significant influence on the expression of spiritual needs. Overall it can be said that none of the examined medical parameters had a noticeable impact on the spiritual needs (Frick et al. 2020).

So far, sociodemographic variables such as gender, age, and religious affiliation had significant effects on the expression of spiritual needs, but none of the medical characteristics. To analyze the impact of the significant sociodemographic variables, a multiple analysis of variance (MANOVA) was performed with the spiritual needs as dependent variables. This analysis showed that *Religious* needs were influenced by gender and age, but mainly by religious affiliation. Female gender showed a weak effect on the *Existential*, *Inner Peace*, and *Giving/Generativity* needs (Frick et al. 2020). Thus, there are probably other indicators for patients' spiritual needs that remain to be characterized.

The research questions formulated in the introduction can be answered as follows:

1. Even in the special environment of an emergency room, time and space to assess the spiritual needs of patients can be found. The response rate of 80% reflects a high acceptance of the survey by the patients.
2. Patients predominantly voiced *Inner Peace* needs and *Giving/Generativity* needs, and to a lesser extent also *Religious* needs and *Existential* needs.

3. Women expressed more *Existential* needs, *Religious* needs, and *Inner Peace* needs than men. *Religious* needs were higher in patients with religious affiliations, especially in Muslim patients. The younger patients had significantly less *Inner Peace* needs and in trend less *Religious* needs than the other age groups.
4. Neither the affected organ system, the urgency of treatment (reflected by the ESI) nor the experience of pain or any of the other examined medical parameters had significant influence on the expression of spiritual needs in the surveyed sample of emergency room patients.

Positioning the Findings in the Research Context

The emergency room is often the first contact point between patient and hospital and is intended to make a quick and efficient decision how to proceed with patients (Fleischmann 2016). It is remarkable that despite little time and complex organizational structures it was possible to conduct an assessment of spiritual needs in emergency patients. Many patients were willing to complete the survey and sometimes the assessment was followed by longer conversations about these needs. One definition of spiritual care is the "recognition of the role of patients' religion and/or spirituality in illness and attention to religious/spiritual concern" (Balboni et al. 2011). Consequently, the assessment itself is a form of spiritual care that gives patients the possibility to speak about their distress. As the field notes show, the assessment has been perceived as helpful by those patients who were grateful for the conversation that left them relieved and calmer than before.

The most significant needs were *Inner Peace* needs and *Giving/Generativity* needs. This is consistent with other studies using the SpNQ in patients with chronic diseases, cancer, and elderly living in nursing/residential homes (Büssing et al. 2010, 2011; Erichsen and Büssing 2013). Generative acts like passing on one's life experience, giving away something of oneself or consoling someone can create the feeling that one's life is meaningful and of value to others (Büssing et al. 2015). In patients with chronic diseases, actively giving shows an association with higher life satisfaction and can be interpreted as the patients' wish to stop being a "passive sufferer" and turn into an active individual with a useful role in life (Murray et al. 2004; Büssing and Koenig 2010).

For the patients interviewed, the most important *Inner Peace* needs were to plunge into beauty of nature and to dwell at a place of quietness and peace. These wishes can be interpreted as the longing to return to a more relaxed emotional state. Spending time in a calm and peaceful environment makes it easier to reach a balanced and peaceful inner state because it works as an external facilitator (Büssing et al. 2013). This shows that the patients want to get away from the stressful atmosphere in the emergency room with its noise, artificial light, pain, and insecurity. To relieve the stress, they long for a place of peace, quietness, harmony, beauty, and nature.

As one may expect, *Religious* needs scored higher in people with religious affiliation. The finding that Muslim patients voiced significantly more *Religious* needs compared to Christian patients has to be interpreted with care. First, there was only a small number of Muslims who took part in the study (n = 24); second, the interviewers were apparently socialized as Christians or at least not Muslims so that the results are likely to be subjected to social biases and need to be verified in future studies. Further, *Religious* needs were less relevant for younger patients compared to older ones. As the end of life gets closer, people are confronted more and more with the challenge to design their life in a different way. The process of somatic ageing, the confrontation with frailty, and the growing proximity of death raise questions about the meaning of life. While physical strength starts to decrease, religion and spirituality contain the opportunity to discover new mental and intellectual potential and to cope with losses and the challenges of ageing (Weyel 2009).

As described, some of the demographic characteristics are related to differences in the expression of spiritual needs. Surprisingly, none of the medical parameters had a significant effect on the intensity of the spiritual needs. Thus, different factors may be considered, that is, anxiety, depressive states, and confidence in manageability of symptoms. One explanation is that it may take time for patients to reflect on their distress, their needs, and their coping strategies to fully comprehend the ongoing situation and find the best way to deal with it. Analyzing and developing coping mechanisms requires sufficient time and rest (Frick et al. 2020).

The literature on spiritual needs in emergency situations is scarce, but in other fields of medicine the impact of illness on spiritual needs has already been studied. In some studies, the results were similar to the present ones, with no significant effect of medical parameters on the expressed spiritual needs. In patients with early and advanced cancer, differences could be found in the expression of spiritual needs depending on the sociodemographic characteristics of the sample (Höcker et al. 2014). Nevertheless, none of the medical characteristics showed a significant influence on the spiritual needs score or its subscales. It was concluded that the spiritual needs might not depend on the cancer stage but appear independently from the course and duration of the illness. Consequently, the needs of patients in early stages of illness and curative treatment should also be taken into account (Höcker et al. 2014). Similarly, in patients with malignant melanoma the course of the illness had no influence on their spiritual needs (Haußmann et al. 2018). When using the SpNQ on patients with chronic diseases, neither symptom scores nor pain disability scores had an effect on specific spiritual needs (Büssing et al. 2013).

Based on these results, one might assume that the course of the illness and other medical characteristics simply do not change the spiritual needs of patients. However, other studies have found an impact of illness on religion/spirituality and spiritual needs. In an assessment of the spiritual needs of patients with chronic pain conditions and cancer, cancer patients expressed significantly more spiritual needs. The fatality of cancer as an illness seemed to have a non-neglectable influence on patients' needs (Büssing et al. 2010). Another study with advanced cancer patients showed a growing importance of religion/spirituality when patients were confronted with their own death and the finiteness of life (Balboni et al. 2007). For hospitalized primary care patients, it could be found that the religious coping was used more often the more severe the illness was felt to be (Ellis et al. 2013). These findings differ with respect to the endpoint, as patients may activate their faith as a resource, and thus may start to pray in times of illness, while their needs may not be triggered by the strength of symptoms but by the resources that are (or are not) available.

It is known that "major life events" raise religious questions and lead to reexamination of existing values and life goals (Weyel 2009). Therefore, it seems very likely for the severity of illness and acuity to have an impact on the development of spiritual needs. Due to the nature of the emergency room, the sample of the present study was very inhomogeneous in regard to the medical characteristics with different affected organ systems, life-threatening illnesses or minor trauma, and diverse comorbidities. To find out more subtle differences and to examine the effect of medical characteristics on the spiritual needs in more detail, a similar study with a larger sample is required.

However diverse the sample may be, all the examined patients shared the same surroundings and atmosphere of the emergency room. The effect of this acute situation might be visible in the relatively high *Inner Peace* need scores of the sample as an expression of the longing to escape from a stressful situation and reach a peaceful state of mind (Büssing et al. 2013).

Due to the organizational structure of the emergency room and the limited time, we cannot exclude that patients could not be approached at a set time and place. They were interviewed at different times before, during, or after treatment and in the waiting room, the hallway, or the consulting rooms. The relatively high number of participants and the 80% response rate are good indicators for the potential of spiritual assessment even in the emergency room.

Conclusion

It was possible to conduct a cross-sectional assessment of spiritual needs even in a hospital's emergency room, and patients were willing to express their needs. Especially the impact of the severity and the course of the illness on the development of spiritual needs should be reevaluated in larger studies.

It is indisputable that many patients have unmet spiritual needs during their hospital stay as an in-patient or ambulant patient. As other studies have found, patients frequently want the health care professionals to address their spiritual needs (Selby et al. 2017; Kruizinga et al. 2018). This requires medical staff to have a basic spiritual care competence to identify patients' spiritual needs and respond to them appropriately (Frick et al. 2019, 2020). As a next step, it would be important to analyze how patients' unmet spiritual needs match with the medical staff's spiritual care competence and health professionals' abilities to react to these needs in the hospital (Frick et al. 2019). In order to provide good spiritual care to patients in need, the necessary processes have to be defined and established. This may include spiritual care training, spiritual assessment, appropriate consideration of spiritual care in billing models and many more (Kruizinga et al. 2018; Frick et al. 2020).

References

Balboni TA, Vanderwerker LC, Block SD, Paulk ME, Lathan CS, Peteet JR, Prigerson HG (2007) Religiousness and spiritual support among advanced cancer patients and associations with end-of-life treatment preferences and quality of life. J Clin Oncol 25(5):555–560. https://doi.org/10.1200/JCO.2006.07.9046

Balboni T, Balboni M, Paulk ME, Phelps A, Wright A, Peteet J et al (2011) Support of cancer patients' spiritual needs and associations with medical care costs at the end of life. Cancer 117(23):5383–5391. https://doi.org/10.1002/cncr.26221

Büssing A, Koenig HG (2010) Spiritual needs of patients with chronic diseases. Religions 1(1):18–27. https://doi.org/10.3390/rel1010018

Büssing A, Balzat HJ, Heusser P (2010) Spiritual needs of patients with chronic pain diseases and cancer—validation of the spiritual needs questionnaire. Eur J Med Res 15:266–273

Büssing A, Lux E, Janko A, Kopf A (2011) Psychosoziale und spirituelle Bedürfnisse bei Patienten mit chronischen Schmerz- und Krebserkrankungen. Deutsche Zeitschrift für Onkologie 43(2):69–73. https://doi.org/10.1055/s-0030-1257626

Büssing A, Janko A, Baumann K, Hvidt NC, Kopf A (2013) Spiritual needs among patients with chronic pain diseases and Cancer living in a secular society. Pain Med 14:1362–1373

Büssing A, Pilchowska I, Surzykiewicz J (2015) Spiritual needs of polish patients with chronic diseases. J Relig Health 54(5):1524–1542. https://doi.org/10.1007/s10943-014-9863-x

Charlson ME, Pompei P, Ales KL, MacKenzie R (1987) A new method of classifying prognostic comorbidity in longitudinal studies: development and validation. J Chronic Dis 40(5):373–383

Edwards A, Pang N, Shiu V, Chan C (2010) The understanding of spirituality and the potential role of spiritual care in end-of-life and palliative care: a meta-study of qualitative research. Palliat Med 8:753–770. https://doi.org/10.1177/0269216310375860

Eiff W, Dodt C, Niehues C, Fleischmann T, Brachmann M (2016) Management der Notaufnahme. Patientenorientierung und optimale Ressourcennutzung als strategischer Erfolgsfaktor, vol 2. Kohlhammer, Stuttgart

Ellis MR, Thomlinson P, Gemmill C, Harris W (2013) The spiritual needs and resources of hospitalized primary care patients. J Relig Health 52(4):1306–1318. https://doi.org/10.1007/s10943-012-9575-z

Erichsen N-B, Büssing A (2013) Spiritual needs of elderly living in residential/nursing homes. Evid Based Complement Alternat Med. https://doi.org/10.1155/2013/913247

Fleischmann T (2016) Schnittstelle Zentrale Notaufnahme. Dtsch Med Wochenschr 141(1):19–23. https://doi.org/10.1055/s-0041-108906

Frick E, Theiss M, Rodrigues Recchia D, Büssing A (2019) Validierung einer deutschsprachigen Spiritual Care-Kompetenz-Skala. Spiritual Care 8(2):193–207. https://doi.org/10.1515/spircare-2018-0066

Frick E, Büssing A, Rodrigues Recchia D, Härtl K, Beivers A, Wapler C, Dodt C (2020) Spirituelle Bedürfnisse von Patienten eines Notfallzentrums. Medizinische Klinik, Intensivmedizin und Notfallmedizin. https://doi.org/10.1007/s00063-020-00653-8

Glenister D, Prewer M (2017) Capturing religious identity during hospital admission: a valid practice in our increasingly secular society? Aust Health Rev 41(6):626–631. https://doi.org/10.1071/AH16139

Gordon BS, Keogh M, Davidson Z, Griffiths S, Sharma V, Marin D, Mayer SA, Dangayach NS (2018) Addressing spirituality during critical illness: a review of current literature. J Crit Care 45:76–81. https://doi.org/10.1016/j.jcrc.2018.01.015

Grossmann FF, Delport K, Keller DI (2009) Emergency severity index. Notfall + Rettungsmedizin 12(4):290–292. https://doi.org/10.1007/s10049-009-1156-7

Han C-Y, Lin C-C, Goopy S, Hsiao Y-C, Barnard A, Wang L-H (2017) Waiting and hoping: a phenomenographic study of the experiences of boarded patients in the emergency department. J Clin Nurs 26(5–6):840–848. https://doi.org/10.1111/jocn.13621

Haußmann A, Schäffeler N, Hautzinger M, Weyel B, Eigentler T, Zipfel S, Teufel M (2018) Religiöse/spirituelle Bedürfnisse und psychosoziale Belastung von Patienten mit malignem Melanom. TumorDiagnostik & Therapie 39(2):116–123. https://doi.org/10.1055/s-0044-100824

Höcker A, Krüll A, Koch U, Mehnert A (2014) Exploring spiritual needs and their associated factors in an urban sample of early and advanced cancer patients. Eur J Cancer Care 23(6):786–794. https://doi.org/10.1111/ecc.12200

Jang T, Kryder GD, Char D, Howell R, Primrose J, Tan D (2004) Prehospital spirituality: how well do we know ambulance patients? Prehosp Disaster Med 19(4):356–361. https://doi.org/10.1017/S1049023X00001989

Kruizinga R, Scherer-Rath M, Schilderman H, Puchalski CM, van Laarhoven H (2018) Toward a fully fledged integration of spiritual care and medical care. J Pain Symptom Manag 55(3):1035–1040. https://doi.org/10.1016/j.jpainsymman.2017.11.015

Murray SA, Kendall M, Boyd K, Worth A, Benton TF (2004) Exploring the spiritual needs of people dying of lung cancer or heart failure: a prospective qualitative interview study of patients and their carers. Palliat Med 18(1):39–45. https://doi.org/10.1191/0269216304pm837oa

Selby D, Seccaraccia D, Huth J, Kurppa K, Fitch M (2017) Patient versus health care provider perspectives on spirituality and spiritual care: the potential to miss the moment. Ann Palliat Med 6(2):143–152. https://doi.org/10.21037/apm.2016.12.03

Wensley C, Botti M, McKillop A, Merry AF (2017) A framework of comfort for practice: an integrative review identifying the multiple influences on patients' experience of comfort in healthcare settings. Int J Qual Health Care 29(2):151–162. https://doi.org/10.1093/intqhc/mzw158

Weyel B (2009) Aszetik: Spiritualität und Religiosität im Alter. In: Kunz R, Klie T, Kumlehn M (eds) Praktische Theologie des Alterns. De Gruyter, Berlin, pp 597–614

Weyrich P, Christ M, Celebi N, Riessen R (2012) Triagesysteme in der Notaufnahme. Medizinische Klinik, Intensivmedizin und Notfallmedizin (1):67–78. https://doi.org/10.1007/s00063-011-0075-9

CHAPTER 20

Spiritual Needs of People with Autism Spectrum Disorder

Jan Christopher Cwik

Introduction

The phenomenon of autism spectrum disorder (ASD) was increasingly focused on psychotherapeutic and psychiatric research in the past, and the number of studies on ASD grew over the last decades (see the meta-analysis of Barger et al. 2013). Initially, autism spectrum symptoms were reported by Sucharewa (1926) in her case report on children with autistic symptoms. However, the fundamental description of autism spectrum symptoms is often ascribed to Kanner (1943) and Asperger (1944), who published their first systematic case reports on patients with autistic symptoms and introduced the concept of autism as a categorical disorder. However, as recently as the publication of the third edition of the Diagnostic and Statistical Manual of mental disorders (DSM-III; American Psychiatric Association [APA] 1980), autism diagnoses were first introduced as codable syndromes. Since then, there were several adaptions

J. C. Cwik (✉)
Department of Clinical Psychology and Psychotherapy, Faculty of Human Sciences, University of Cologne, Köln, Germany
e-mail: jcwik@uni-koeln.de

A. Büssing (ed.), *Spiritual Needs in Research and Practice*,
https://doi.org/10.1007/978-3-030-70139-0_20

to the classification of autistic diagnoses and related symptoms. In 2013, the fifth edition of the DSM (DSM-5; APA 2013) was published. The categorical concept of autistic syndromes was dropped, and the dimensional concept of the autism spectrum disorder (ASD) was introduced as part of the section of neurodevelopment disorders. According to the diagnostic criteria of the DSM-5, the criteria of ASD comprise persistent deficits in (1) social communication and (2) interaction across multiple contexts (e.g., social–emotional reciprocity or nonverbal communicative behaviors used for social interaction) and restricted, repetitive patterns of behavior, interests, or activities (e.g., stereotyped or repetitive motor movements, use of speech or inflexible adherence to routines, or hyper- or hypo-reactivity to sensory input). These symptoms must persist throughout the individual's early developmental period and must cause clinically significant impairment in daily life. Furthermore, the symptoms must not be better explained by intellectual disability or global developmental delay (see APA 2013, 50–51). These criteria are also carried over to the eleventh edition of the International Statistical Classification of Diseases and related health problems (ICD-11; see World Health Organization 2017, 2018).

According to the DSM-5, about 1% of all children, adolescents, and adults fulfill an ASD diagnosis (APA 2013). However, there is also evidence that the rate of ASD is internationally overestimated and encompasses approximately a half to a third of the reported range of rates (Fisch 2012). Although epidemiological studies report lower prevalence rates of about 10–70 cases per 10,000 (Tsai 2014; Rutter 2007), an increase of the incidence of ASD of the factor of 7.5–15 within the last five decades has been reported (Rutter 2007). However, this increase is likely related to the development and availability of diagnostic instruments (Rutter 2007; Ouellette-Kuntz et al. 2014). Furthermore, the prevalence rates will likely decrease due to changes in the diagnostic criteria from DSM-IV to DSM-5 (Kim et al. 2014; Tsai 2014). The meta-analysis results of Barger et al. (2013) showed that males suffer about 4.5 times more often from ASD than females. Furthermore, prevalence rates of ASD are higher in White children than children of other ethnicities (Zahorodny et al. 2014).

ASD is associated with a significant impairment of quality of life. In a study in the United Kingdom, 370 people with an ASD diagnosis were investigated regarding their subjective quality of life (Mason et al. 2018). As a result of this study, adults with an ASD diagnosis reported a significantly lower quality of life than adults of the general population, whereas younger people with ASD reported a higher quality of life than older people with ASD. Furthermore, meta-regressive results illustrated that the quality of life of people with ASD is associated with social functioning (Kim and Bottema-Beutel 2019). Also, the daily living skills of people with ASD were significantly associated with a higher quality of life of people with ASD (Kamp-Becker et al. 2010). Given the significant impairment and burdens of people with ASD in daily life and the relatively low quality of life, people with ASD could benefit from a psychotherapeutic treatment to improve their social functioning, daily living skills, and quality of life.

Religiosity and Spirituality as Resources in Psychotherapy

Identifying patients' unique resources is a crucial point of several psychotherapeutic concepts and is a mechanism of action for the therapeutic process (Willutzki and Teismann 2013; Fiedler 2011). According to the meta-analysis results of 897 approach-independent psychotherapy studies, a central mechanism of psychotherapeutic action is the identification and utilization of unique resources of patients (Grawe et al. 2001). However, for identifying resources, it is essential that both the patient and the therapist are congruent (both can identify a resource) regarding a potential resource, whereas incongruence hinders a successful identification (Willutzki 2000). Thus, it is necessary to sensitize therapists for potential resources (Willutzki 2000).

Such a resource is the religiosity and spirituality of patients. Study results illustrated the general importance of the resource of religiosity and spirituality for patients (Haußmann et al. 2018). Nevertheless, psychotherapists' sense of religiosity and spirituality is moderate (Shafranske and Malony 1990; Hofmann and Walach 2011; Hofmann 2011). Accordingly, patients would benefit if psychotherapists would be more sensitive to this specific resource (Vieten et al. 2013).

Religiosity and Spirituality and ASD

Religiosity and Spirituality of Relatives of Children with ASD

Religiosity and spirituality are relatively well examined in psychotherapy and psychiatry (Bonelli and Koenig 2013; Rew and Wong 2006; Wong et al. 2006; Zimmer et al. 2016). However, religiosity and spirituality are investigated in the context of ASD to a lesser extent. Nevertheless, due to the bio-psycho-social limitations that are associated with ASD, religiosity and spirituality have been seen with ASD (Swinton and Trevett 2009). Fortunately, this perspective has faded into the background, and research in this area increases continuously (Kaye and Raghavan 2002), albeit most research focuses on qualitative analyses surveyed from parents of children with ASD. One of these studies showed that Irish parents of children with ASD look upon their religiosity and spirituality as an essential resource to face the burdens associated with the ASD diagnosis of their children (Coulthard and Fitzgerald 1999). Other studies illustrated that higher manifestations of religious and spiritual practices and beliefs are associated with increased well-being of parents of children with ASD (Ekas et al. 2009; Huws et al. 2016). Other studies also identified religiosity and spirituality as a resilience factor (Bayat 2007) or coping-mechanism (Luther et al. 2005; Gray 2006) for parents of children with ASD. Furthermore, these results were shown across religious orientations (Jegatheesan et al. 2010; Jegatheesan 2013; Shaked 2005; Das et al. 2017; Pandya 2018).

Religiosity and Spirituality in Adults with ASD

Whereas there is some evidence regarding the relevance of religiosity and spirituality as coping and resilience factors in family members of people with ASD, research of these aspects in people with ASD is rare. Visuri (2012) investigated the attitudes regarding religiosity and spirituality of four adults with ASD using qualitative interviews. The results showed that the interviewed people described God as a passive person and could not name God's specific intentions. Furthermore, the interviewees reported that God would not respond to prayers, but ghosts and guardian angels would favorably interact with humans. Crespi et al. (2019) investigated the associations between spirituality and autism symptoms in a sample of healthy adults without fulfilling ASD diagnostic criteria. Participants filled out self-rating questionnaires to rate the extent of spirituality and autism symptoms. The results of the study illustrated that there is a significant negative association between spirituality and autism symptoms.

Furthermore, the authors report a significant negative association between faith in God and autism symptoms. However, considering that the authors investigated a sample that did not fulfill the ASD criteria, these results should be transferred to ASD with caution. Additionally, the spirituality in this study focused on faith in God, whereas other facets of spirituality were not investigated. Hills et al. (2019) conducted an interview study with people with severe ASD, also called nonverbal autism, because people with this form of ASD are unable to communicate verbally. The results of this study showed that also people with this severe ASD appraise spirituality as an important source for their well-being. Thus, the interviewees also reported of spiritual practices in their everyday life. These results indicate that religiosity and spirituality could be relevant for people with ASD, but could their relevance be different compared with the general population?

In his theoretical consideration, Deeley (2009) discussed two potential explanations of why people with ASD exhibit religiosity and spirituality to a lower extent than the general population. He considers that one of these factors is the deficit of people with ASD to mentalize perspectives, opinions, or beliefs of others—the so-called theory of mind. As the second factor, Deeley discusses that people with ASD are especially interested in nonsocial activities so that religiosity and spirituality are less relevant for people with ASD. However, Deeley points out that these considerations are solely theoretical due to a lack of evidence and empirical research in this field.

Spiritual and Religious Attitudes in Dealing with Illness and Spiritual Needs in Adults with Autism Spectrum Disorder

As illustrated, the reported studies investigated the relevance of religiosity and spirituality in relatives of children with ASD or adults with ASD symptoms in the broadest sense. However, a concrete quantitative investigation of religiosity and spirituality in a sample of adults fulfilling the criteria of ASD is missing. Thus, Cwik and Büssing (2019) conducted a cross-sectional study to collect quantitative data of the spiritual needs of adults with ASD. Parts for the results were reported recently (Cwik and Büssing 2019). The aims of the study were to investigate:

1. Which dimensions of spirituality and gratitude are relevant for adult people with ASD?
2. Are there age- or gender-specifics in adult people with ASD regarding spirituality that are comparable with the general population?

3. Are there significant associations between spirituality and self-efficacy, social connections, and life satisfaction in adult people with ASD?

The results of the study should provide additional knowledge regarding spirituality as a potential resource for adult people with ASD that could be relevant for support programs or psychotherapy.

The data were collected by using an online survey (SoSciSurvey; Leiner 2014). Participants were recruited in online forums, self-help groups, and social networks. After giving their informed consent, participants were able to fill out the self-rating questionnaires.

Overall, $N = 201$ adults with ASD took part in this study. Participants were at an average 37.4 ± 12.4 [18–63] years old. Most participants (66%) were female, had a higher education entrance qualification (65%; secondary school certificate 22%, others 13%), were employed (52%), and were living alone (42%) or living with their partner (39%). The majority of participants reported being diagnosed with Asperger's syndrome (88%), followed by a general ASD diagnosis (5%), and other forms of autism (7%). Approximately one out of four stated having faith in God or Allāh (30%), 15% participants were undecided, and the majority (57%) stated to be faithless.

To measure spiritual needs as well as the usage of spiritual and religious practices in everyday life in adults with ASD, and the associations with quality of life, the following questionnaires were used (note: internal consistencies of measures for the current sample of people with ASD were measured with McDonald's omega (McDonald 1970, 1999) [ω]): The Spiritual Needs Questionnaire (SpNQ) (Büssing et al. 2010, 2018) was used in a 14-item version that refrains from linguistically complicated items. All items are rated on a four-point scale, ranging from zero (not at all) to three (very strong). Higher scores indicate greater spiritual needs.

Frequency of different forms of spiritual practices was measured with the 17-item SpREUK-P (Büssing et al. 2012). Items are rated on a four-point scale ranging from zero (never) to three (regularly). As facets of spiritual and religious practices, the following five subscales were measured: (1) religious practices ($\omega = 0.87$), (2) prosocial/humanistic practices ($\omega = 0.65$), (3) existentialistic ($\omega = 0.78$), (4) gratitude/awe ($\omega = 0.68$), and (5) spiritual mind/body practices ($\omega = 0.79$).

Life satisfaction was measured with the 10-item Brief Multidimensional Life Satisfaction Scale (BMLSS-10 (Büssing et al. 2009). All items of the

BMLSS-10 are scored on a six-point scale, ranging from zero (terrible) to six (delighted). Means scored were transferred to a 100% scale.

Sources of meaning in life were measured with five items of the Sources of Meaning and Meaning in Life Questionnaire (SoME) ($\omega = 0.84$) (Schnell and Becker 2007). These items are rated on a six-point self-rating scale, ranging from zero (totally disagree) to five (totally agree).

Self-efficacy was measured with the 10-item General Self-Efficacy scale (GSE; $\omega = 0.89$) (Schwarzer and Jerusalem 1999; Jerusalem and Schwarzer 2014). Each item is rated on a four-point scale, ranging from one (not at all true) to four (exactly true).

Besides these questionnaires, some additional measures for the assessment of the quality of life of people with ASD were used in the study. Participants were asked to rate to what extent they spend their leisure time with friends, going to the cinema, and going out alone. These three items were all rated on a scale from zero (not at all) to three (much). Subsequently, participants were asked regarding their job-related situation (zero = having no job or one = having a job/going to school). Finally, a score of independence was calculated by summing up all four items ranging from zero (low independence) to 10 (high independence).

The results of the study showed that people with ASD generally have spiritual needs and use religious and spiritual practices (see Table 20.1). Accordingly, spiritual and religious needs and practices could be potential

Table 20.1 Range, means, and standard deviations of measures in adult people with ASD

	Min	*Max*	*Mean*	*Standard deviation*
SpNQ-14: Religious needs	0	3	0.46	0.74
SpNQ-14: Existential needs	0	3	1.32	0.79
SpNQ-14 Inner Peace needs	0	3	2.11	0.81
SpNQ-14: Giving/Generativity needs	0	3	1.45	0.92
SpREUK-P SF17: Religious practices	0	100	15.33	23.17
SpREUK-P SF17: Prosocial/humanistic practices	0	100	65.77	18.07
SpREUK-P SF17: Existentialistic practices	0	100	69.47	23.63
SpREUK-P SF17: Gratitude/awe	0	100	49.98	20.98
SpREUK-P SF17: Spiritual mind/body practices	0	100	20.05	24.11
BMLSS-10: Life satisfaction	0	100	52.81	19.01
SoME: Meaning in life	0	30	14.71	7.95
GSE: Self-efficacy expectation	10	36	22.33	5.67
Independence	0	7	2.90	1.28

resources for people with ASD and should be assessed at the beginning of potential psychotherapy (Büssing and Frick 2015). However, considering the results of studies on other people with chronic illnesses, people with ASD report fewer spiritual needs and religious and spiritual practices (Büssing et al. 2016; Büssing and Recchia 2016).

A closer look at the reported spiritual needs shows that people with ASD particularly had strong needs for *Inner Peace*. This could be due to the perceived burdens of everyday life that people with ASD undergo. People with ASD also reported moderate manifestations of *Existential* needs and *Giving/Generativity* needs, whereas *Religious* needs scored low. This is in line with the results of studies on patients with posttraumatic stress disorder (Glavas et al. 2017), chronic illness (Büssing et al. 2018), or cancer (Büssing et al. 2010) that also showed that patients report high needs for *Inner Peace*. Overall, people with ASD reported higher psychosocial and spiritual needs than people with somatic diseases (Büssing et al. 2018). These results could also reflect the degree of suffering in social interactions; one could mention that people with ASD develop psychosocial and spiritual needs due to their psychosocial limitations. Considering the low levels of *Religious* needs of people with ASD, participants unsurprisingly reported less frequent religious practices and spiritual mind/body practices. In contrast, existentialistic practices and prosocial/humanistic practices were relatively frequently reported. This is in line with the results of higher *Inner peace*, *Existential*, and *Giving/Generativity* needs. Interestingly, faith in God or Allāh was reported by merely one out of four participants. This could also be an explanation for the relatively low manifestations of religious and spiritual needs and practices.

The conducted correlation analyses showed that particularly *Religious* needs of people with ASD are associated with sources of meaning and meaning of life (see Table 20.2). Furthermore, *Existential* needs showed a weak negative association with satisfaction with life, whereas none of the assessed spiritual needs was significantly associated with general self-efficacy or independence in the investigated people with ASD. Furthermore, only *Inner Peace* need correlated marginally with age ($rS = 0.14$, $p = 0.047$) and none of the spiritual practices (SpREUK-P SF17). Accordingly, older people with ASD report higher needs for *Inner Peace*. Interestingly, Gratitude/Awe as a measure of a person's ability to stop in wondering awe with subsequent feelings of gratitude was strongly related with sources of meaning (Table 20.2).

Table 20.2 Correlations between spiritual needs, frequency of spiritual practices, and indicators of quality of life

	Spiritual needs				*Frequency of spiritual practices*					*Quality of life indicators*			
	Religious	*Existential*	*Inner Peace*	*Giving / Generativity*	*Religious*	*Prosocial-humanistic*	*Existential*	*Gratitude/ Awe*	*Spiritual Mind-Body*	*Life satisfaction*	*Sources of meaning*	*Self-efficacy expectation*	*Independence*
Religious needs	1.000	**0.509****	0.199**	**0.345****	**0.776****	0.169	0.288**	0.282**	0.164	0.019	**0.393****	0.056	0.114
Existential needs		1.000	**0.377****	**0.403****	**0.365****	0.231**	**0.518****	0.289**	0.280**	-0.200**	0.214**	0.043	0.127
Inner Peace needs			1.000	0.162	0.122	0.044	**0.347****	0.182**	**0.384****	-0.095	0.088	-0.027	0.015
Giving/ Generativity needs				1.000	0.259**	0.245**	0.204**	0.080	0.196**	-0.038	0.187**	0.085	0.109
Religious practices					1.000	0.081	0.161	**0.334****	0.194**	0.068	**0.440****	0.017	0.111
Prosocial-humanistic practices						1.000	0.167	0.108	0.130	-0.028	0.229**	0.122	-0.012
Existential practices							1.000	0.168	**0.327****	-0.163	0.214**	0.085	0.011
Gratitude/ awe								1.000	0.212**	0.315**	**0.562****	0.276**	0.171
Spiritual mind–body practices									1.000	0.069	0.232**	0.051	0.010

**$p < 0.01$ (Spearman rank correlation coefficient); moderate to strong correlations are highlighted (bold)

To explore the associations between the relatively high correlations between spiritual needs as well as spiritual and religious practices and sources of meaning and meaning in life, a stepwise linear regression analysis with the SoME sum score as a dependent variable was conducted. In the first step, all measures of spiritual needs and spiritual and religious practices were entered. In the second step, age and gender of participants were entered. Finally, formal education, faith, relationship status, autism diagnosis, and extracurricular activities were entered. This model explained 42% of the variance of sources of meaning and meaning in life ($R^2 = 0.42$, $p < 0.001$). In the final model, only Religious practices ($p = 0.006$), Existentialistic practices ($p = 0.025$), and Gratitude/Awe ($p < 0.001$) were significantly associated with sources of meaning and meaning in life, whereas none of the spiritual needs variables were significantly associated. Also, neither the remaining spiritual and religious practices nor the other demographic variables were significantly associated with sources of meaning and meaning in life.

Finally, it was investigated whether spiritual needs, as well as religious and spiritual practices differ between genders of people with ASD. The results showed that there were no significant group-differences of spiritual needs between women and men. Furthermore, regarding most of the religious and spiritual practices, there were no significant group-differences of religious and spiritual practices between women and men with ASD. Only regarding the Gratitude/Awe, women with ASD reported significantly higher scores than men with ASD ($p = 0.029$).

Critical Considerations Regarding Religiosity and Spirituality in the Field of ASD

The reported results illustrated the importance of assessing spirituality and religiosity as potential resources for people with ASD. However, as the results of the study of Cwik and Büssing (2019) also showed, faith and spiritual needs, and spiritual and religious practices are not very common in people with ASD. Their results are in the broadest sense in line with qualitative results, showing that mothers of children with ASD, who are members of a congregation, do not identify their religion as a resource in facing their burdens (Kuhaneck et al. 2010). In turn, this is in line with the results of Cwik and Büssing (2019), showing that spiritual needs and spiritual and religious practices showed predominantly no significant associations with measures of quality of life.

Conclusions

In conclusion, the results provide quantitative evidence that religiosity and spirituality could be relevant to the everyday life of adult people with ASD. Participants reported of spiritual needs, as well as spiritual and religious practices, and the analyses showed that these aspects are associated with several measures of quality of life. However, the results of the study also showed that religious and spiritual practices and needs are less pronounced compared with other samples.

In summary, spirituality and religiosity in people with ASD can be a resource for some individuals, whereas for others it is no resource or could be debilitating. Thus, there is a need for a systematic assessment and evaluation of spiritual needs and religious and spiritual practices as part of the medical history in people with ASD (Büssing and Frick 2015). Nevertheless, even if religious and spiritual practices and needs could be relevant for the therapeutic process for people with ASD, psychotherapy should never become religious or spiritual guidance (Pfeifer 2017). Finally, the results of the study of Cwik and Büssing (2019) suggest that the 14-item version of the SpNQ can be a reliable tool to assess spiritual needs in people with ASD systematically.

Acknowledgments I would like to thank all participants who took part in the study that was the basis for this chapter.

References

American Psychiatric Association (1980) Diagnostic and statistical manual of mental disorders, 3rd edn. American Psychiatric Association, Washington, DC

American Psychiatric Association (2013) Diagnostic and statistical manual of mental disorders, 5th edn. American Psychiatric Association, Washington, DC

Asperger H (1944) Die "Autistischen Psychopathen" im Kindesalter. Arch Psychiatr Nervenkr 117:76–136. https://doi.org/10.1007/BF01837709

Barger BD, Campbell JM, McDonough JD (2013) Prevalence and onset of regression within autism spectrum disorders: a meta-analytic review. J Autism Dev Disord 43(4):817–828. https://doi.org/10.1007/s10803-012-1621-x

Bayat M (2007) Evidence of resilience in families of children with autism. J Intellect Disabil Res 71(9):702–714. https://doi.org/10.1111/j.1365-2788.2007.00960.x

Bonelli RM, Koenig HG (2013) Mental disorders, religion and spirituality 1990 to 2010: a systematic evidence-based review. J Relig Health 52(2):657–673. https://doi.org/10.1007/s10943-013-9691-4

Büssing A, Frick E (2015) Psychosoziale und spirituelle Bedürfnisse chronisch Kranker. In: Büssing A, Surzykiewicz J, Zimowski Z (eds) Dem Gutes tun, der leidet. Springer, Berlin, Heidelberg. https://doi.org/10.1007/978-3-662-44279-1_1

Büssing A, Recchia DR (2016) Spiritual and non-spiritual needs among German soldiers and their relation to stress perception, PTDS symptoms, and life satisfaction: results from a structural equation modeling approach. J Relig Health 55(3):747–764. https://doi.org/10.1007/s10943-015-0073-y

Büssing A, Fischer J, Haller A, Heusser P, Ostermann T, Matthiessen PF (2009) Validation of the brief multidimensional life satisfaction scale in patients with chronic diseases. Eur J Med Res 14(4):171–177. https://doi.org/10.1186/2047-783X-14-4-171

Büssing A, Balzat H-J, Heusser P (2010) Spiritual needs of patients with chronic pain diseases and cancer – validation of the Spiritual Needs Questionnaire. Eur J Med Res 15(6):266–273. https://doi.org/10.1186/2047-783X-15-6-266

Büssing A, Reiser F, Michalsen A, Baumann K (2012) Engagement of patients with chronic diseases in spiritual and secular forms of practice: results with the shortened SpREUK-P SF17 questionnaire. IMCJ 11(1):28–38

Büssing A, Franczak K, Surzykiewicz J (2016) Frequency of spiritual/religious practices in Polish patients with chronic diseases: validation of the Polish version of the SpREUK-P questionnaire. Religions 55(1):67–84. https://doi.org/10.1007/s10943-014-9967-3

Büssing A, Rodrigues Recchia D, Koenig H, Baumann K, Frick E (2018) Factor structure of the Spiritual Needs Questionnaire (SpNQ) in persons with chronic diseases, elderly and healthy individuals. Religions 9(1):13–13. https://doi.org/10.3390/rel9010013

Coulthard P, Fitzgerald M (1999) In God we trust? Organised religion and personal beliefs as resources and coping strategies, and their implications for health in parents with a child on the autistic spectrum. Ment Health Relig Cult 2(1):19–33. https://doi.org/10.1080/13674679908406329

Crespi B, Dinsdale N, Read S, Hurd P (2019) Spirituality, dimensional autism, and schizotypal traits: the search for meaning. PLoS ONE 14(3):e0213456. https://doi.org/10.1371/journal.pone.0213456

Cwik JC, Büssing A (2019) Spiritualität und Religiosität und ihr Zusammenhang mit Lebenszufriedenheit bei Personen mit Autismus-Spektrums-Störung. Spiritual Care 8(3):251–261. https://doi.org/10.1515/spircare-2018-0096

Das S, Das B, Nath K, Dutta A, Bora P, Hazarika M (2017) Impact of stress, coping, social support, and resilience of families having children with autism: a

North East India-based study. Asian J Psychiatr 28:133–139. https://doi.org/10.1016/j.ajp.2017.03.040

Deeley Q (2009) Cognitive style, spirituality, and religious understanding: the case of autism. J Relig Disabil Health 13(1):77–82. https://doi.org/10.1080/15228960802581479

Ekas NV, Whitman TL, Shivers C (2009) Religiosity, spirituality, and socioemotional functioning in mothers of children with autism spectrum disorder. J Autism Dev Disord 39(5):706–719. https://doi.org/10.1007/s10803-008-0673-4

Fiedler P (2011) Ressourcenorientierte Psychotherapie. In: Frank R (ed) Therapieziel Wohlbefinden. Springer, Berlin, Heidelberg. https://doi.org/10.1007/978-3-642-13760-0_2

Fisch GS (2012) Nosology and epidemiology in autism: classification counts. Am J Med Genet C Semin Med Genet 160 C(2):91–103. https://doi.org/10.1002/ajmg.c.31325

Glavas A, Jors K, Bössing A, Baumann K (2017) Spiritual needs of PTSD patients in Croatia and Bosnia-Herzegovina: a quantitative pilot study. Psychiatr Danub 29(3):282–290. https://doi.org/10.24869/psyd.2017.282

Grawe K, Donati R, Bernauer F (2001) Psychotherapie im Wandel: Von der Konfession zur Profession, 5th edn. Hogrefe, Göttingen

Gray DE (2006) Coping over time: the parents of children with autism. J Intellect Disabil Res 50(12):970–976. https://doi.org/10.1111/j.1365-2788.2006.00933.x

Haußmann A, Schäffeler N, Hautzinger M, Weyel B, Eigentler T, Zipfel S, Teufel M (2018) Religiöse/spirituelle Bedürfnisse und psychosoziale Belastung von Patienten mit malignem Melanom. TumorDiagnostik und Therapie 39:116–123. https://doi.org/10.1055/s-0044-100824

Hills K, Clapton J, Dorsett P, Andersen K (2019) Spirituality in the context of nonverbal autism: a research process – analysis and findings. J Disabil Relig 23(4):365–386. https://doi.org/10.1080/23312521.2019.1682104

Hofmann L (2011) Spirituelle oder religiöse Orientierung und deren Auswirkung auf die psychotherapeutische Tätigkeit. In: Büssing A, Kohls N (eds) Spiritualität transdisziplinär – Wissenschaftliche Grundlagen im Zusammenhang mit Gesundheit und Krankheit. Springer, Berlin, Heidelberg, New York, pp 173–196

Hofmann L, Walach H (2011) Spirituality and religiosity in psychotherapy – a representative survey among German psychotherapists. Psychother Res 21(2):179–192. https://doi.org/10.1080/10503307.2010.536595

Huws JC, Jones RSP, Ingledew DK (2016) Parents of children with autism using an email group: a grounded theory study. J Health Psychol 6(5):569–584. https://doi.org/10.1177/135910530100600509

Jegatheesan B (2013) An ethnographic study on religion, spirituality, and maternal influence on sibling relationships in a Muslim family with a child with autism. RDS Int J 9(1):5–19

Jegatheesan B, Miller PJ, Fowler SA (2010) Autism from a religious perspective: a study of parental beliefs in South Asian Muslim immigrant families. Focus Autism Other Dev Disabil 25(2):98–109. https://doi.org/10.1177/1088357610361344

Jerusalem M, Schwarzer R (2014) Allgemeine Selbstwirksamkeitserwartung (SWE). Beschreibung der psychometrischen Skala. https://psycharchives.org/bitstream/20.500.12034/320/1/PT_9001003_SWE_Autorenbeschreibung.pdf. Accesses 17 Sept 2020

Kamp-Becker I, Schröder J, Remschmidt H, Bachmann CJ (2010) Health-related quality of life in adolescents and young adults with high functioning autism-spectrum disorder. GMS Psycho-Soc-Med 7.:Doc03. https://doi.org/10.3205/psm000065

Kanner L (1943) Autistic disturbances of affective contact. Nerv Child 2:217–250

Kaye J, Raghavan SK (2002) Spirituality in disability and illness. J Relig Health 41:231–242. https://doi.org/10.1023/A:1020284819593

Kim SY, Bottema-Beutel K (2019) A meta regression analysis of quality of life correlates in adults with ASD. Res Autism Spectr Disord 63:23–33. https://doi.org/10.1016/j.rasd.2018.11.004

Kim YS, Fombonne E, Koh Y-J, Kim S-J, Cheon K-A, Leventhal BL (2014) A comparison of DSM-IV pervasive developmental disorder and DSM-5 autism spectrum disorder prevalence in an epidemiologic sample. J Am Acad Child Adolesc Psychiatry 53(5):500–508. https://doi.org/10.1016/j.jaac.2013.12.021

Kuhaneck HM, Burroughs T, Wright J, Lemanczyk T, Darragh AR (2010) A qualitative study of coping in mothers of children with an autism spectrum disorder. Phys Occup Ther Pediatr 30(4):340–350. https://doi.org/10.3109/01942638.2010.481662

Leiner DJ (2014) SoSci Survey (Version 2.4.00-i) [Computer Software].

Luther EH, Canham DL, Cureton VY (2005) Coping and social support for parents of children with autism. J Sch Nurs 21(1):40–47. https://doi.org/10.1622/1059-8405(2005)021[0040:cassfp]2.0.co;2

Mason D, McConachie H, Garland D, Petrou A, Rodgers J, Parr JR (2018) Predictors of quality of life for autistic adults. Autism Res 11(8):1138–1147. https://doi.org/10.1002/aur.1965

McDonald RP (1970) The theoretical foundations of principal factor analysis, canonical factor, and alpha factor analysis. Br J Math Stat Psychol 23(1):1–21. https://doi.org/10.1111/j.2044-8317.1970.tb00432.x

McDonald RP (1999) Test theory: a unified treatment. Lawrence Erlbaum Associates, Inc., Mahwah, NJ

Ouellette-Kuntz H, Coo H, Lam M, Breitenbach MM, Hennessey PE, Jackman PD, Lewis MES, Dewey D, Bernier FP, Chung AM (2014) The changing prevalence of autism in three regions of Canada. J Autism Dev Disord 44(1):120–136. https://doi.org/10.1007/s10803-013-1856-1

Pandya SP (2018) Spirituality to build resilience in primary caregiver parents of children with autism spectrum disorders: a cross-country experiment. Int J Dev Disabil 64(1):53–64. https://doi.org/10.1080/20473869.2016.1222722

Pfeifer S (2017) Religiöse Patienten und säkulare Therapeuten – ein ethisch-professionelles Spannungsfeld. Spiritual Care 6(1):21–29. https://doi.org/10.1515/spircare-2016-0123

Rew L, Wong YJ (2006) A systematic review of associations among religiosity/spirituality and adolescent health attitudes and behaviors. J Adolesc Health 38(4):433–442. https://doi.org/10.1016/j.jadohealth.2005.02.004

Rutter M (2007) Incidence of autism spectrum disorders: changes over time and their meaning. Acta Paediatr 94(1):2–15. https://doi.org/10.1111/j.1651-2227.2005.tb01779.x

Schnell T, Becker P (2007) Fragebogen zu Lebensbedeutung und Lebenssinn (LeBe). Hogrefe, Göttingen

Schwarzer R, Jerusalem M (1999) Skalen zur Erfassung von Lehrer- und Schülermerkmalen. Dokumentation der psychometrischen Verfahren im Rahmen der wissenschaftlichen Begleitung des Modellversuchs Selbstwirksame Schulen. Freie Universität Berlin, Berlin

Shafranske EP, Malony HN (1990) Clinical psychologists' religious and spiritual orientations and their practice of psychotherapy. Psychother Theory Res Pract Train 27(1):72–78. https://doi.org/10.1037/0033-3204.27.1.72

Shaked M (2005) The social trajectory of illness: autism in the ultraorthodox community in Israel. Soc Sci Med 61(10):2190–2200. https://doi.org/10.1016/j.socscimed.2005.04.022

Sucharewa GJ (1926) Die schizoiden Psychopathien im Kindesalter. Monatsschr Psychiatr Neurol 60(3-4):235–247. https://doi.org/10.1159/000190478

Swinton J, Trevett C (2009) Religion and autism: initiating an interdisciplinary conversation. J Relig Disabil Health 13(1):2–6. https://doi.org/10.1080/15228960802606193

Tsai LY (2014) Impact of DSM-5 on epidemiology of autism spectrum disorder. Res Autism Spectr Disord 8(11):1454–1470. https://doi.org/10.1016/j.rasd.2014.07.016

Vieten C, Scammell S, Pilato R, Ammondson I, Pargament KI, Lukoff D (2013) Spiritual and religious competencies for psychologists. Psychol Relig Spiritual 5(3):129–144. https://doi.org/10.1037/a0032699

Visuri I (2012) Could everyone talk to god? A case study on Asperger's syndrome, religion, and spirituality. J Relig Disabil Health 16(4):352–378. https://doi.org/10.1080/15228967.2012.731888

Willutzki U (2000) Ressourcenorientierung in der Psychotherapie – eine "neue" Perspektive? In: Hermer M (ed) Psychotherapeutische Perspektiven am Beginn des 21. Jahrhunderts. DGVT-Verlag, Tübingen, pp 193–212
Willutzki U, Teismann T (2013) Ressourcenaktivierung in der Psychotherapie. Hogrefe, Göttingen
Wong YJ, Rew L, Slaikeu KD (2006) A systematic review of recent research on adolescent religiosity/spirituality and mental health. Issues Ment Health Nurs 27(2):161–183. https://doi.org/10.1080/01612840500436941
World Health Organization (2017) ICD-11 beta draft. https://icd.who.int/dev11/l-m/en.
World Health Organization (2018) ICD-11 for mortality and morbidity statistics. https://icd.who.int/browse11/l-m/en#/http%3a%2f%2fid.who.int%2ficd%2f entity%2f437815624. Accesses 17 Sept 2020
Zahorodny W, Shenouda J, Howell S, Rosato NS, Peng B, Mehta U (2014) Increasing autism prevalence in metropolitan New Jersey. Autism 18(2):117–126. https://doi.org/10.1177/1362361312463977
Zimmer Z, Jagger C, Chiu C-T, Ofstedal MB, Rojo F, Saito Y (2016) Spirituality, religiosity, aging and health in global perspective: a review. SSM-Population Health 2:373–381. https://doi.org/10.1016/j.ssmph.2016.04.009

CHAPTER 21

Spiritual Needs of Persons with Down Syndrome

Arndt Büssing and Janusz Surzykiewicz

Introduction

Persons with Down syndrome (DS) have a genetic disorder (with three copies of chromosome 21) that cannot be "repaired" or corrected. Apart from the obvious "visible" symptoms, they have specific physical and mental impairments, on the one hand, and risks for several health problems, on the other hand. The respective symptoms and their intensity may vary and

A. Büssing (✉)
Professorship Quality of Life, Spirituality and Coping, Faculty of Health, Witten/Herdecke University, Herdecke, Germany

IUNCTUS—Competence Center for Christian Spirituality, Philosophical-Theological University of Münster, Münster, Germany
e-mail: Arndt.buessing@uni-wh.de

J. Surzykiewicz
Faculty of Philosophy and Education, Katholische Universität Eichstätt-Ingolstadt, Eichstätt, Germany

Faculty of Education, Cardinal Stefan Wyszynski University in Warsaw, Warsaw, Poland
e-mail: Janusz.Surzykiewicz@ku.de

A. Büssing (ed.), *Spiritual Needs in Research and Practice*,
https://doi.org/10.1007/978-3-030-70139-0_21

have differential relevance during the phases of life (i.e., heart defects, hip dislocations, diabetes, coeliac disease, sleep apnea, risk of leukemia). Their cognitive impairments range from mild to moderate, while strong impairments are rather rare (Bull et al. 2011). Behavioral problems may relate to impulsive behavior and judgment difficulties, but also reduced attention span and slow learning abilities. Nevertheless, several persons with DS can live a healthy life with a supportive family. Adequate schooling and support allows development of life skills and (to varying degrees) social integration. Today, the life expectancy of persons with DS has increased to 50–60 years on average. Nevertheless, due to the higher risk of various health problems, intensive support, assistive devices and treatments (inclusively physical, speech-language, occupational and behavioral therapies) are needed, and social networks are crucial for the whole family.

While the everyday, health-related and psychosocial needs of people with Down syndrome have already been studied from various perspectives (Fidler et al. 2005; Buckley et al. 2006; Daunhauer et al. 2014; Amadó et al. 2016; Zimpel 2016), the spiritual-religious area remains poorly explored (Gaventa and Peters 2001; Swinton 2001a, b, 2002; Wong et al. 2006; Young 2007; Watts 2011; Baldwin et al. 2015). At the same time, spirituality was recognized as an important factor for the life satisfaction of this group of people (Crompton and Jackson 2004; Shogren and Rye 2005; Skotko et al. 2011; Glicksman 2011; Gaventa and Coulter 2014; Büssing et al. 2017). However, there is still insufficient research on the role of spirituality as a resource for ensuring the quality of life of people with intellectual disabilities and especially with DS. It is possible that this problem is also methodologically related, as this group has not been reached with standardized surveys so far and, further, the findings are often from a second-person perspective. Consequently, it has not been possible to gain generally valid insights. Attempts have been made to provide evidence-based data and findings in this area as well. Life satisfaction (as a multidimensional construct) was found to be connected with spirituality (as another multidimensional construct) among people with DS (Crompton and Jackson 2004), whereby spiritual aspects in particular were confirmed as an important factor in well-being.

Which role may spiritual concerns play in the life of persons with DS? Is it a resource providing hope, orientation and hold? It is often an argument that spirituality is foremost a cognitive construct difficult to "understand" (i.e., the theoretical doctrines and beliefs of religions)—particularly by persons with lower intellectual abilities. However, this might be a prejudice. First, the multidimensional construct "spirituality" has also emotional, relational and experiential aspects and these might be of stronger relevance for persons with DS. Second, also persons with DS have a vital spiritual life. A book of two men with DS was entitled *Count Us In* and described their perspective on religion and God (Kingsley and Levitz 1994). In an interview with a male person with DS one may find explicit statements about complex perceptions such as awe and gratitude, and attitudes toward praying, church attendance and meaning in life (Büssing and Broghammer-Escher 2019). The *Little Sisters Disciples of the Lamb* is a contemplative religious community in France that welcomes also persons with DS into consecrated life (Viet 2019). One of these religious sisters with DS stated: "I have tried to know Jesus by reading the Bible and the Gospel. I was born with a disability called Down syndrome. I am happy. I love Life. I pray, but I am sad for the children with Down syndrome who will not feel this same joy of living" (Viet 2019). One of the non-DS co-sisters stated that the sisters with DS have a "great spiritual strength" and that "they are souls of prayer, they are very spiritual, very close to Jesus" (Viet 2019). Thus, also persons with DS may value faith as an important source, may rely on the Transcendent, have a vital prayer life, and may have mystical experiences and perceptions—like others, too. The Superior of the aforementioned congregation underlines that "their souls are not disabled!" and that "they bring joy to society and, above all, they bring love to the world. A world that needs it so much" (Viet 2019).

These are exceptional examples of inclusion, while in other cases their life situation might be more difficult. Phases of depression and frustration about their life may nevertheless arise. However, a meta-analysis from 2011 did not find a higher prevalence of depression in persons with DS (Walker et al. 2011). The review authors suggested that their many vulnerabilities and exposition to several stressors could facilitate phases of depression that seem to be often ignored.

There is evidence that a person's spirituality, in particular religious involvement (in terms of participation) and religious activity (in terms of its centrality in life) may have emotionally stabilizing effects (especially in difficult phases of life). Whether this is also true for persons with DS is unclear. While it was stated that particularly persons with special needs should be supported in their spiritual concerns, it is largely unknown which specific spiritual needs they have and how these could be supported (Swinton 2002; Liu et al. 2014). Often there are only statements about persons with DS and what they may or should require, while their own statements are rare.

Methodological Aspects to Assess the Spiritual Needs of Persons with Down Syndrome

To value their own perceptions and views of persons with DS, a cross-sectional survey was initiated. The intentions and aims of the study were explained to the participants and they had to sign an informed consent document (further, their parents or legal guardians). Most German interviewees asked for help with reading and filling out the questionnaire (83%), and thus all statements and the underlying scorings were explained by an interviewer who completed the questionnaire on behalf. The items were taken from standardized questionnaires in use (i.e., SpNQ, SpREUK-P, AKU), and adapted grammatically and linguistically with respect to the specific sample. The thematic focus was on experiential, emotional, and behavioral topics. Apart from this quantitative approach, also ten structured, guided interviews were performed to clarify that the items were understood and what the interviewees associate with these statements (Büssing et al. 2017).

The following topics were addressed: experience of gratitude, awe, beauty, and joy in life (five items), awareness of others' needs (two items), conscious interactions (three items), relational needs (two items), experience of a transcendent presence (three items), religious activities (two items), talking about fears and worries (one item), and reflection of meaning in life (one item). The pilot testers with DS gave positive feedback that their views were appreciated, and they were proud when they had responded to all statements ("with success").

Life Satisfaction and Indicators of Spirituality of Persons with Down Syndrome from Germany

In Germany, 65 persons with DS were interviewed (Büssing et al. 2017); more than half were female and their mean age was 29 ± 9 [16–51] years. Half of them were living with their parents. Most assessed their life satisfaction as very good (using a 5-grade smiley scale), while three persons perceived it as weak or bad; 94% perceived that their heart is "filled with great joy", 6% either not or seldom only. A majority of them is going out with friends often (39%) or very often (26%).

Positive life experiences and feelings of gratefulness related to nature were perceived often or very often (84% and 83% respectively) and these were intended to be shared with others (i.e., the girlfriend or caregiver), indicating an aspect of relational spirituality. Feelings of wondering awe were perceived less often (49%). Thinking of others in need (63%) and concrete helping when others need it (80%) were further important topics. This awareness of others and the subsequent intentions to help are again an indicator of relational spirituality in terms of connectedness. Similarly, conscious interactions with others (83%) and with nature (77%) were important to most of them, underlining that conscious awareness of an interconnectedness is of relevance to them. Explicit relational needs were expressed by most enrolled persons, that is, to "have someone on hand who is always on my side" (93%), to have someone one could turn to "in a loving attitude" (93%), or someone to talk about fears and worries (81%). Because such a close relational partner is not always available, they also referred to a (private) Guardian Angel (67%) and to God who was felt "at my side" (71%). Even when there might be no physical "proof" for this, the emotional (and spiritual) longing for such an external source of close connection that is guiding and protecting and always available to them, was striking. In line with this, private prayers to communicate with God (65% often to very often) were of stronger relevance than the going to church (28% often to very often). Here, the lack of opportunities to attend the service of a religious community could be discussed.

One statement of a male person connected "faith and confidence" with rather mystical considerations: "About faith and confidence, and purpose of life is almost like the water of life. Like a spring. […] Like a spring of life, exactly, is the __ is also the meaning in life. Because, the water continues to flow, and also the meaning in life continues to flow." (Büssing et al. 2017) Here, the young man has the awareness that personal meaning in life is nothing one may *have*, but that it is constantly changing and one has to be open to the current situation, open to the flowing water, to nature around and how one relates with it.

Of special interest was the finding that their life satisfaction was moderately related with the feeling that God is at one's side ($r = 0.42$), which would indicate that the emotional perception of God's presence as a source of emotional/spiritual support contributes to their well-being, particularly when close friends and loving relations (that were longed for) are not available. Further associations between life satisfaction and praying ($r = 0.26$) or going out with friends ($r = 0.26$) were weak. This aforementioned relational context that contributes to their life satisfaction is further underlined by the finding that those living with their parents who may give them stability had significantly higher life satisfaction. In the interviews, the wish for stable partnership and also of being allowed to have one's own family and own children appeared (Büssing et al. 2017). This was the cause of conflicts with their legal guardians and parents and caused depressive defiance if no admission could be made.

Life Satisfaction and Indicators of Spirituality of Persons with Down Syndrome from Poland

Using the same questionnaire and procedure, 38 persons with DS from Poland were enrolled. Here, 53% were female and 47% male; their mean age was 25 ± 10 [15–55] years. Most were living with their parents (76%). Their life satisfaction was assessed as very good (using a 5-grade smiley scale), while four perceived it as weak or bad; 74% perceived that their heart is "filled with great joy", 26% not or only seldom. A majority is only seldom out with friends (50%) or not at all (16%).

Positive life experiences were perceived often or even very often (76%), while feelings of gratefulness or feelings of wondering awe were perceived less often (61% and 55%, respectively). Thinking of others in need and helping them when they need it were relevant topics, too (76% and 71%, respectively). Similarly, conscious interactions with others (79%) and with nature (84%) were important to most of them. Explicit relational needs were expressed by a majority of enrolled persons with DS, that is, to "have someone on hand who is always on my side" was stated by 95%, to have someone one could turn to "in a loving attitude" (79%), or someone to talk about fears and worries (82%). Polish persons with DS also referred to a (private) Guardian Angel (85%) and to God who was felt "at my side" (79%). Private prayers to communicate with God (84% often to very often) are of same relevance than their intention to go to church (87% often to very often).

In this smaller group of persons with DS from Poland, life satisfaction was strongly related with trust in one's Guardian Angel ($r = 0.59$) and moderately with the feeling that God is at one's side ($r = 0.42$). Further, life satisfaction was strongly related to feelings of wondering awe ($r = 0.52$), and moderately with praying ($r = 0.46$), going to church ($r = 0.35$) and going out with friends ($r = 0.49$).

Differences Between Polish and German Persons with Down Syndrome

Due to cultural and religious differences between Catholic Poland and rather secular Germany, both groups of persons with DS significantly differ with respect to their frequency of praying (1.6 ± 1.1 vs. 2.4 ± 0.8 [ranging from 0 to 3]) and going to church (1.2 ± 0.9 vs. 2.5 ± 0.9 [0–3]), which were lower in the German sample ($p < 0.0001$; Mann-Whitney-U test). Nevertheless, both groups have a similarly high perception that God is with them ("at my side"). Their relational needs are similarly strong, in terms of having a concrete person at their side with whom one may talk about fears and worries or with whom one may have a loving relationship (Fig. 21.1). The latter need was significantly lower in Polish persons with DS. Further, the ability of going out with friends was significantly higher in the German sample (1.9 ± 0.9 vs. 1.3 ± 0.9 [0–3]; $p = 0.007$; Mann-Whitney-U test); also their life satisfaction was higher (4.3 ± 1.0 vs. 3.9 ± 1.1 [0–3]; $p = 0.026$; Mann-Whitney-U test), and the perception that the heart is filled with great joy (2.5 ± 0.7 vs. 2.0 ± 0.9 [0–3]; $p = 0.001$; Mann-Whitney-U test).

The correlation pattern of persons with DS from Poland is different from that of persons from Germany. In Polish persons with DS, the best predictors of their life satisfaction were the frequency of going to the cinema (as an indicator of autonomy), praying (as an indicator of

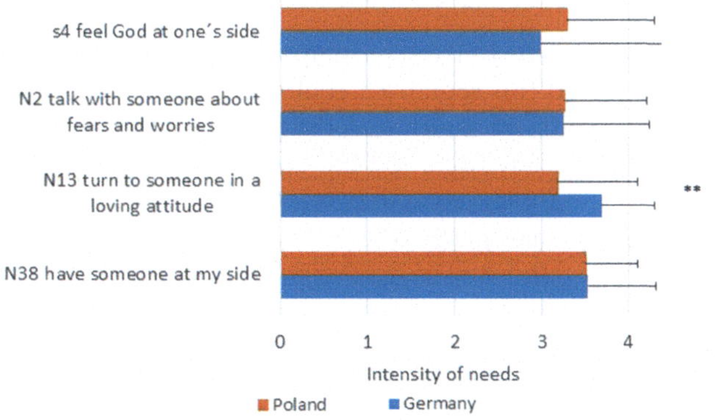

Fig. 21.1 Comparison of relational needs in persons with DS from Poland and Germany (Note: $^{**}p = 0.001$—Mann-Whitney-U test)

connectedness with God), the need to turn to someone in a loving attitude (as an indicator of relational needs) and the perception that the heart is "filled with great joy" (as an indicator of intrinsic happiness). These four variables would explain in the respective regression model 55% of variance in life satisfaction (as depending variable), with praying as the weakest predictor. In the German sample, the prediction model was much weaker. The perception that the heart is "filled with great joy" and the intention to go to church are the sole significant variables explaining 21% of variance in their life satisfaction scores. In none of these prediction models, the frequency of time with friends or perceptions of awe or gratefulness contributed to their life satisfaction.

Thus, both groups of persons with DS from culturally and religiously different countries have similar relational needs and longings, both with respect to concrete others and in terms of God and their trust in a "private" Guardian Angel that is available for them. The main differences are their life satisfaction, intrinsic happiness and autonomy, which were higher in the German group. The difference for this inner happiness between both groups is large (Cohen's d = 0.82) and thus relevantly different, while the effects sizes for life satisfaction and their autonomy to go out with friends was small (Cohen's d = 0.40) and thus not of outstanding relevance. It is unclear whether Polish persons with DS are utilizing their religiosity to compensate their lower quality of life or whether their religiosity is an independent source.

Consequences

The needs for social inclusion and participation were clearly perceived during the interviews and this remains a challenging task. Similar topics were also found in a qualitative study enrolling 12 persons with DS by Scott et al. (2014). In their view, a "good life" relates to relationships, community participation, independence and hopes for the future. However, in the study among German persons with DS, half of them were working in sheltered workshops, and stay in residential communities that give them a secure space to live, while they nevertheless lack "real" participation outside their protected living areas. Some have "outside" jobs and can participate more easily, while others cannot. Due to the "variability of performance among individuals with DS" not all can be easily included, and only a minority of adult persons with DS are contracted with regular jobs (Bertoli et al. 2011). Participation "in all aspects of society as full persons with all their special abilities and disabilities" seems to be difficult to realize (Büssing et al. 2017). This is also true for participation in religious communities. Even when several of these communities intend to invite persons with special needs, the concrete inclusion continues to be a challenge. A framework for such an inclusion in faith communities was described by Goldstein and Ault (2015).

Having close friends and/or partners was seen as important by the enrolled persons with DS (Fig. 21.1). Having friends means to be able to talk about fears and worries and to cope with stressors, while lacking close friends who can emotionally understand and support them will aggravate their feelings of being "different" and thus their perception of loneliness. To address these needs, Jobling et al. (2000) developed an intervention program to help young adults with DS to explore the types of friendships and the related emotional relationships.

Even when there are several inclusion barriers and obvious unmet psychosocial and spiritual needs, most of the enrolled persons with DS stated a high life satisfaction. Also in a study from Skotko et al. (2011) enrolling 284 people with DS, a majority (>95%) stated to be "happy with their lives", that they "like who they are" and "how they look". It was touching that they encouraged others to "value them, emphasizing that they share similar hopes and dreams as people without DS" (Skotko et al. 2011).

More detailed analyses revealed important practical fields of action for actively promoting the subjective quality of life of people with Down syndrome. As other studies show, people with intellectual disabilities are very interested in friendships and trusting relationships (Andrzejczak et al. 2010; Gaventa 2012; Gaventa and Coulter 2014; Carter 2013; Carter et al. 2015). This not only addresses the well-known social isolation of people with special needs, which is clearly opposed to the explicitly expressed desire for connectivity, but also spaces in which people with special needs are allowed to experience themselves as actors and helpers instead of being stigmatized as needy, weak, ill or disabled (Bittles and Glasson 2004; Vogel et al. 2006; McNair and Carter 2010; Markowetz 2016; Sokołowska 2019). It is necessary to optimize support for such involvement and to create opportunities for people with DS to participate in taking on responsibility. It can be assumed that one of their particular strengths lies in their apparent "friendly helpfulness", which is not only emotionally conditioned. Their prosocial attitudes with their typical characteristics, such as emotional responsiveness, trustfulness, need for sensitive emotional sounds and moods can be expressed very positively in the form of noncognitive and speech-free, nonverbal help potentials. These spiritually bound prosocial attitudes can thus also be developed into participation resources for people with DS (Pillay 2010; Mergen 2014; Taylor et al. 2014; Barnoy et al. 2017).

Another central finding regarding spiritual aspects as resources for life satisfaction and well-being is the central importance of religiously connoted spirituality. At the item level, this includes the concrete practice of religious practices (including prayer, going to church) as well as faith, trust and solidarity with religious advocates (e.g., Guardian Angels). The results show that also persons with DS may have religious–spiritual transcendence perceptions. The results of the available research on spirituality or religiosity in people with DS refer mostly to their personal, individual relationship with God. In many cases, this corresponds more or less to general interpersonal communication or emotionality with similar characteristics of giving thanks, asking, demanding, wishing, etc., and can have both positive and negative effects on life satisfaction (Swinton 2001a, b, 2002; Young 2007; Zhang 2010).

Particularly with regard to actional aspects of faith, simple ritualized and concrete spiritual offers and rituals can provide good support (Anderssohn 2007). Especially common worship services and prayers are associated with an increased joy of life and contentment in persons with special needs and help to prevent negative emotional states, for example by making religious meeting places more open and proactive for all people (Johnstone et al. 2012; Liu et al. 2014; Taylor et al. 2014; Gaventa and Coulter 2014). Appropriate action days and individual events, but also the introduction of routines in everyday church life (e.g., pick-up services) can not only raise awareness and sensitivity in the church congregation, but also create important places for interaction and inclusion (Vogel et al. 2006; Taylor et al. 2014; Carter et al. 2015).

Conclusions

Persons with special needs may require special attention—when they want it. Responding to the spiritual needs of persons with DS should respect their desire for self-determination and autonomy in order to avoid encroachment. Persons with DS may be "different" in terms of some of their behavior and physical characteristics, but they share similar desires and hopes as others. Due to the heterogeneity of their abilities and restrictions, the individual person is in the forefront and not a label ("Down syndrome"). Addressing their spiritual needs means to value their individual perceptions, feelings and intentions. Whether all of their spiritual needs and longings can be met and "fulfilled" remains unclear. To recognize that the spirituality of persons with DS is rather emotion, experience and relation oriented opens new perspectives to challenge our view of what spirituality may mean in a performance-oriented society.

The spiritual needs approach proves fruitful and ensuring specific access to people with DS and their quality of life, in understanding the "function" of their spirituality. The promotion of spirituality as a basic life resource for all and especially for people with special needs is consequently recognized as an important premise for inclusion efforts (Hatton et al. 2004; Young 2007; Egan 2010; Carter 2013; Liégeois 2014). Spirituality and religiosity are regarded as important prerequisites for social and health-related quality of life, whereby, in the light of research, essential patterns of justification should be emphasized here: spirituality is perceived by people with Down syndrome themselves as an important part of their quality of life (Schulz 2005; Glicksman 2011; Terrell-Lee 2015; Loynes and O'Harra 2015). A religious–spiritual life of people with DS generally indicates quality of life as a concrete inclusive potential. However, with regard to the corresponding support options, it is necessary to examine the needs of each person individually, where their spiritual needs lie and how they can be met without possibly overburdening them. Accordingly, religious education and pastoral structures must be created, in which people with DS or mental disability can move together with others and, when desired, also independently (Taylor et al. 2014; Lech 2014).

The developing of independence by people with special needs represents a concrete expectation of modern societies and their citizens. In order to strengthen people with different levels of physical and psychological competence on their path through life, it is necessary to open up opportunities in different ways and to support them in overcoming or removing obstacles (Swinton 2002; Swinton et al. 2011; Anderssohn 2011). Above all, the areas of inclusion, the search for meaning and corresponding development represent an important research desideratum (Buckley et al. 2006; Zhang 2010; Zhang and Wu 2012). Intercultural and interreligious expertise and the overcoming of communication barriers are also crucial for this (Loynes and O'Harra 2015; Crotty and Doody 2016).

References

Amadó A, Serrat E, Vallès-Majoral E (2016) The role of executive functions in social cognition among children with down syndrome: relationship patterns. Front Psychol 7:1363. https://doi.org/10.3389/fpsyg.2016.01363

Anderssohn S (2007) Gott ist die bunte Vielfalt für mich – Einblicke in die Religiosität von Menschen mit geistiger Behinderung – Perspektiven für die integrative Pädagogik. Neukirchener Verlag, Neukirchen-Vluyn

Anderssohn S (2011) Gott ist die bunte Vielfalt für mich – Religiöse Entwicklung zwischen "Autonomie" und "Sozialisation" – Perspektiven für die integrative Arbeit. In: Wuckelt A, Pithan A, Beuers C (eds) Und schuf dem Menschen ein Gegenüber… – Im Spannungsfeld zwischen Autonomie und Angewiesen sein, Forum für Heil- und Religionspädagogik 6. Comenius Institut, Münster, pp 72–87

Andrzejczak J, Śmigiel R, Szemplińska A (2010) Wspolnota zamieszkania Arka (L'Arche) miejscem doświadczenia dorosłości osob z zespołem Downa. In: Kaczmarek B (ed) Trudna dorosłość osob z zespołem Downa. Oficyna Wydawnicza Impuls, Kraków

Baldwin PJ, Evans J, Etherington N, Nichols M, Wright V, McDougall J (2015) Youth with disabilities talk about spirituality: a qualitative descriptive study. Qual Rep 20(7):941–958

Barnoy S, Biton A, Itzhaki M (2017) Social inclusion of children with down syndrome: Jewish and Muslim mothers' knowledge, attitudes, beliefs, and behavioral intentions. J Pediatr Nurs 35:50–56

Bertoli M, Biasini G, Calignano MT, Celani G, De Grossi G, Digilio MC, Fermariello CC, Loffredo G, Luchino F, Marchese A, Mazotti S, Menghi B, Razzano C, Tiano C, Zambon Hobart A, Zampino G, Zuccalàl G (2011) Needs and challenges of daily life for people with Down syndrome residing in the city of Rome, Italy. J Intellect Disabil Res 55(8):801–820. https://doi.org/10.1111/j.1365-2788.2011.01432.x

Bittles AH, Glasson EJ (2004) Clinical, social and ethical implications of changing life expectancy in Down syndrome. Dev Med Child Neurol 46(4):282–286

Buckley S, Bird G, Sacks B, Archer T (2006) A comparison of mainstream and special education for teenagers with Down Syndrome: implications for parents and teachers. Down Syndr Res Pract 9(3):54–67

Bull MJ, The Committee on Genetics (2011) Health supervision for children with Down syndrome. Pediatrics 128:393–406

Büssing A, Broghammer-Escher S (2019) Sinn des Lebens ist fast wie das Wasser des Lebens – Interview mit Timm. Spiritual Care 8:319–322

Büssing A, Broghammer-Escher S, Baumann K, Surzykiewicz K (2017) Aspects of spirituality and life satisfaction in persons with Down syndrome. J Disabil Religion 21:14–29. https://doi.org/10.1080/23312521.2016.1270179

Carter EW (2013) Supporting inclusion and flourishing in the religious and spiritual lives of people with intellectual and developmental disabilities. Inclusion 1:64–75

Carter EW, Kleinert HL, LoBianco TF, Sheppard-Jones K, Butler LN, Tyree MS (2015) Congregational participation of a national sample of adults with intellectual and developmental disabilities. Intellect Dev Disabil 53(6):381–393

Crompton M, Jackson R (2004) Spiritual well-being of adults with Down syndrome. The Down Syndrome Education Trust, Southsea, Hampshire

Crotty G, Doody O (2016) Transcultural care and individuals with an intellectual disability. J Intellect Disabil 20(4):386–396

Daunhauer LA, Fidler DJ, Hahn L, Will E, Lee NR, Hepburn S (2014) Profiles of everyday executive functioning in young children with Down syndrome. Am J Intellect Dev Disabil 119(4):303–318

Egan R (2010) Health promotion and spirituality: making the implicit explicit. Keeping Up to Date 34:1–4. http://www.hauora.co.nz/assets/files/Hauora%20and%20KUTD/Keeping%20Up%20to%20Date%2034.pdf. Accessed 29 Aug 2020

Fidler DJ, Philofsky A, Hepburn SL, Rogers SJ (2005) Nonverbal requesting and problem-solving by toddlers with Down syndrome. Am J Ment Retard 110(4):312–322

Gaventa B (2012) Lessons in community building from including the "other": caring for one an-other. J Religion Disabil Health 16:231–247

Gaventa WC, Coulter D (2014) Spirituality and intellectual disability: international perspectives on the effect of culture and religion on healing body, mind, and soul. Routledge, London

Gaventa W, Peters R (2001) Spirituality and self-actualization: recognizing spiritual needs and strengths of persons with cognitive limitations. In: Tymchuk AJ, Lakin C, Luckasson R (eds) The forgotten generation: the status and challenges of adults with mild cognitive limitations. Paul H. Brooks Publishing Company, Baltimore

Glicksman S (2011) Supporting religion and spirituality to enhance quality of life of people with intellectual disability: a Jewish perspective. Intellect Dev Disabil 49(5):397–402

Goldstein P, Ault MJ (2015) Including Individuals with disabilities in a faith community: a framework and example. J Disabil Religion 19:1–14

Hatton C, Turner S, Shah R, Rahim N, Stansfield J (2004) Religious expression, a fundamental human right: the report of an action research project on meeting the religious needs of people with learning disabilities. The Mental Health Foundation, London

Jobling A, Moni KB, Nolan A (2000) Understanding friendship: young adults with Down syndrome exploring relationships. J Intellect Develop Disabil 25:235–245. https://doi.org/10.1080/13269780050144299

Johnstone B, Yoon DP, Cohen D, Schopp LH, McCormack G, Campbell J, Smith M (2012) Relationships among spirituality, religious practices, personality factors, and health for five different faith traditions. J Relig Health 51(4):1017–1041

Kingsley J, Levitz M (1994) Count Us in: Growing Up With Down Syndrome. Harvest Books

Lech W (2014) Współpraca środowisk katechetycznych w wychowaniu religijnym osób z niepełnosprawnością intelektualną w nowych dokumentach programowych katechezy. Colloquia Theologica Ottoniana 1:203–224

Liégeois A (2014) Quality of life without spirituality? A theological reflection on the quality of life of persons with intellectual disabilities. J Disabil Religion 18(4):303–317

Liu EX, Carter EW, Boehm TL, Annandale NH, Taylor CE (2014) In their own words: the place of faith in the lives of young people with autism and intellectual disability. Intellect Dev Disabil 52:388–404

Loynes B, O'Harra J (2015) How can mental health clinicians, working in intellectual disability services, meet the spiritual needs of their service users? Adv Ment Health Intellect Disabil 9(1):9–18

Markowetz R (2016) Inklusion im Förderschwerpunkt geistige Entwicklung. Kohlhammer Verlag, Stuttgart

McNair J, Carter EW (2010) Special issue: inclusive Christian religious education (Part 1 and 2). J Religion Disabil Health 14:111–112

Mergen W (2014) Menschen mit Down-Syndrom–eXXXtra-begabte Botschafter der LIEBE: Das Down-Syndrom aus spiritueller Sicht. Neobooks, Berlin

Pillay D (2010) Spiritual and organised religion in supporting parents of children with Down syndrome and intellectual disability. Thesis, Edith Cowan University, Crawley

Schulz E (2005) The meaning of spirituality for individuals with disabilities. Disabil Rehabil 27(21):1283–1295

Scott M, Foley KR, Bourke J, Leonard H, Girdler S (2014) "I have a good life": the meaning of well-being from the perspective of young adults with Down syndrome. Disabil Rehabil 36:1290–1298. https://doi.org/10.3109/09638288.2013.854843

Shogren KA, Rye MS (2005) Religion and individuals with intellectual disabilities: an exploratory study of self-reported perspectives. J Religion Disabil Health 9(1):29–53

Skotko BG, Levine SP, Goldstein R (2011) Self-perceptions from people with Down syndrome. Am J Med Genet A 155A(10):2360–2369. https://doi.org/10.1002/ajmg.a.34235

Sokołowska A (2019) Korzyści i straty z asystentury osobom z niepełnosprawnością intelektualną w L'Arche w oczach asystentów poznańskiej wspólnoty. Niepełnosprawność-zagadnienia, problemy, rozwiązania 2(31):122–163

Swinton J (2001a) A space to listen: meeting the spiritual needs of people with learning disabilities. Mental Health Found 3(6):1–4

Swinton J (2001b) Spirituality in mental health care: rediscovering a forgotten dimension. Jessica Kingsley, London

Swinton J (2002) Spirituality and the lives of people with learning disabilities. Tizard Learn Disabil Rev 7:29–35

Swinton J, Mowat H, Baines S (2011) Whose story am I? Redescribing profound intellectual disability in the Kingdom of God. J Religion Disabil Health 15(1):5–19

Taylor CE, Carter EW, Annandale NH, Boehm TL, Logeman AK (2014) Welcoming people with developmental disabilities and their families: a practical guide for congregations. Vanderbilt Kennedy Center, Nashville, TN

Terrell-Lee T (2015) Toward a therapeutic use of spirituality among individuals with mild to moderate intellectual sisabilities. Walden University Scholar Works, Walden

Viet C (2019) Religious sisters with Down syndrome: the joy of shared contemplative life. Vatican News. https://www.vaticannews.va/en/world/news/2019-07/stories-religious-sisters-with-down-syndrome.html. Accessed 18 Aug 2020

Vogel J, Polloway EA, Smith JD (2006) Inclusion of people with mental retardation and other developmental disabilities in communities of faith. Ment Retard 44(2):100–111

Walker JC, Dosen A, Buitelaar JK, Janzing JG (2011) Depression in Down syndrome: a review of the literature. Res Dev Disabil 32(5):1432–1440. https://doi.org/10.1016/j.ridd.2011.02.010

Watts G (2011) Intellectual disability and spiritual development. J Intellect Develop Disabil 36:238–245

Wong YJ, Rew L, Slaikey KD (2006) A systematic review of recent research on adolescent religiosity/spirituality and mental health. Issues Ment Health Nurs 27:161–183

Young A (2007) Theology and Down syndrome –reimaging disability in late modernity. Baylor University Press, Waco

Zhang KC (2010) Spirituality and disabilities: implications for special education. Intellect Dev Disabil 48(4):299–302

Zhang KC, Wu DI (2012) Nurturing the spiritual well-being of children with special needs. Support Learn Br J Learn Support 27(3):119–122. https://doi.org/10.1111/j.1467-9604.2012.01528.x

Zimpel AF (2016) Trisomie 21 – Was wir von Menschen mit Down-Syndrom lernen können. 2000 Personen und ihre neuropsychologischen Befunde. Vandehoeck und Rupprecht, Göttingen

CHAPTER 22

Spiritual Needs of Adolescents with Chronic Diseases

Arndt Büssing, Justine Hussong, Jörg Große-Onnebrink, and Alexander von Gontard

Background

Children and adolescents can be affected by chronic illness, such as asthma, allergies, diabetes, rheumatoid arthritis, neurological disorders, etc. (Louis-Jacques and Samples 2011; Voll et al. 2013). Chronic illness is an

A. Büssing (✉)
Professorship Quality of Life, Spirituality and Coping, Faculty of Health, Witten/Herdecke University, Herdecke, Germany

IUNCTUS—Competence Center for Christian Spirituality, Philosophical-Theological University of Münster, Münster, Germany
e-mail: Arndt.buessing@uni-wh.de

J. Hussong • A. von Gontard
Department of Child and Adolescent Psychiatry, Saarland University Hospital, Homburg, Germany
e-mail: justine.hussong@uks.eu; alexander.gontard@uks.eu

J. Große-Onnebrink
Department of General Pediatrics, Pediatric Respiratory Medicine Unit, University Hospital Münster, Münster, Germany
e-mail: joerg.grosse-onnebrink@ukmuenster.de

A. Büssing (ed.), *Spiritual Needs in Research and Practice*,
https://doi.org/10.1007/978-3-030-70139-0_22

umbrella term, which can be defined by duration and impact of illness. The prevalence varies according to the definitions of chronic disease: if defined by duration of over 3 months, 10–20% are affected; if defined by a duration of over 12 months, the prevalence is 13%; 7% of children are limited in their daily activities and 1–2% are severely disabled with daily impairment; and 20–30% of children with chronic illness have comorbid psychological disorders, and even 50–70% when the central nervous system is involved (Wallander and Varni 1998; von Hagen and Schwarz 2009). Overall, internalizing disorders such as depression, anxiety, and posttraumatic stress disorders predominate, while externalizing disorders such as conduct disorders and ADHD are less common.

Risk factors for psychological disorders include disease-specific factors, such as central nervous system involvement, physical handicap and long duration. Treatment factors such as invasive procedures can increase the risk for posttraumatic stress disorders. Child factors such as low self-esteem and increased stress play a role, as well as family factors such as dysfunctional interaction, conflicts, lack of social support, and parental depression (LeBlanc et al. 2003).

Worldwide, approximately 10–20% of children are affected by clinically relevant mental health disorders (Fuchs et al. 2013). Even under most conservative estimates, 15% of children and adolescents have psychological disturbances with daily incapacitation. But are these disorders actually increasing? Bor et al. (2014) tackled this question in their carefully conducted review and found that for toddlers and children, there was no major increase of psychological disorders. However, adolescents show an increasing risk for internalizing disorders such as anxiety and depression, especially girls.

Dealing with chronic illness requires active coping in addition to dealing with developmental tasks during adolescence. Adolescence is defined as the transitional stage of physical and psychological human development generally occurring during the period from puberty to legal adulthood (i.e., 10–18 years) (Louis-Jacques and Samples 2011). Due to economic dependence on parents, adolescence is prolonged in many societies. Adolescence, again, can be subdivided into early adolescence (ages 10–13 years), middle adolescence (14–16 years), and late adolescence (17–21 years). During each substage, adolescents have to deal with typical normative developmental tasks (Louis-Jacques and Samples 2011).

Coping has been defined as the cognitive and behavioral efforts to manage external and internal demands that are appraised as taxing or exceeding the resources of a person (Lazarus and Folkman 1984). Compas et al. (2012) defined three different modes of coping in adolescents: primary or active coping (efforts to act on the source of stress or one's emotions), secondary control or accomodative coping (adaptation to source of stress, reappraisal, positive thinking, acceptance), and disengagement or passive coping (avoidance or denial of stress, leading to poor adjustment). Primary and secondary coping are the most successful modes, while passive coping leads to poor adjustment. Some adolescents are better able to cope with their chronic illness than others. For example, a systematic review on children with serious pediatric disease has shown that both children and parents can develop posttraumatic growth (PTG) (Picoraro et al. 2014). In adults, PTG consists of five elements: a greater appreciation of life, improved interpersonal relationships, greater personal strength, recognition of new possibilities and spiritual and/or religious growth. Although not as distinct as in adults, children can develop all five domains as a result of the severe impact as chronic disease. Children with PTG appear wiser and more mature than other children that have not had to deal with such difficult situations.

Spirituality is generally seen as a resource to cope in times of distress and illness (Pargament 1997, 2011). Particularly, such difficult times in life can be crucial in deciding to additionally rely on other sources of help. With respect to the locus of health control (Rotter 1966; Levenson 1972), these resources can be either external (i.e., medical doctors, psychologists, pastors, God) or intrinsic (i.e., self-efficacy, sense of coherence, conscious and healthy way of living). While there are various studies that underline that spirituality is a resource for coping, there are studies that show that it is also relevant for younger persons with chronic diseases (Damsma Bakker et al. 2018). The topic of spirituality is also relevant for children and adolescents (von Gontard 2013). However, it was also shown that not all aspects of spirituality are similarly relevant for healthy younger persons, particularly not for those who would not regard themselves as religious, but may relate to other, more secular aspects of spirituality (Büssing et al. 2012). Nevertheless, a wide spectrum of empirical studies has shown positive effects of spirituality on mental disorders, for example, depression. Spirituality can be a protective factor against depression (Barkin et al. 2015; Miller 2013), particularly when this resource is available ("central") in the life of children and adolescents. Religiosity also may have an effect on reducing depression (Miller and Gur 2002); however, in secular societies several adolescents have turned away from institutional religiosity and thus this resource might not be relevant to them. Further, spiritual experiences, forgiveness, and religious coping are related to less depression (Desrosiers and Miller 2007). In contrast to the many studied effects on mental health, there are only a limited number of studies on spirituality and physical health outcomes (Cotton et al. 2006). To our knowledge, no studies have compared adolescents' spirituality with respect to mental and physical chronic illness.

Meanwhile, there are several recommendations that assessing childrens' or adolescents' spiritual needs is important (Shelly 1982; Hufton 2006; McSherry and Smith 2007; Bull and Gillies 2007; Bull 2016); however, not all refer to epidemiologic data. Bull and Gillies (2007) addressed the spiritual needs of five hospitalized children using pictures to facilitate storytelling. A concept analysis of Petersen (2014) focused on dying childrens' spirituality and their spiritual needs. Feudtner et al. (2003) intended to assess the spiritual care needs of children and asked pastors instead of the children. To our knowledge, there are no studies that have systematically assessed adolescents' spiritual needs with a validated instrument.

Therefore, we intended to assess spiritual needs of adolescents with chronic diseases and long-term treatment in a standardized way, using the adolescent version of the SpNQ (see Chap. 8). We focused on the question which psychosocial, existential, and spiritual needs are of relevance for them. Are there differences between adolescents with somatic or psychosomatic/psychiatric diseases, and between female and male adolescents?

Description of the Sample

To address this, we analyzed data sets of 200 adolescents (62% female, 38% male) with a mean age of 15.6 ± 1.8 [11–22] years. With respect to the underlying causes of treatment, 52% had somatic diseases (i.e., diabetes, cystic fibrosis, asthma) and 48% were treated for psychosomatic/psychiatric conditions (i.e., depression, anxiety disorders, eating disorders, obesity) in both pediatric/psychosomatic/psychiatric hospitals and ambulant treatment centers.

Both groups differ significantly for their life satisfaction, which was lower in adolescents with psychosomatic/psychiatric conditions (BMLSS: 69 ± 18 vs. 59 ± 27 [ranging from 0 to 100]; $p < 0.0001$, Mann-Whitney-U test [MWU]) and perceived impairment due to disease-related symptoms, which was lowest in adolescents with somatic diseases (VAS: 38 ± 24 vs. 48 ± 25 [0–100]; $p = 0.002$, MWU test). Their treatment satisfaction showed no significant differences between both groups. However, self-efficacy expectation was higher in adolescents with somatic diseases (GSE:

19 ± 5 vs. 15 ± 6 [0–40]; p < 0.0001, MWU test). As the GSE's scale range is from 10 to 40, these scores are in the lower mid-range; in a representative sample of younger persons (16–40 years), the GSE score is around 30.8 ± 5.4 (Hinz et al. 2006).

Intensity of Adolescents' Spiritual Needs

As described in Chap. 8, *Attention/Positive Confirmation* needs scored highest, followed by *Inner Peace* needs and *Existential/Giving needs*, while *Religious* needs were of lowest relevance for the adolescents. Here, female adolescents had significantly higher *Attention/Positive Confirmation* needs (p = 0.001, MWU test) and *Existential/Giving* needs (p = 0.038, MWU test) than male persons (Fig. 22.1a). This is at least in line with the observations that young girls and women are much more talkative than boy and young men, who are rather reserved about their emotional reactions. Further, women use emotion-focused coping strategies more often than men (Wu et al. 2018). With respect to the underlying treatment conditions, *Attention/Positive Confirmation* needs and *Existential/Giving* needs were significantly higher in adolescents with psychosomatic/psychiatric conditions compared to those with somatic ones, while their *Religious/Praying* needs and *Inner Peace* needs did not significantly differ (Fig. 22.1b). Detailed analyses revealed that within the subgroup of female patients (n = 120) persons with psychosomatic/psychiatric conditions had significantly higher *Attention/Positive Confirmation* needs than girls with somatic diseases (1.95 ± 0.86 vs. 2.29 ± 0.73; p = 0.018, MWU test), while *Existential/Giving* needs were only higher in trend (p = 0.053, MMWU test). In male adolescents (n = 76), there were no significant differences between both disease groups (data not shown). For all other needs, there were no significant within-gender differences.

Belief in God as a Resource

In this sample, 41% believe in God, 38% do not, and 21% were undecided about it. Here, believing in God was related to significantly higher *Religious* needs (1.15 ± 0.90) as compared to those who are unclear about it (0.42 ± 0.63) and nonbelievers (0.04 ± 0.17); these differences are statistically significant (F = 56.7, p < 0.0001, ANOVA). Thus, although *Religious* needs scored rather low in the general sample, this does not mean that these needs are not relevant—they are relevant for 41% of the

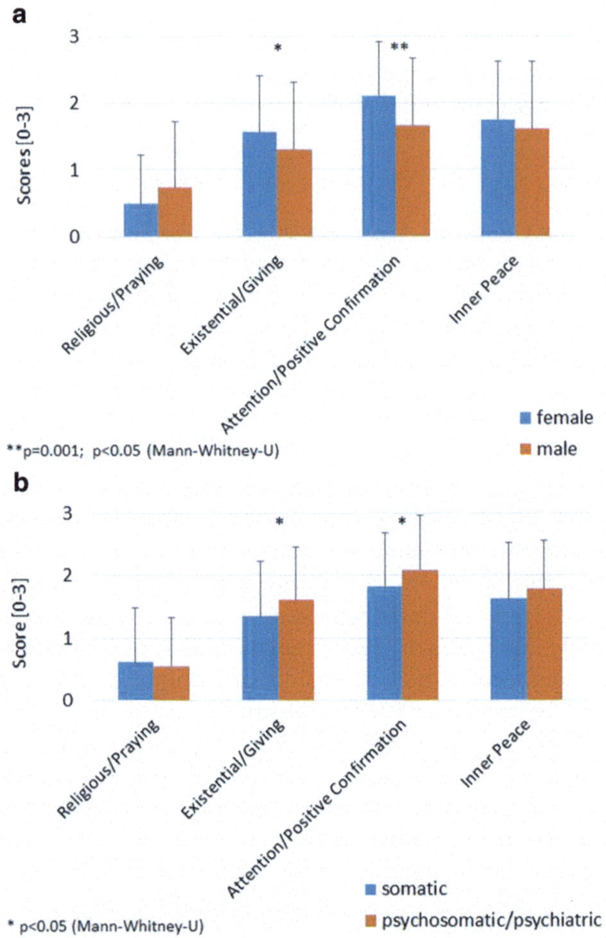

Fig. 22.1 Expression of spiritual needs in adolescents depending on treatement condition (**a**) and gender (**b**)

sample. These persons communicate in their prayer, which can be seen also as a coping strategy to deal with fears and worries. However, the need to talk with someone (meant as a concrete person) about fears and worries (item N2) was not significantly different between the three believing categories.

However, *Attention/Positive Confirmation* needs scored highest in the undecided group (2.18 ± 0.81) compared to the believers (2.03 ± 0.87) and nonbelievers (1.72 ± 0.87); these differences are significant, too ($F = 4.5$, $p = 0.012$). Maybe these undecided persons are aware that they require more concrete resources of support than belief in a "distant" God. For *Existential/Giving* needs and *Inner Peace* needs, no differences related to their belief in God were observed (data not shown).

Talking with Someone about Fears and Worries

The need to talk with someone about fears and worries (item N2) was remarkable as the difference between both treatment groups was more prominent. This need was in fact higher in persons with psychosomatic/psychiatric diseases than persons with somatic diseases (1.47 ± 1.08 vs. 1.86 ± 1.00; $p = 0.010$, MWU test); most of them were already in psychotherapeutic treatment. For this need, female adolescents with psychosomatic/psychiatric conditions had higher scores than their somatic counterparts in trend (1.61 ± 1.07 vs. 1.98 ± 0.92; $p = 0.051$; MWU test), while for male adolescents no significant differences were observed. This fits to the observation that particularly female adolescents use such talks with their peers to cope with their problems and stressors. Further, the psychiatric conditions of adolescent girls (internalizing disorders such as depression, anxiety) may differ from those of boys at that age (including externalizing symptoms as conduct disorder, ADHD). The kind of disorder may also affect the need to talk about the symptoms with peers. Girls' needs to talk about their fears and worries were particularly related to their need of having someone who is always at their side (N38: $r = 0.47$, Spearman rho), that someone assures how to proceed with the difficult situation (in a positive way) (N44: $r = 0.45$), that the situation is improving for the better (N43: $r = 0.41$), and to talk with someone about meaning in life (N11: $r = 0.40$). The communicative aspect is clearly in the forefront of female adolescents' needs for such relieving talks. For male adolescents, their need to talk about their fears and worries was particularly related with their need to be assured that life is meaningful and of value (N27: $r = 0.50$), and with the *Attention/Positive Confirmation* needs too (N38: $r = 0.57$; N44: $r = 0.48$), and that the situation is improving for the better (N43: $r = 0.42$).

Two items were particularly interesting because of their strong relevance for the adolescents with chronic or long-lasting conditions: the need to have someone who is always at their side (N38: 2.14 ± 1.08) and that the situation is improving for the better (N43: 2.16 ± 1.09). Only 14% stated that they do not have such a need for someone at their side (59% with somatic diseases; 64% males) and 13%, however, do not have the need that their situation is improving for the better (63% with somatic diseases; 52% males). Thus, there is an interplay of gender and underlying treatment conditions ("disease groups") that may have an influence on the readiness to talk about their needs, those who are more aware of their needs and those who are rather unclear about it or who may be too shy to talk, for example, about relationships.

Associations between Spiritual Needs and Life Satisfaction, Disease-Related Symptoms, and Self-Efficacy Expectation

In female and male adolescents, their spiritual needs are differentially related to life satisfaction, disease-related symptoms, and self-efficacy expectation. While for both, girls and boys, their *Attention/Positive Confirmation* needs and *Inner Peace* needs are similarly (weakly) negatively related to multidimensional life satisfaction, girls' perception of daily life impairment through disease-related symptoms was moderately positively correlated to *Attention/Positive Confirmation* needs, *Existential/Giving* needs and *Inner Peace* needs (Table 22.1). In contrast, boys' impairment through disease-related symptoms was weakly related to *Attention/Positive Confirmation* needs, but not with *Existential/Giving* needs *or Inner Peace* needs. For both genders, *Religious* needs were weakly associated with disease-related symptoms (Table 22.1). Girls' self-efficacy expectation correlated weakly negative with *Existential/Giving* needs and *Attention/Positive Confirmation* needs, while in boys, no significant associations with their self-efficacy expectation were observed.

This means, reduced life satisfaction is for both genders a relevant cause, while low self-efficacy expectation is of relevance predominantly for female adolescents. For female adolescents their symptoms are causes to state various spiritual needs, and they particularly require attention and positive confirmation, while for boys their symptom burden calls for attention and positive confirmation too, but not in general for relational and communicational needs or states of inner peace. This does not mean that boys do not regard these as important, but that there is no clear association, which was obvious in girls with chronic conditions.

Table 22.1 Correlations analyses in female and male adolescents

		Religious/ Praying needs	*Existential/ Giving needs*	*Attention/ Positive Confirmation needs*	*Inner Peace needs*
Females (n = 121)	Life satisfaction (BMLSS)	-0.108	-0.161	-0.279*	-0.245*
	Disease-related symptoms (VAS)	0.217*	**0.301***	**0.450***	**0.306***
	Self-efficacy expectation (GSE)	-0.082	-0.235*	-0.217*	-0.117
	Praying (SpREUK-P)	**0.655***	0.181*	0.196*	0.067
	Reflection on meaning in life (SpREUK-P)	002	**0.508***	**0.324***	**0.508***
Males (n = 76)	Life satisfaction (BMLSS)	-0.104	-0.194	-0.226*	-0.297*
	Disease-related symptoms (VAS)	0.270*	0.066	0.273*	0.067
	Self-efficacy expectation (GSE)	0.099	-0.122	-0.057	-0.092
	Praying (SpREUK-P)	**0.675***	0.283*	**0.362***	0.055
	Reflection on meaning in life (SpREUK-P)	0.089	**0.378***	0.221	**0.349***

*p < 0.05 (Spearman rho); moderate-to-strong correlations were highlighted (bold)

Associations between Spiritual Needs and Praying and Reflection on the Meaning in Life

Praying is an important indicator of religiosity. Most of the adolescents never prayed privately (59%), 18% rarely, 13% often, and 10% very often. In Northwestern Europe, a decline of subjective importance of religion, relevance of service attendance, and praying is to be acknowledged in the youth with a Christian background, while this is not seen in youth with a Muslim faith (Simsek et al. 2019). There were no significant gender-related differences between the engagement scores of praying. Reflecting on the meaning of life is an indicator of existential practices. Here, 21% were never reflecting on this, 33% rarely, 24% often, and 21% very often. Girls had significantly higher engagement scores for this reflection on meaning in life than boys ($p = 0.028$; MWU test).

Religious/Praying needs were strongly related with the frequency of private praying (item p1 of the SpREUK-P questionnaire), both in female and male adolescents (Table 22.1). In girls, *Existential/Giving* needs and *Attention/Positive Confirmation* needs were marginally only related with praying. In contrast, in boys their *Attention/Positive Confirmation* needs were much stronger related with their praying frequency, and their *Existential/Giving* needs at least weakly. For both groups, their *Inner Peace* needs were not related with praying.

The frequency of their reflection on the meaning of life (item p10 of the SpREUK-P questionnaire) was strongly related with *Existential/Generativity* needs and *Inner Peace* needs and moderately with *Attention/Positive Confirmation* needs in girls, while these associations were moderately and weakly related only in boys (Table 22.1).

Predictors of Adolescents' Spiritual Needs

The spiritual needs of adolescents with chronic conditions were differentially expressed and were related to different influencing variables. Therefore, stepwise regression analyses were performed to identify predictors of these needs. The respective findings are summarized in the following.

Religious/Praying needs were predicted best by frequency of private praying (Beta = 0.53, $p < 0.0001$) and belief in God (Beta = 0.29, $p < 0.0001$). Gender, disease, life satisfaction, self-efficacy expectation, affections of daily life through disease-related symptoms, and reflecting on meaning in life had no independent effect in this model, which would explain 55% of variance (50% by praying alone). This means, the individual religiosity of the person is the main reason for expressing these needs. The symptom burden can nevertheless be the cause of intensifying praying (for health and help) but is probably not the main reason (see Table 22.1).

Existential/Generativity needs were predicted by reflecting on meaning in life (Beta = 0.36, $p = 0.001$), affections of daily life through disease-related symptoms (Beta = 0.18, $p = 0.010$) and age (Beta = 0.16,

$p = 0.021$). Gender and disease had no independent effect in this model, which would predict 24% of variance (19% by reflection alone). Here, the pattern of predictors points to an ability to consider the question of meaning in life, which might be triggered by disease-related symptoms; this ability is probably influenced by age and thus life experience.

Attention/Positive Confirmation needs were predicted best five variables, by affections of daily life through disease-related symptoms alone (Beta = 0.36, $p < 0.0001$), reflection on meaning in life (Beta = 0.16, $p = 0.018$), female gender (Beta = 0.18, $p = 0.007$), age (Beta = 0.16, $p = 0.015$), and belief in God (Beta = 0.16, $p = 0.015$). Disease, life satisfaction and self-efficacy expectation, and praying had no significant effect in this model, which would explain 31% of variance (19% by affections of daily life through disease-related symptoms). Obviously, the symptom burden is the main trigger of these needs, with further influences of ability to reflect (+4% explained variance). Girls of higher age seem to have these needs a bit stronger than boys or persons of younger age.

Inner Peace needs were predicted best by reflection on meaning in life (Beta = 0.37, $p < 0.0001$), and further by age (Beta = 0.18, $p = 0.010$) and symptoms (Beta = 0.15, $p = 0.037$). Gender, disease, life satisfaction, self-efficacy expectation, and belief in God had no independent effect in this model, which would explain 24% of variance (19% by reflection alone). It seems that what may give meaning in life is also suited to provide states of inner peace; this ability to reflect might be a coping strategy that could be more available (and trained) in persons of higher age. In adults with chronic diseases or in the elderly, *Inner Peace* needs were particularly expressed by a low quality of life and negative mood states (Offenbaecher et al. 2013; Erichsen and Büssing 2013; Höcker et al. 2014). The underlying cause of this might be different in adolescents and persons of higher age.

In none of these predictor models general life satisfaction or self-efficacy expectation had a significant independent influence. The low relevance of self-efficacy expectation is important as it is generally seen as a resource to cope with problems and difficult phases in life, as an ability to manage these and find adequate solutions (Bandura 1977; Schwarzer and Jerusalem 2002). The adolescents investigated herein have rather low self-efficacy scores; maybe several of them have experienced that their own abilities to manage their health problems is limited and they are dependent on the help of external others. In this case, it is not surprising that this resource is not of outstanding relevance. However, it showed a weak negative association with *Existential/Giving* needs and *Attention/Positive Confirmation* needs in girls only, but not in boys. This means several girls do not expect that they have the abilities to cope with their health problems, and thus they express the respective needs.

Outlook

A major strength of this study is the large sample size and the use of standardized instruments, while a limitation is that it includes a heterogeneous group of conditions, differing in severity and impact. However, a direct comparison of chronic physical illness and psychiatric disorders has not been performed so far.

For the clinical situation, it would be important to identify young patients with spiritual needs and to ask them in the context of an anamnesis how these needs could be supported: for example, with respect to their coping strategies when they have a strong symptom burden, in addition to questions about their psychological/physical well-being. Addressing their spiritual needs would allow considering additional offers such as praying, meditation, nature experiences, and contact options with their peers group (including online formats). Here, intervention studies are needed.

Conclusions

Adolescents with chronic conditions or long-lasting treatments have unmet spiritual needs that are important to them. These have to be carefully addressed and supported. Bull and Gillies (2007) were very clear with their recommendation that healthcare professionals have to recognize children's spiritual needs and "that it is part of their duty of care to attempt to identify and meet such needs". Whether the support of their spiritual needs will really change their situation, remains unclear. At least addressing these needs is the signal that talking about their fears, worries, and unmet needs is possible.

Acknowledgments We are grateful to all those who have helped to recruit the adolescents who have filled the questionnaire, particularly Laura Sieber and Charlotte Roch.

References

Bandura A (1977) Self-efficacy: toward a unifying theory of behavioral change. Psychol Rev 84:191–215

Barkin SH, Miller L, Luthar SS (2015) Filling the void: spiritual development among adolescents of the affluent. J Relig Health 54:844–861

Bor W, Dean AJ, Najman J, Hayatbaksh R (2014) Are child and adolescent mental health problems increasing in the 21st century? Aust N Z J Psychiatry 48:606–616

Büssing A, Kerksieck P, Föller-Manici A, Baumann K (2012) Aspects of spirituality and ideals to help in adolescents from Christian academic high schools. Int J Child Spiritual 17:99–116

Bull A (2016) Assessing and communicating the spiritual needs of children in hospital. A new guide for healthcare professionals and chaplains. Jessica Kingsley Publishers, London

Bull A, Gillies M (2007) Spiritual needs of children with complex healthcare needs in hospital. Paediatr Nurs 19:34–38

Compas BE, Jaser SS, Dunn MJ, Rodriguez EM (2012) Coping with chronic illness in childhood and adolescence. Annu Rev Clin Psychol 8:455–480

Cotton S, Zebracki K, Rosenthal SL, Tsevat J, Drotar D (2006) Religion/spirituality and adolescent health outcomes: a review. J Adolesc Health 38:472–480

Damsma Bakker AA, van Leeuwen RRR, Roodbol PFP (2018) The spirituality of children with chronic conditions: a qualitative meta-synthesis. J Pediatr Nurs 43:e106–e113

Desrosiers A, Miller L (2007) Relational spirituality and depression in adolescents girls. J Clin Psychol 63:1021–1037

Erichsen NB, Büssing A (2013) Spiritual needs of elderly living in retirement/nursing homes evidence-based complementary and alternative medicine. Article ID913247. https://doi.org/10.1155/2013/913247

Feudtner C, Haney J, Dimmers MA (2003) Spiritual care needs of hospitalized children and their families: a national survey of pastoral care providers' perceptions. Pediatrics 111(1):e67–72

Fuchs M, Bösch A, Hausmann A, Steiner H (2013) "The child is father or man"—review von relevanten Studien zur Epidemiologie in der kinder- und Jugendpsychiatrie. Zeitschrift für Kinder und Jugendpsychiatrie und Psychotherapie 41:45–57

Hinz A, Schumacher J, Albani C, Schmid G, Brähler E (2006) Bevölkerungsrepräsentative Normierung der Skala zur Allgemeinen Selbstwirksamkeitserwartung. Diagnostica 52:26–32

Höcker A, Krüll A, Koch U, Mehnert A (2014) Exploring spiritual needs and their associated factors in an urban sample of early and advanced cancer patients. Eur J Cancer Care 23:786–794

Hufton E (2006) Parting gifts: the spiritual needs of children. Journal of Child Health Care 10(3):240–250

Lazarus R, Folkman S (1984) Stress, appraisal and coping. Springer, Wien and New York

LeBlanc LA, Goldsmith T, Patel DR (2003) Behavioral aspects of chronic illness in children and adolescents. Pediatr Clin N Am 50:859–878

Levenson H (1972) Distinctions within the concept of internal-external control: development of a new scale. Proceedings of the 80th Annual Convention of the American Psychological Association 7:261–262

Louis-Jacques J, Samples C (2011) Caring for teens with chronic illness: risky business? Curr Opin Pediatr 23:367–372

McSherry W, Smith J (2007) How do children express their spiritual needs? Paediatr Nurs 19:17–20

Miller L (2013) Spiritual awakening and depression in adolescents: a unified pathway or "two sides of the same coin". Bull Menn Clin 77:332–348

Miller L, Gur M (2002) Religiosity, depression and physical maturation in adolescent girls. J Am Acad Child Adolesc Psychiatry 41:206–214

Offenbaecher M, Kohls N, Toussaint LL, Sigl C, Winkelmann A, Hieblinger R, Walther A, Büssing A (2013) Spiritual needs in patients suffering from fibromyalgia. Evidence-based complementary and alternative medicine. Article ID 178547. https://doi.org/10.1155/2013/178547

Pargament KI (1997) The psychology of religion and coping: theory, research, practice. Guilford, New York

Pargament KI (2011) Religion and coping: the current state of knowledge. In: Folkman S (ed) Oxford handbook of stress, health, and coping. Oxford University Press, New York

Petersen CL (2014) Spiritual care of the child with cancer at the end of life: a concept analysis. Journal of Advanced Nursing 70(6):1243–1253

Picoraro JA, Womer JW, Kazak AE, Feudtner C (2014) Posttraumatic growth in parents and pediatric patients. J Palliat Med 17:209–218

Rotter J (1966) Generalized expectations for internal versus external control reinforcement. Psychol Monogr 80:1–27

Schwarzer R, Jerusalem M (2002) Das Konzept der Selbstwirksamkeit. In Jerusalem M, Hopf D (eds) Selbstwirksamkeit und Motivationsprozesse in Bildungsinstitutionen. Zeitschrift für Pädagogik 44(Beiheft):28–53

Shelly JA (1982) The spiritual needs of children: a guide for nurses, parents and teachers. InterVarsity Press, Westmont

Simsek M, Fleischmann F, van Tubergen F (2019) Similar or divergent paths? Religious development of Christian and Muslim adolescents in Western Europe. Soc Sci Res 79:160–180

Voll RE, Krumm B, Cregger B, Shaw RJ (2013) Psychische Störungen bei chronischen Erkrankungen und ihre Rehabilitation. In: Lehmkuhl G, Poustka F,

Holtmann M, Steiner M (eds) Lehrbuch der Kinder- und Jugendpsychiatrie. Hogrefe, Göttingen, pp 1232–1267

von Gontard A (2013) Spiritualität von Kindern und Jugendlichen. Kohlhammer, Stuttgart

von Hagen C, Schwarz HP (eds) (2009) Psychische Entwicklung bei chronischer Krankheit im Kindes- und Jugendalter. Kohlhammer, Stuttgart

Wallander JL, Varni JW (1998) Effects of pediatric chronic physical disorder on child and family adjustment. J Child Psychol Psychiatry 39:29–46

Wu Q, Slesnick N, Zhang J (2018) Understanding the role of emotion-oriented coping in women's motivation for change. J Subst Abus Treat 86:1–8. https://doi.org/10.1016/j.jsat.2017.12.006

CHAPTER 23

Spiritual Needs in Postwar Population Posttrauma Patients in Croatia and Bosnia-Herzegovina

Andrijana Glavas and Klaus Baumann

Traumatized Postwar Populations

During the so-called Balkan war in former Yugoslavia during the early 1990s, many people in Croatia and Bosnia-Herzegovina were exposed to gravely traumatizing events. More than 25 years after the end of the war, the populations are still suffering from its material, physical and psychosocial consequences. The aftermaths and wounds of the war crimes are still present and have not been worked through or coped with successfully in many cases. Many people who survived traumatizing war events have developed mental and physical diseases, including a higher mortality rate (Filipp and Aymanns 2010) and long-standing consequences of social imbalance. Two frequent diseases—but not the only ones—have been

A. Glavas • K. Baumann (✉)
Caritas Science and Christian Social Work, Faculty of Theology, Albert-Ludwigs University, Freiburg, Germany
e-mail: andrijana.glavas@theol.uni-freiburg.de; klaus.baumann@theol.uni-freiburg.de

A. Büssing (ed.), *Spiritual Needs in Research and Practice*,
https://doi.org/10.1007/978-3-030-70139-0_23

posttraumatic stress disorder (PTSD) and enduring personality change after catastrophic experience.

There are various factors that favor the development of PTSD and others that protect against it. One thing is the traumatic event itself; other factors concern individual resources and vulnerabilities and protective as well as risk factors of the social environment. Any critical life event and even more severe diseases stimulate and challenge religious and spiritual needs and practices, including existential questions about the meaning of life in general and of this disease in particular. Trauma by definition fundamentally shakes the feelings of safety of persons and their roots in life by the experience of utmost helplessness and impotence. They frequently feel depressed, hardly self-efficacious, tending to substance abuse and suicidality. Obviously, also religious faiths and spiritual orientations as part of the roots in life are shaken and impaired by the experience of trauma in most cases (Baumann 2018). Starting treatment of patients with posttraumatic disorders as early as possible with qualified psychotherapy and pharmaceuticals is crucial to alleviate the condition. In addition to this necessary treatment, therapeutic interventions should discover, activate and strengthen the patients' resources and protective factors in a holistic approach, part of which may be religious and spiritual resources (Reddemann and Dehner-Rau 2007). Such treatment intends to prevent from chronification and to facilitate—hopefully—posttraumatic growth.

In fact, finding meaning in life and in disease are among the strongest resources for coping with disease and trauma (Knuf 2008) and can be considered predictors of posttraumatic growth (McFarlane and Van der Kolk 2000). In clinical contexts, the dimension of religious, spiritual and personal beliefs is about getting more attention (Klein et al. 2011). What about the postwar posttrauma patients in Croatia and Bosnia-Herzegovina and their religious and spiritual needs, resting aware that in general many victims of trauma avoid treatment (Kantor et al. 2017)? What role do these needs have for postwar trauma patients in the context of their experience of, and coping with, their disorder?

Patients in Psychiatric and Psychotherapeutic Treatment in Bosnia-Herzegovina and Croatia

As part of a larger study, in this chapter we will pull together data of spiritual needs of in-patients, day care and ambulant patients diagnosed with PTSD (ICD 10 F43.1) or with enduring personality change after catastrophic experience (ICD 10 F62.0) from Bosnia-Herzegovina (Sarajevo and Tuzla University Hospitals) and from Croatia (Rijeka University Hospital), surveyed in keeping with the present version of the Helsinki declaration and European data protection rules after approval of the respective Ethics committees (Glavas et al. 2017, 2020).

The nine-page questionnaire contained the SpNQ-20 (Büssing et al. 2018), translated into Croatian by the first author (a native speaker) for its first use in both countries. The SpNQ-20's four scales address *Religious* needs, *Inner Peace* needs, *Existential* needs, and *Giving/Generativity* needs. In our survey, the internal consistency of the 20-items was very high (Cronbach's $\alpha = 0.93$) and high for the subscales Religious Needs with six items (Cronbach's $\alpha = 0.88$), Existential Needs with six items (Cronbach's $\alpha = 0.82$), the *Giving/Generativity* needs including four items (Cronbach's $\alpha = 0.86$), and low for the Inner Peace needs scale with four items (Cronbach's $\alpha = 0.54$).

In addition, four items were asking for *Family Support* needs, concerning aspects of connection with, and integration into one's own family—and showed good reliability in our sample (Cronbach's $\alpha = 0.74$). Two additional items addressing self-perception as a religious and/or spiritual person allow the differentiation of four groups, depending on their self-assessments as more (+) or less (-) religious and more (+) or less (-) spiritual.

Over two-thirds of the sample of returned questionnaires (N = 164) were from male patients, who were also the majority in active war fighters. Most patients were married, had children and had a middle-to-higher education. Interestingly, there was a considerable amount of new diagnoses of PTSD among younger patients (age 18–44 years) who—in part—were born after the Balkan war. With the participation of two clinics in Bosnia-Herzegovina with its predominantly Muslim population and one clinic in Croatia (predominantly Catholics) this sample constituted a majority of Muslim participants. Of the participants, 76% (n = 120) reported themselves to be religious and/or spiritual, for example, 34% regarded themselves as R+S+, 8% as R+S-, 34% as R-S+ and 24% as R-S-.

How Strong Are Spiritual Needs in this Sample?

Items of the *Religious* needs scale scored lowest, yet still comparatively often (Table 23.1). Especially the need to turn to a higher power (i.e. to pray) was strongest with 84%. All the other "religious needs" were

Table 23.1 Frequency and Strength of spiritual needs

		%	N
Religious needs	N23 to turn to a higher presence	84.0	162
	N22 to read religious/spiritual books	80.8	162
	N21 to participate in religious ceremonies	80.9	163
	N20 to pray on one's own	71.4	161
	N19 to be prayed for	73.6	163
	N18 to pray with someone	71.1	163
Giving/Generativity needs	N26 to share one's own life experiences	88.4	164
	N27 to know that one's life was meaningful and valuable	80.2	162
	N15 to be able to comfort/solace someone	77.3	163
	N14 give away something from yourself	76.5	162
Inner peace needs	N6 to plunge into the beauty of nature	86.4	162
	N7 to dwell in a quiet and peaceful place	86.0	164
	N8 to find inner peace	95.7	164
	N2 to talk with someone about fears and worries	94.7	153
Existential needs	N4 to reflect back on one's life	85.9	164
	N5 to resolve unsolved problems	89.0	164
	N10 to find meaning in one's illness/suffering	88.4	164
	N11 to talk with someone about the question of meaning in life?	88.4	164
	N12 to speak with someone about the possibility of life after death	78.5	163
	N16 to forgive someone from a distinct period of your life	73.4	162
	N17 that someone forgives you	74.1	162
Social/Family Support needs	N25 to be connected to one's family[a]	91.4	163
	N30 to receive support from one's family[a]	93.7	159
	N13 to turn lovingly to someone else[a]	76.4	153
	N28 to be more involved by your own family[a]	87.1	163

Note: Numbers and percentages refer to scores of "moderate" (2) or "strong" (3)

[a]In addition to the four main scales of SpNQ

important to no less than 70% of the patients. As to *Existential* needs, the vast majority—from 86% to 89%—felt the need to resolve unsolved problems, to find meaning in their illness, to ask for the meaning of their lives and to reflect back on their lives. Though *Giving/Generativity* needs were considerably strong, too, most important to the patients were *Inner Peace* needs, closely followed by needs for *Social/Family Support*. Most important were the needs to find inner peace and to talk with someone about their fears and worries (with 96% and 95%, respectively). It is noteworthy and remarkable that these latter needs were reported so strongly in the context of the clinical treatment setting—either because they find a treatment responsive to these needs or less.

Intensity of Spiritual Needs in the Sample

Table 23.2 shows the comparative strength (in contrast to the frequency dealt with before) of the four SpNQ scales and of the additional family support scale. Compared to men, female patients score significantly higher for *Religious* needs, *Existential* needs and *Social/Family Support* needs, in trend for *Giving/Generativity* needs, but not for *Inner Peace* needs.

Interestingly, the younger participants of our survey (18–44 years) had significantly higher mean scores than the middle group (51–55), while the oldest group (56+ years) differed significantly with stronger existential needs (data not shown).

Table 23.2 Strength of spiritual needs in subgroups

		Religious needs (N = 157)	*Existential needs (N = 160)*	*Inner Peace needs (N = 164)*	*Giving/ Generativity needs (N = 160)*	*Social Support needs (N = 162)*
All persons	Mean	2.27	2.21	2.47	2.27	2.42
	SD	0.84	0.65	0.46	0.77	0.68
Gender						
Men	Mean	2.16	2.13	2.45	2.20	2.34
	SD	0.88	0.65	0.46	0.81	0.71
Women	Mean	2.50	2.38	2.52	2.44	2.58
	SD	0.72	0.64	0.46	0.67	0.58
F value		5.28	4.71	0.87	3.31	4.02
p value		**0.02**	**0.03**	0.35	0.07	**0.04**
Religion						
Catholics	Mean	1.77	1.97	2.47	2.03	2.09
	SD	0.97	0.63	0.45	0.74	0.73
Muslims	Meant	2.42	2.26	2.47	2.34	2.50
	SD	0.74	0.66	0.47	0.79	0.65
F value		16.40	4.74	0.02	3.88	9.25
P value		**<0.001**	**0.03**	0.96	0.06	**<0.001**

Note: Significant differences were highlighted (bold)

Of course, we are interested in the comparison of Spiritual needs between the different religious denominations of Muslims and Catholics (and eventually others). There are especially and significantly strong differences only with regard to *Religious, Existential,* and *Social/Family Support* needs, all stronger in the Muslim participants, while *Inner Peace* needs are equally strong between both groups (Table 23.2).

Spiritual Needs Are Strongly Present in Posttrauma Patients of the Postwar Societies in Bosnia-Herzegovina and Croatia

The consequences of the Balkan war in the first part of the 1990s are permeating all the layers of the postwar societies in Croatia and Bosnia-Herzegovina, including economic and social problems for many people in the respective countries. Meanwhile, 25 years after the war, veterans and their problems are no longer in the focus of public interest or of everyday life's preoccupations. This may make it even harder for new patients to present to their doctors with their posttraumatic symptoms (Kantor et al. 2017). Nevertheless, we got an astonishingly big subsample of younger patients (age 18–44 years) that confirms that it was not only active participants who have been traumatized. Without being able to present their details, most of the patients of the present sample were exposed to multiple traumata during the Balkan war. They are still suffering from severe mental and/or physical impairments. With regard to the youngest patients, we can even reflect on the possibility of intergenerational transmission.

In spite of good medical and psychological care for the veterans, while there is empirical evidence in Croatia that cardiovascular diseases are the main cause of death in the general population, among veterans the prevalent cause is neoplasms or cancer (Republika Hrvatska; https://branitelji.gov.hr/istaknute-teme/istrazivanje-pobola-i-smrtnosti-hrvatskih-branitelja/805, retrieved 15 September 2020). One of the hypothesized reasons is the stress to which they were exposed during the war as well as the perpetuation of that stress in posttraumatic diseases they suffer from. The traumatic experiences have continuously stressed and deeply shaken their basic beliefs and assumptions about the world, themselves and their lives, and threatened their lives and integrity with violence and death (Löffler et al. 2012; Baumann 2018).

The results of our survey show moderate-to-strong spiritual and religious needs in the majority of patients with posttraumatic diseases. All of the scales achieve comparatively high mean values, the strongest of which, however, are *Inner Peace* needs and *Family/Social Support* needs. These seem to imply that there is a lot of inner unrest or even turmoil in many of the patients, which they hope, among others, to settle in a safe family environment. In addition, these respondents desire to give and to be sure that their lives have been meaningful. These results resemble those of a German study with chronic diseases and cancer (Büssing et al. 2010).

In our sample, younger patients (age 18–44 years) reported stronger Religious needs than the other groups while the oldest groups (age 56+ years) marked stronger *Existential* needs. Both trends deserve more attention rather than trying a precocious interpretation. Female patients showed significantly stronger *Religious, Existential* and *Family/Social Support* needs than men. It seems they experience their illness and cope with it differently from men (Meyer 2008). Mladina and Huber's (2002) study on war survivors in Bosnia reported empirical evidence that women have drawn more strongly on religious aspects in their coping with PTSD symptoms.

Not really surprisingly, Muslim respondents expressed significantly stronger *Religious* needs, for example, for praying alone or together with others. They also differed significantly from Catholic patients in more intense *Giving/Generativity* needs as well as for *Family/Social Support* needs. Another interesting significant difference between the two religious denomination groups is found among those who scored neither religious nor spiritual (R-S-), who make up for 24% of the sample. Significantly more Muslim patients reported themselves R-S- than Catholic ones ($p = 0.04$). And there was an age difference, too: Though younger patients also tended to score higher in *Religious* needs, there were also more R-S- persons among them ($p < 0.01$) than in the other age groups. The higher scores for Religious needs are correlated with young Muslim patients, but also the bigger number of persons with R-S-. This could indicate the polar development among young people toward a more religious and a more secular orientation. In our opinion, these results are hints and indications for further attention and deserve more detailed analysis in future studies.

Finally, we intend to highlight two details of the SpNQ results in this sample: Two items scored highest in our sample, even higher than the *Family/Social Support* needs: The needs "To find inner peace" (N8: 96%) and "To talk with someone about fears and worries" (N4: 95%). Flashbacks, panic attacks and anxieties as parts of posttrauma symptoms undermine inner peace continuously. This is but one side of the coin. The need to talk with someone is expressed so strongly by almost all who responded to this item even though they have been surveyed during their treatments. Most patients need to talk and want to talk. Does their treatment—stationary, day care, ambulant—provide sufficient opportunity to respond to this need in the medical system in general (Maio 2015, 2020), in psychiatry and psychotherapy (see Chap. 17), and in particular for these traumatized patients? Note that the need to talk with someone about worries and fears was responded to by 153 of 164 patients, the least number of patients (along with the need to "turn lovingly to someone else", important to 74% of them). For those who answered this item, this was an important need. Those who did not respond seem to have been undecided if they can dare talk about their special posttraumatic worries and fears with anybody—another indication how painful their psychological condition might be.

Conclusions

The overall result of our survey shows strong spiritual needs in all the realms (scales) of the SpNQ and of *Family Support* needs. This strong presence of spiritual needs in posttraumatic disorders does not imply that they are adequately or satisfactorily met or dealt with, be this in private life, in family, in the communities or, last not least, in the health care system. Spiritual care ought not to be focused on the terminal phase of life, that is, in palliative care, but become a qualified part of any health care system and subsystem. The data presented in this chapter provide plain evidence of strong spiritual needs of posttrauma patients; for sure, they need to be enriched and then further analyzed.

In addition, patients are experts in their own matters, too, and ought to be part of further research looking for the best ways how to do justice to, and how to meet their spiritual needs in the complexity of their health conditions and personalities, in keeping with the professional ethics and boundaries in the health care system. A patient-centered (holistic) approach in health care, in our opinion, cannot but take these patient realities seriously, with the goal to alleviate their patients' burdens of their critical health condition. As a result, for patients with posttraumatic stress disorder or with enduring personality change after catastrophic experience, and for their families, realistic hope for posttraumatic growth may increase.

Acknowledgment We are grateful to all the participants of our survey and to the medical staff of the participating wards for psychiatry and psychotherapy of the university clinics of Tuzla, Sarajevo and Rijeka for their effective and generous support without which it would not have been possible to conduct this survey.

References

Baumann K (2018) Religiosität bzw. Spiritualität und Traumabewältigung. In: Baumann K, Bendel R, Maruhukiro D (eds) Flucht, Trauma, Integration; Nachkriegseuropa und Ruanda/Burundi im Vergleich. Lit Verlag, Berlin-Münster-Wien-Zurich, pp 17–28

Büssing A, Balzat HJ, Heusser P (2010) Spiritual needs of patients with chronic pain diseases and cancer—validation of the spiritual needs questionnaire. Eur J Med Res 15:266–273

Büssing A, Recchia DR, Koenig H, Baumann K, Frick E (2018). Factor Structure of the Spiritual Needs Questionnaire (SpNQ) in Persons with Chronic Diseases, Elderly and Healthy Individuals. Religions 9(1):13. https://doi.org/10.3390/rel9010013

Filipp SH, Aymanns P (2010) Kritische Lebensereignisse – eine erste Annäherung. In: Kritische Lebensereignisse und Lebenskrisen. Von Umgang mit den Schattenseiten des Lebens. Kohlhammer, Stuttgart

Glavas A, Jors K, Büssing A, Baumann K (2017) Spiritual needs of PTSD patients in Croatia and Bosnia-Herzegovina: a quantitative pilot study. Psychiatr Danub 29(3):282–290

Glavas A, Büssing A, Baumann K (2020) Religiöse und spirituelle Bedürfnisse bei traumatisierten Patienten in Sarajevo. Spiritual Care (ahead of print: 16 June 2020). https://doi.org/10.1515/spircare-2019-0042

Kantor V, Knefel M, Lueger-Schuster B (2017) Perceived barriers and facilitators of mental health service utilization in adult trauma survivors: a systematic review. Clin Psychol Rev 52:52–68

Klein C, Bert H, Balck F (eds) (2011) Gesundheit – Religion – Spiritualität. Konzepte, Befunde und Erklärungsansätze. Juventa, Weinheim

Knuf A (2008) Spiritualität, Genesung und psychiatrische Arbeit. Soziale Psychiatrie 4:20–23

Löffler S, Bogausch A, Knappe R, Joraschky P, Pöhlmann K (2012) Wachstum oder Wunde? Sinnfindung und Traumabewältigung bei Patienten mit Posttraumatischer Belastungsstörung. Z Psychosom Med Psychother 58:192–204

Maio G (2015) Den kranken Menschen verstehen. Für eine Medizin der Zuwendung. Herder, Freiburg

Maio G (ed) (2020) Von Angesicht zu Angesicht. Zur Bedeutung der persönlichen Begegnung in der Medizin. Herder, Freiburg

McFarlane AC, Van der Kolk BA (2000) Trauma und seine Herausforderung an die Gesellschaft. In: Van der Kolk BA, McFarlane AC, Weisaeth L (eds) Traumatic stress. Grundlagen und Behandlungsansätze. Theorie, Praxis und Forschung zu posttraumatischem Stress sowie Traumatherapie. Junfermann, Paderborn, p 48

Meyer P (2008) Gender, Trauma, Sucht. Flucht vor der Erinnerung. Deutsches Ärzteblatt 11:522–523

Mladina V, Huber HP (2002) Live after war: coping with war trauma. Psychologische Beiträge 44(4):616–626

Reddemann L, Dehner-Rau C (2007) Trauma. Folgen erkennen, überwinden und an ihnen wachsen. Ein Übungsbuch für Körper und Seele. Trias, Stuttgart

Republika Hrvatska. Ministarstvo hrvatskih branitelja. Istraživanje pobola i smrtnosti hrvatskih branitelja. https://branitelji.gov.hr/istaknute-teme/istrazivanje-pobola-i-smrtnosti-hrvatskih-branitelja/805. Accessed 15 Sep 2020

CHAPTER 24

Spiritual Needs and Life Satisfaction of Refugees in Bavaria

Kathrin Maier and Janusz Surzykiewicz

Background

According to the United Nations High Commissioner for Refugees (2010), a refugee is "any person who is outside their country of origin and unable or unwilling to return there or to avail themselves of its protection, owing to well-founded fear of persecution for reasons of race, religion, nationality, membership of a particular social group (an additional ground not found in the UNHCR Statute), or political opinion" (Goodwin-Gill 2014).

K. Maier (✉)
Department of Educational Psychology in Social Work, Catholic University of Applied Sciences Munich, Munich, Germany
e-mail: Kathrin.Maier@ksh-m.de

J. Surzykiewicz
Faculty of Philosophy and Education, Katholische Universität Eichstätt-Ingolstadt, Eichstätt, Germany

Faculty of Education, Cardinal Stefan Wyszynski University in Warsaw, Warsaw, Poland
e-mail: Janusz.Surzykiewicz@ku.de

A. Büssing (ed.), *Spiritual Needs in Research and Practice*,
https://doi.org/10.1007/978-3-030-70139-0_24

Refugees are forced to leave their homeland and country, often without a chance to return back. Many refugees in transit experience harsh and dangerous living conditions, low nutrition health support, difficulties in meeting their basic needs, separation from family and social networks, exclusion from education or employment, instability and fear for the future, reduced access to healthcare, and sometimes hostility from the host society (Schouler-Ocak et al. 2016; Schick et al. 2018; Goodkind et al. 2020). In consequence, most refugees experience emotional, psychological, and social difficulties, as well as economic and environmental instability and societal fragility (Benson et al. 2012; Bekteshi and Kang 2018; Mallett and Hagen-Zanker 2018; Borho et al. 2020). And even when people's functional needs, such as food, security, work, and education are met through relocation, they may still be disadvantaged by social, cultural, or religious losses (Betts et al. 2020). Refugees are thus confronted with many uncertainties that threaten their resources. Alienation, lack of meaning, and lack of life satisfaction are expected outcomes during such drastic and pervasive changes toward a new life, a new culture, and a new society (Çetin 2019; Esses et al. 2017; von Werthern et al. 2018; Pandya 2018; Fennig 2020; Byrow et al. 2020; Nesterko et al. 2020). In fact, acculturative stress predicted lower levels of well-being and more psychological symptoms (Adam and Ward 2016; Echterhoff et al. 2020; Jasperse et al. 2011; Stuart et al. 2016). Refugees can thus be seen as a specifically vulnerable group for developing mental health problems and suffering from low subjective well-being (Hashemi et al. 2019). At the same time, there is a necessity and public interest to assure well-being and life satisfaction of those seeking protection and refugee. This must be taken into account as a fundamental prerequisite for social stability (Karaman and Ricard 2016; Woods and Pulla 2016; Naja et al. 2016; Silove et al. 2017; Omata 2017; Hodge 2015, 2018; Schick et al. 2018).

To tackle these issues, numerous recent studies have focused on the relationship between trauma, serious post-migration problems, conditions for individual adaptation processes, as well as social support systems and their impact on mental health in refugees and asylum seekers. Yet in contrast, research on more existential or sociocultural needs of refugees and their associations to life satisfaction and mental health is largely missing. On the other hand, societal and cultural systems, religious beliefs, and various everyday demands and needs play a significant role in a person's perceived life satisfaction and mental health condition. This is especially true for refugees and migrants who are confronted with deep structural losses. Thus, a systematic exploration of the refugees' backgrounds outside the discourse of trauma would enable to identify factors and mechanisms to promote well-being (Harrop et al. 2006). Such an approach would not only help to identify factors of psychosocial adaptation to support refugees to assure their mental health needs, it would also help to uncover commonly overlooked key resources of mental health which were the refugees' strength during their forced migration and resettlement (Tempany 2009; Tippens 2017; Nesterko et al. 2020; Betts et al. 2020; Renner et al. 2020).

In this context, research on psychological and spiritual needs might be an interesting approach. Various studies from within self-determination theory indicated that the satisfaction of a limited set of basic psychological needs—namely, autonomy, competence, and relatedness, also with reference to the religious context—was already sufficient for human flourishing (Deci and Ryan 1991; Ryan and Deci 2000, 2017). Psychological needs thus play a crucial role in human well-being and development, by giving meaning and understanding to a situation, providing a sense of self-esteem, mastery, and control, as well as a sense of belonging and connectedness (Deci and Ryan 2000). Yet the fulfillment of these needs—and thus the promotion of well-being—was shown to be directly related to societal affordances and social conditions (Ryan et al. 2019; Ryan and Deci 2017; DeHaan et al. 2016).

Refugee's Needs and Their Religion and Spirituality

Challenges, needs, and struggles that refugees have to cope with vary depending on the cultural, religious, and social beliefs in which they appear. Therefore, existential and psychological struggles should be focused to better understand risk factors, complications in specific psychosocial functioning, as well as accompanying mental difficulties (Diener et al. 2010; Alemi et al. 2014; AbdAleati et al. 2016; Ryan and Deci 2017; Çetin 2019). This is particularly important in case of refugees from nations where religion plays a central role in culture and social life. Coming from such nations and cultural backgrounds, people frequently process their difficulties, disruptions in lives, or associated traumas through the prism of religious (e.g., Islamic or Christian) norms (Eltaiba 2014).

In the last decade, a wide array of studies focused on whether religious and spiritual beliefs and needs rather support or hinder refugees in their migration and settlement process in a host country (McSherry 2010;

Diener et al. 2011; Acquaye 2017; Omata 2017; Newman and Graham 2018; Sabouni 2019; Byrow et al. 2020; Spatrisano et al. 2020; Krause and Schmidt 2020). Overall, religion and spirituality seem to reveal beneficial effects for refugees. Religious faith and practices are a source of cultural continuity that keeps refugees in contact with their home countries, people, language, and traditions. Religiosity and spirituality provide a sense of belonging and support that help refugees to sustain their hope and to develop an attitude of acceptance for the current and future situation. In addition, a religious belief system activates resilience and provides a prominent way to cope with challenges, psychological difficulties, and unmet needs (Dorais 2007; Snodgrass et al. 2017; Abraham et al. 2018; Sabouni 2019). In addition, religious faith plays a central role in preserving the identity of refugees, regardless of the ethnic identity and dominant religious affiliations in the host country. Their spirituality and religion may offer refugees a framework for cognitive, emotional, and social-behavioral representations that may provide guidance and strategies for adjustment to life demands and needs. Being involved in religious and spiritual activities secures an affiliate group, promotes feelings of social inclusion, and enables a gradual adjustment to the new existential environment (Shoeb et al. 2007; Horstmann and Jung 2015; Pulla and Woods 2016; Wilkinson et al. 2017; Bekteshi and Kang 2018; Oishi and Diener 2014; Çetin 2019). The experience of social belonging was shown to be a supportive factor for well-being in refugees (Çetin 2019; Abraham et al. 2018).

Life Satisfaction, Well-Being, and Religion

Despite different conceptualizations of mental health and well-being, the most common approaches either focus on the presence of positive attributes (e.g., happiness, satisfaction with life), or the absence of negative attributes (e.g., depressive symptoms, diagnosis of a psychiatric illness). Subjective well-being indicates how a person evaluates the overall quality of his or her life (Diener 2006). This appraisal includes a cognitive account, referring to the perceived fulfillment of one's own expectations and goals in the life span, termed life satisfaction. There is also an affective component that balances between positive and negative affect (Diener et al. 1985; Diener 2006). Along with subjective well-being and happiness, life satisfaction can be also understood as an indicator of quality of life (Veenhoven 2015). Numerous studies have focused on the construct of life satisfaction and relevant influencing factors.

Among others, religion and spirituality were shown to have beneficial effects on well-being, both in its cognitive and affective components (Graham and Crown 2014; Arabzadeh et al. 2017; VanderWeele 2017; Grant and Oman 2018; Oman 2018; Kim-Prieto and Miller 2018; Long et al. 2019; Edinger-Schons 2019; Villani et al. 2019). However, effect sizes are often low (Kim-Prieto and Miller 2018). Positive associations were found across various populations like youth, adults, and elderly (Johnstone et al. 2012; Gull and Dawood 2013; AbdAleati et al. 2016) as well as across religions and cultures (Kim-Prieto and Miller 2018). Across religions, subjective well-being was highly related to church attendance (Lim 2015; Jenks 2020) as well as positive religious coping styles (Abu-Raiya and Pargament 2015; Adam and Ward 2016). In addition, religious oneness-beliefs promoted life satisfaction, regardless of religious affiliations (Diener and Clifton 2002; Edinger-Schons 2019). Turning to culture, Graham and Crown (2014), for example, reported an overall positive association between religiosity and subjective well-being, including about 160 nations. The strength of impact was moderated by the extent to which a culture valued religion or not (Tay and Diener 2011; Gebauer et al. 2012; Hayward and Elliott 2014) as well as by cross-national differences concerning the general level of religiosity in the population (Okulicz-Kozaryn 2010). Other respective moderators were support for spiritual practice, societal hostility toward religion, and feeling for respect (Diener et al. 2011; Lun and Bond 2013). Thus, beside overall effects, results on the contribution of spirituality and religion to well-being on a more detailed level also show inconsistent and varying findings (Lim and Putnam 2010; Ellison and Henderson 2011; Dimitrova and Aydinli-Karakulak 2016; Safak-Ayvazoglu and Kunuroglu 2019; Hashemi et al. 2019).

Turning to refugees, studies indicated religious beliefs as a coping resource to buffer against the negative impact of acculturative stress on well-being (Ano and Vasconcelles 2005; Sanchez et al. 2012; Gladden 2012; Adam and Ward 2016; Hakim et al. 2017; Abraham et al. 2018; Acquaye et al. 2018; Acquaye 2017; Areba et al. 2018; Shaw et al. 2019; Muruthi et al. 2020). In addition, religious identity demonstrated a positive association on psychological well-being through social support, less perceived discrimination, and more social connectedness with the host community (Hashemi et al. 2019). Further studies on refugee populations showed positive associations between indicators of spirituality or religion and psychosocial well-being (Tippens 2017; Pandya 2018; Çetin 2019). Other studies in contrast revealed negative associations between religion and well-being. Promoting religious struggles along with ruminative dialogues as well as feelings of religious guilt were also shown to be a potential obstacle for the acculturation process in the host society (Dimitrova and Aydinli-Karakulak 2016; Ikizler and Szymanski 2018; Areba et al. 2018).

Refugees in Germany and Their Spiritual Needs and Life Satisfaction

In 2019, 1.8 million persons seeking protection were registered in the Central Register of Foreigners in Germany (in Bavaria 213,120 persons). The three countries of origin, Syria (41%), Afghanistan (11%), and Iraq (10%) together accounted for the majority of all protection seekers with recognized protection status. An analysis of asylum applications in 2019 from the perspective of religious affiliation showed that at 62% members of Islam made up the largest share of first-time applicants, followed by Christian believers at 20%. In third place followed persons of the Jesidic faith with 5%, 4% non-denominational, 5% Jewish, and 9% other/unknown (BAMF 2020).

Background of a Cross-Sectional Quantitative Study

We intended to assess how spiritual needs of refugees in Germany relate to their life satisfaction. Based on previous findings that acculturative stress is related to lower levels of life satisfaction and more psychological symptoms (Adam and Ward 2016), spirituality might be an important resource for refugees to adapt to the foreign country and culture, and thus assessment of their spiritual needs would be crucial.

First, spirituality was shown to be an important coping resource in the context of chronic illness (Büssing et al. 2013; Nejat et al. 2017; Choi and Hastings 2019), deleterious life circumstances (Dill 2017), life stressors (Pargament 2009), and major life events (Lancaster and Palframan 2009). This also applies to refugees suffering from traumatic events or forced migration (Zbidat et al. 2020; Markova et al. 2020). As such, spirituality may relate to higher life satisfaction in daily life (Marques et al. 2013; Habib et al. 2018; Villani et al. 2019; Garssen et al. 2020) as well as in the face of life challenges like chronic illnesses (Abu et al. 2018; Cruz et al. 2016; Lin et al. 2018; Maier and Surzykiewicz 2020). The positive link between spirituality and mental health indicators such as life satisfaction was also revealed for refugees (Roh et al. 2014; Pandya 2018; Çetin 2019).

Second, previous findings indicated a positive relationship between the satisfaction of psychological needs and life satisfaction in different aspects of daily life (Unanue et al. 2017; Jin and Kim 2017; Guo 2018). Results also supported a respective link between increased need-satisfaction and fewer psychological symptoms (Weinstein et al. 2016) as well as higher life satisfaction among refugees (Davison et al. 2020).

Third, a limited number of findings already focused on spiritual needs and relationships to life satisfaction, predominantly in the field of chronical and serious illnesses (Hermann 2007; Büssing et al. 2010, 2015, 2018; Narayanasamy 2010) and stressors in life (Büssing and Recchia 2016). Yet, to date, no respective study was found for refugee populations.

Following these results, we expected an association between spiritual needs and life satisfaction in refugees. As refugees in Germany are not a homogenous population, sociodemographic influences on the proposed relationship were expected. Beside religious affiliation and religious status (Abu-Raiya and Pargament 2015; Villani et al. 2019; Edinger-Schons 2019), numerous studies particularly highlighted the impact of culture and nationality in the context of life satisfaction (Oishi et al. 1999; Gebauer et al. 2012; Emerson et al. 2018; Dorahy et al. 2000; Fennig 2020). Among them, some studies even set a specific focus on cultural or multinational aspects in the link between spirituality/religion and indicators of life satisfaction (Okulicz-Kozaryn 2010; Lun and Bond 2013; Abu-Raiya et al. 2018).

Based on these findings, our study proposed a moderator model on the association between spiritual needs (*Religious*, *Existential*, *Inner peace*, and *Giving/Generativity* needs) and life satisfaction, including refugees' home countries (Mashreq countries, Maghreb states, other African countries, and Afghanistan) as a moderator variable.

Participants of This Study

The sampling took place in Bavaria, especially in the regions around Munich and Ingolstadt. Sampling was respondent-driven, starting with a nonrandom convenience sample of people who then recruited other people from the refugee population and so on. The convenience sample was based on key people in refugee institutions, refugee centers and refugee camps who were asked to distribute the questionnaire among their clients and to active other relevant and accessible networks. With respect to the hard-to-reach population, the survey was a paper-based questionnaire that took approximately 20 min to complete. The questionnaires were offered in English, Arabic, Farsi, German, and French.

Cross-sectional data from 744 refugees were collected. For this analysis, data of 682 refugees could be used. Among them 68.6% were male and 26.4% female, while 34 participants did not report their gender. Their mean age was 28.2 ± 8.6 [14–67] years. Most refugees came from the Mashreq countries (54%), in particular from Syria (43%), 17% from the Maghreb states (Algeria, Libya, Morocco, Tunisia), 18% from other African countries, and 11% from Afghanistan; 51% were already approved for asylum, 26% were still waiting for their approval, and 23% did not declare their current asylum status. With respect to their countries of origin, 69% of refugees from Mashreq countries including civil-war refugees from Syria, 23% from Maghreb states, 34% from other African countries, and 37% from Afghanistan were approved for asylum. Regarding the peoples' religious affiliation, 74% were Muslims and 20% Christians, 3% were followers of other religions, 1% had no religious affiliation, and 3% did not declare their religious affiliation. Refugees from the Mashreq countries (81%), Afghanistan (95%), and the Maghreb states (97%) were predominantly Muslims, refugees from other African countries were mostly Christians (65%); 52% came alone, 28% with partner and/or children, and 20% did not provide this information.

Measures

Frequently applied and validated scales were used to ensure adequate measurement of each study variable.

Life satisfaction was measured as a dependent variable. Here the single-item measure "Please indicate how satisfied you are all in all with your life" was used. The response format was a percentage scale, in increments of 10, ranging from 0% (extremely poor) to 100% (extremely good).

Spiritual needs were conceptualized using the Spiritual Needs Questionnaire (SpNQ; Büssing et al. 2010, 2018). As this instrument has so far also applied to stressed (healthy) persons, it was the assumption that the instrument seemed suitable also for refugees (who suffer from high levels of stress). In the original scale validation, the items were grouped into four dimensions of spiritual needs with Cronbach's alpha ranging from 0.71 to 0.92. These subscales were also applied for the present study:

Religious needs, that is, the need to pray or to read spiritual/religious books (Cronbach's alpha = 0.80); *Existential* needs, that is, the need to find meaning in illness and/or suffering or to reflect upon one's previous life (Cronbach's alpha = 0.83); *Inner Peace* needs, that is, the need to find inner peace or to plunge into the beauty of nature (Cronbach's alpha = 0.78); *Giving/Generativity* needs, that is, the need to give solace to someone or to feel connected with family (Cronbach's alpha = 0.78). Cronbach's alpha for the total 27-item score of spiritual needs was 0.92. The items were coded on a 4-point scale from disagreement to agreement, ranging from 1 (not at all) to 4 (very strong). Responses were added to a mean score.

Spiritual Needs and Life Satisfaction Within the Group of Refugees

In the whole sample, refugees' life satisfaction was moderate (48.61 ± 22.42) and their spiritual needs moderately high. Spiritual needs of the 27-item version scored high and were expressed as "strong" needs (Table 24.1). Highest mean scores were found in refugees from Maghreb states (3.06 ± 0.55), followed by other African countries (2.72 ± 0.59),

Table 24.1 Means, standard deviations, standard errors, and correlations between life satisfaction and spiritual needs

Variable	*1*	*2*	*3*	*4*	*5*	*Mean*	*SD*	*SE*
1 Life satisfaction						48.61	22.42	0.86
2 Spiritual needs Score (27-item mean)	0.184**					2.62	0.59	0.02
3 Existential needs	0.151**	0.835**				2.40	0.79	0.03
4 Giving/ generativity needs	0.180**	0.834**	0.624**			2.78	0.64	0.02
5 Inner peace needs	0.143**	0.658**	0.315**	0.500**		2.75	0.67	0.03
6 Religious needs	0.136**	0.833**	0.701**	0.614**	0.324**	2.58	0.78	0.03

$^{**}p < 0.01$; $^{*}p < 0.05$ (Pearson)

indicating a "strong" needs expression. Mean scores of spiritual needs for refugees from Afghanistan (2.52 ± 0.52) and Mashreq countries (2.47 ± 0.53) were expressed as between "somewhat strong" and "strong". Considering the refugees' religious affiliations, the 27-item score of spiritual needs from Muslims (2.63 ± 0.57) and Christians (2.66 ± 0.60) were each expressed as between "somewhat strong" and "strong". With respect to the different dimensions of spiritual needs, Christians expressed stronger *Existential* needs (F [1, 640] = 8.33, $p < 0.01$; $M_{\text{Christ.}} = 2.60$ vs. $M_{\text{Muslim}} = 2.37$), while Muslims expressed higher *Inner Peace* needs (F [1, 640] = 7.74, $p < 0.01$; $M_{\text{Muslim}} = 2.81$ vs. $M_{\text{Christ}} = 2.63$). Refugees who were still waiting for their asylum had higher *Existential* needs (F [1, 527] = 23.98, $p < 0.001$; $M_{\text{Waiting}} = 2.51$ vs. $M_{\text{Approved}} = 2.19$) and higher *Religious* needs (F [1, 527] = 6.38, $p < 0.05$; $M_{\text{Waiting}} = 2.58$ vs. $M_{\text{Approved}} = 2.42$). There were no significant differences with respect to gender. Regarding the correlations between the study variables, spiritual needs were moderately to strongly interrelated, while their associations with life satisfaction were weak (Table 24.1).

Home Country as Moderator of the Link Between Spiritual Needs and Life Satisfaction

The proposed moderation model was tested for the 27-item score of spiritual needs as well as each of the four spiritual needs dimensions. Therefore, a series of two-step hierarchical linear regressions was conducted. In the first step of the hierarchical regression, spiritual needs (27-item *Score* of spiritual needs, *Religious* needs, *Existential* needs, *Inner Peace* needs, *Giving/Generativity* needs, respectively) as well as the refugees' home countries (Mashreq countries, Maghreb states, other African states, and Afghanistan) were entered as predictors. This step allowed us to examine the unique effects of the study's main variables on refugees' life satisfaction. In the second step, we additionally added the interaction terms between the home countries and spiritual needs as additional predictors. This was to explore whether the link between spiritual needs and life satisfaction was influenced (e.g., moderated) by the refugees' home countries. A significant increase of the model's explained variance (ΔR^2_{corr}) indicated a moderator effect.

A moderator effect of the refugees' home countries on the link between spiritual needs and life satisfaction could be revealed for the total score of spiritual needs (Table 24.2), as well as for each of the four dimensions of

Table 24.2 Hierarchical linear regression analysis of the proposed mediator model for spiritual needs

	B	$SD_{(B)}$	*t*	*p*	R^2_{korr}	*F*	*df*	*Sig(F)*
Outcome variable: life satisfaction								
Model 1					0.114	21.69	4, 677	<0.001
Spiritual needs score (27-item score)	3.29	0.88	3.76	<0.001				
Other African countries	-7.01	1.66	-4.24	<0.001				
Maghreb states	10.90	1.77	6.17	<0.001				
Mashreq countries	3.88	1.28	3.03	0.003				
Model 2					0.128	15.28	7, 674	<0.001
Spiritual needs score (27-item score)	3.69	1.02	3.62	<0.001	Change Statistics Model 2			
Other African countries	-5.08	1.70	-2.98	0.003	ΔR^2	ΔF	*df*	$\Delta Sig(F)$
Maghreb states	6.61	2.03	3.26	0.001	0.023	6.08	3, 674	<0.001
Mashreq countries	5.15	1.31	3.93	<0.001				
Other African countries x Spiritual needs	-2.45	1.69	-1.45	0.148				
Maghreb states x Spiritual needs	7.48	1.78	4.22	<0.001				
Mashreq countries x Spiritual needs	-1.73	1.33	-1.30	0.195				

Note: The continuous variable (spiritual needs) was mean-centered, the categorical variable (home countries) was effect-coded with Afghanistan as reference category

spiritual needs (data not shown). A detailed result presentation will be limited to the total score of spiritual needs only.

To probe the interaction effects, conditional effects of the predictor on the outcome variable at different levels of the moderator were analyzed. Fig. 24.1 shows conditional effects in the moderator model.

First, ***conditional effects of spiritual needs*** on life satisfaction were calculated at each level of the moderator, for example, the different refugees' home countries. Higher life satisfaction was linked to higher spiritual needs for refugees from Maghreb states only ($B_{\text{SPIR, z-score}} = 11.17$, $p < 0.001$). For refugees from Mashreq countries, Afghanistan, and other African states, no relationship between spiritual needs and life satisfaction could be revealed.

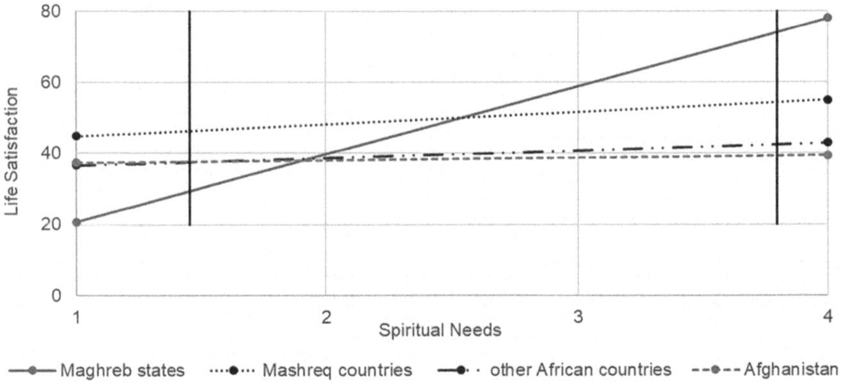

Fig. 24.1 Visualization of the conditional effects in the moderator model. The black vertical lines indicate the low (two standard deviations below the mean) and high levels of spiritual needs (two standard deviations above the mean), which were used to calculate the conditional effects of home countries on life satisfaction.

Second, *conditional effects of the refugees' home countries* on life satisfaction were calculated at high (two standard deviations above the mean) and low levels of spiritual needs (two standard deviations below the mean). In case of high levels of spiritual needs, refugees from Maghreb states reported a significant higher life satisfaction compared to refugees from Mashreq countries ($B_{Mashreq} = -19.88$, $p < 0.001$), Afghanistan ($B_{Afghan.} = -34.87$, $p < 0.001$), and other African countries ($B_{African} = -31.55$, $p < 0.001$). Life satisfaction was also higher for refugees from Mashreq countries compared to refugees from other African countries ($B_{African} = -11.67$, $p < 0.05$) and Afghanistan ($B_{Afghan.} = -14.99$, $p < 0.05$). No difference in life satisfaction was found between refugees from other African countries and Afghanistan. In case of low levels of spiritual needs, refugees from Mashreq countries reported a significantly higher life satisfaction compared to refugees from Maghreb states ($B_{Maghreb} = -16.95$, $p < 0.01$). No further differences in life satisfaction between refugees' home countries were revealed.

In addition to this global analysis on spiritual needs, moderator effects were also analyzed for each of the four dimensions of spiritual needs. Overall, the reported findings of the 27-item score of spiritual needs can be also found in the single dimensions of the construct (data not shown):

Referring to the *conditional effects of spiritual needs* on life satisfaction for the refugees' different home countries, a positive relationship for refugees from the Maghreb states was consistently found for each dimension of the spiritual needs score. In addition, higher life satisfaction was reported for refugees from the Mashreq countries in case of higher *Existential* needs. Focusing on the *conditional effects of the refugees' home countries* on life satisfaction at high levels of spiritual needs (two standard deviations above the mean), refugees from Maghreb states report significant higher life satisfaction than refugees from all other countries. This applied to all dimensions of spiritual needs. In addition, life satisfaction of refugees from Mashreq countries was higher compared to refugees from other African countries and Afghanistan for high levels of *Existential* needs and *Inner Peace* needs, while no respective difference was found for high levels of *Religious* needs and *Giving/Generativity* needs. In case of low levels of spiritual needs (two standard deviations below the mean), findings indicated higher life satisfaction of refugees from Mashreq countries compared to refugees from other African countries for *Existential* needs, compared to refugees from other African countries and Afghanistan for *Religious* needs as well as compared to refugees from other African countries, Maghreb states, and Afghanistan for *Giving/Generativity* needs.

Discussion of Findings

Based on the cultural heterogeneity of this population as well as previous findings on the impact of culture on the relationship between spirituality and life satisfaction (Abu-Raiya et al. 2018), the refugees' countries of origin were included as a moderator variable into the analysis. Our findings supported the moderation effect, revealing that the relationship between spiritual needs and life satisfaction was influenced by refugees' home countries. Thus, higher levels of spiritual needs did not systematically imply higher levels of life satisfaction. This link could only be revealed for people from Maghreb states and Mashreq countries. Refugees from Mashreq countries expressed higher life satisfaction in case of higher *Existential* needs and felt less satisfied when *Existential* needs were low. Considering the contribution of *Existential* needs to life satisfaction, this dimension expresses the need to find answers to questions about the meaning of life, challenging life events, and finally death. A spiritual reflection on these existential questions (Delgado 2005; Eisenmann et al. 2016) can provide hope, meaning, and comfort, especially in the face of difficult life situations by encouraging an individual toward situation adjustment and to believe in his or her personal mastery at it (Pargament 1997; Laubmeier et al. 2004; Linley and Joseph 2011; Neimeyer and Burke 2014). Referring to Maslow's hierarchy of needs (Maslow 1943) and respective studies on the needs of refugees (Bouaiti et al. 2016; Davison et al. 2020), existential reflections thus can be viewed as a basic need dimension among spiritual needs of refugees. These considerations also might explain why other spiritual needs dimensions did not relate to higher life satisfaction in this population group. Refugees from Maghreb states also experienced higher life satisfaction in case of higher spiritual needs. This applied to each dimension of spiritual needs as well as spiritual needs in total. Yet, *Existential* needs in this group showed a significantly weaker association to life satisfaction compared to *Religious, Giving/ Generativity*, and *Inner Peace* needs. This finding further supports the suggestion of a hierarchical structure of spiritual needs. Based on satisfied *Existential* needs, which enable attributions of meaning and sense, other spiritual needs seem to be present: *Religious* needs might encourage specific means, like praying or attending the service, in order to adapt and cope with the present, meaningful challenges. In a similar way, a focus on the next generation as expressed in *Giving/Generativity* needs as well as needs for *Inner Peace* in terms of harmony and love might act as additional motivational forces and encourage a person to actively deal with difficult or challenging circumstances (Emmons 2000). Such an active involvement in terms of active religious or spiritual coping is linked to higher well-being and life satisfaction (Abu-Raiya and Pargament 2015; Adam and Ward 2016).

Life satisfaction of refugees from other African countries and Afghanistan in contrast was unrelated to spiritual needs. In addition, life satisfaction of these two groups seemed the lowest overall and was systematically lower compared to life satisfaction of refugees from Mashreq countries. This was especially true for the dimensions of religious and generativity needs. Referring to previous findings, some studies also indicated missing or even negative links between spirituality or spiritual needs and life satisfaction (Abu-Raiya and Pargament 2015; Büssing and Recchia 2016; Copolov et al. 2017; Areba et al. 2018). In a review of 272 cross-sectional studies, Koenig (2012) reported 63% positive relationships between indicators of spirituality and lower depression, 6% with negative associations indicating higher depression, and 22% with no associations. With respect to well-being, out of 326 peer-reviewed studies, 79% reported positive associations and less than 1% a negative relationship between indicators of spirituality and well-being (Koenig 2012). Negative associations are especially found if a person's spirituality is linked to negative or passive instead of active religious coping styles (Cummings and Pargament 2010).

Overall, belief systems seem to have an impact on a person's well-being and life satisfaction. However, they are embedded and confounded with a vast array of other contributing factors. Posselt et al. (2018) performed a systematic review of peer-reviewed quantitative and qualitative findings on psychological well-being among refugees and asylum seekers. They identified relevant factors for psychological well-being, such as social support, faith, religion, and spirituality, cognitive strategies, education and training opportunities, employment and economic activities, behavioral strategies, political advocacy, and environmental conditions. Another meta-analysis has shown a consistent, though modest, association between indicators of spirituality or religiousness respectively and mental health, including distress, well-being, mental health, negative and positive mood, and life satisfaction (Garssen et al. 2020). The results of our study are in line with these meta-analytic findings. The importance of regarding refugees' national backgrounds with different value systems, religious affiliations, worldviews, and cultural traditions was shown to be an important factor in understanding and explaining the association between indicators of spirituality such as spiritual needs and a person's life satisfaction.

Implications for Practical Considerations

First, the so far neglected category of spiritual needs was shown to be an important resource to enhance life satisfaction and well-being in refugees. This is in line with previous results on the relationship between spirituality and life satisfaction in refugees (Pandya 2018; Çetin 2019) and complements findings on the importance of psychological needs-satisfaction in the promotion of refugees' well-being (Weinstein et al. 2016; Davison et al. 2020).

Second, the importance and necessity of incorporating religion and spirituality into social work and clinical practice with refugees was increasingly recognized in recent years (George and Ellison 2015; Hodge 2019). Respective spiritual-sensitive approaches in counseling need to be expanded to also include the dimension of spiritual needs and spiritual need-satisfaction. Offering spirituality-based counseling about unmet spiritual needs might enable refugees to build up new hope perspectives regarding chances for better times in their lives, which in turn would enhance their overall life satisfaction.

Third, there is no overall link between spiritual needs and the promotion of life satisfaction and well-being of refugees. Our findings thus call for culture-specific and culturally competent approaches in spirituality-sensitive counseling, depending on the refugees' specific cultural requirements. A person's religion and spirituality not only offer an explanatory framework to understand a refugee's culture of origin, for example, with respect to a person's values system or worldview (Eltaiba 2014; Hashemi et al. 2019), but the cultural background conversely also seems to influence and shape a person's spiritual needs.

Turning back to our findings, life satisfaction from refugees of the Maghreb states might be enhanced by addressing and promoting their spiritual needs in terms of turning toward and satisfying their *Religious* needs, *Existential* needs, *Inner Peace* needs, and *Giving/Generativity* needs, while refugees from Mashreq countries only seemed to benefit from supporting their *Existential needs* dimension. However, this does not argue against the importance of their other needs being addressed. Spiritual needs-sensitive interventions for refugees from Afghanistan and other African countries in contrast seem not be beneficial at all in order to promote life satisfaction. Future research is needed to focus on a deeper understanding of underlying mechanisms and influencing variables to further break down these preliminary insights.

References

AbdAleati NS, Zaharim NM, Mydin YO (2016) Religiousness and mental health: systematic review study. J Relig Health 55:1929–1937

Abraham R, Lien L, Hanssen I (2018) Coping, resilience and posttraumatic growth among Eritrean female refugees living in Norwegian asylum reception centers: a qualitative study. Int J Soc Psychiatry 64:359–366

Abu HO, Ulbricht C, Ding E, Allison JJ, Salmoirago-Blotcher E, Goldberg RJ, Kiefe CI (2018) Association of religiosity and spirituality with quality of life in patients with cardiovascular disease: a systematic review. Qual Life Res 27(11):2777–2797

Abu-Raiya H, Pargament KI (2015) Religious coping among diverse religions: commonalities and divergences. Psychol Relig Spiritual 7(1):24–33

Abu-Raiya H, Ayten A, Tekke M, Agbaria Q (2018) On the links between positive religious coping, satisfaction with life and depressive symptoms among a multinational sample of Muslims. Int J Psychol 54(5) https://doi.org/10.1002/ijop.12521

Acquaye HE (2017) PTSD, optimism, religious commitment, and growth as post-trauma trajectories: a structural equation modeling of former refugees. Prof Couns 7(4):330–348

Acquaye HE, Sivo SA, Jones KD (2018) Religious commitment's moderating effect on refugee trauma and growth. Couns Values 63(1):57–75

Adam Z, Ward C (2016) Stress, religious coping and wellbeing in acculturating Muslims. J Muslim Mental Health 10(2):3–26. https://doi.org/10.3998/jmmh.10381607.0010.201

Alemi Q, James S, Cruz R, Zepeda V, Racadio M (2014) Psychological distress in Afghan refugees: a mixed-method systematic review. J Immigr Minor Health 16(6):1247–1261

Ano GG, Vasconcelles EB (2005) Religious coping and psychological adjustment to stress: a meta-analysis. J Clin Psychol 61(4):461–480

Arabzadeh M, Naiemi G, Pirsagh F (2017) Prediction of life satisfaction in students based on Islamic lifestyle and spiritual intelligence. Rooyesh-e-Ravanshenasi 6(1):25–44

Areba EM, Duckett L, Robertson C, Savik K (2018) Religious coping, symptoms of depression and anxiety, and well-being among Somali college students. J Relig Health 57(1):94–109

BAMF (2020) Das Bundesamt in Zahlen 2019. Asyl, Migration und Integration. https://www.bamf.de/SharedDocs/Anlagen/DE/Statistik/BundesamtinZahlen/bundesamt-in-zahlen-2019.pdf?__blob=publicationFile&v=3. Accessed 5 Oct 2020

Bekteshi V, Kang SW (2018) Contextualizing acculturative stress among Latino immigrants in the United States: a systematic review. Ethn Health 25(6):897–914

Benson GO, Sun F, Hodge DR, Androff DK (2012) Religious coping and acculturation stress among Hindu Bhutanese: a study of newly-resettled refugees in the United States. Int Soc Work 55(4):538–553

Betts A, Omata N, Sterck O (2020) Self-reliance and social networks: explaining refugees' reluctance to relocate from Kakuma to Kalobeyei. J Refugee Stud 33(1):62–85

Borho A, Viazminsky A, Morawa E, Schmitt GM, Georgiadou E, Erim Y (2020) The prevalence and risk factors for mental distress among Syrian refugees in Germany: a register-based follow-up study. BMC Psychiatry 20(1):1–13

Bouaiti EA, Kessouati J, Gartoum M, Elbaite A, Elkandry S, Sair K, Mrabet M (2016) Exploring refugee camp needs: an empirical investigation of Maslow's theory in Za'atari Camp in 2013. IOSR J Dental Med Sci 15(9):117–124

Büssing A, Recchia DR (2016) Spiritual and non-spiritual needs among German soldiers and their relation to stress perception, PTDS symptoms, and life satis-

faction: results from a structural equation modeling approach. J Relig Health 55(3):747–764
Büssing A, Balzat HJ, Heusser P (2010) Spiritual needs of patients with chronic pain diseases and cancer. Validation of the spiritual needs questionnaire. Eur J Med Res 15(6):266–273
Büssing A, Janko A, Baumann K, Hvidt NC, Kopf A (2013) Spiritual needs among patients with chronic pain diseases and cancer living in a secular society. Pain Med 14:1362–1373
Büssing A, Pilchowska I, Surzykiewicz J (2015) Spiritual needs of Polish patients with chronic diseases. J Relig Health 54(5):1524–1542
Büssing A, Recchia D, Koenig H, Baumann K, Frick E (2018) Factor structure of the spiritual needs questionnaire (SpNQ) in persons with chronic diseases, elderly and healthy individuals. Religions 9(1):13–23
Byrow Y, Pajak R, Specker P, Nickerson A (2020) Perceptions of mental health and perceived barriers to mental health help-seeking amongst refugees: a systematic review. Clin Psychol Rev 75:101812. https://doi.org/10.1016/j.cpr.2019.101812
Choi SA, Hastings JF (2019) Religion, spirituality, coping, and resilience among African Americans with diabetes. J Religion Spirituality Soc Work Soc Thought 38(1):93–114
Copolov C, Knowles A, Meyer D (2017) Exploring the predictors and mediators of personal wellbeing for young Hazaras with refugee backgrounds in Australia. Aust J Psychol 70(2):122–130
Cruz JP, Colet PC, Alquwez N, Inocian EP, Al-Otaibi RS, Islam SMS (2016) Influence of religiosity and spiritual coping on health-related quality of life in Saudi haemodialysis patients. Hemodial Int 21(1):125–132
Cummings JP, Pargament KI (2010) Medicine for the spirit: religious coping in individuals with medical conditions. Religions 1(1):28–53. https://doi.org/10.3390/rel1010028
Davison CM, Watt H, Michael S, Bartels SA (2020) "I don't know if we'll ever live in harmony": exploring the unmet needs of Syrian adolescent girls protracted displacement in Lebanon. Res Square. https://doi.org/10.21203/rs.3.rs-49006/v1
Deci EL, Ryan RM (1991) A motivational approach to self: integration in personality. In: Dienstbier RA (ed) Current theory and research in motivation, Nebraska symposium on motivation, 1990: perspectives on motivation, vol 38. University of Nebraska Press, pp 237–288
Deci EL, Ryan RM (2000) The "what" and "why" of goal pursuits: human needs and the self-determination of behavior. Psychol Inquiry 11:227–268
DeHaan CR, Hirai T, Ryan RM (2016) Nussbaum's capabilities and self-determination theory's basic psychological needs: relating some fundamentals of human wellness. J Happiness Stud 17:2037–2049

Delgado C (2005) A discussion of the concept of spirituality. Nurs Sci Q 18:157–162

Diener E (2006) Guidelines for national indicators of subjective wellbeing and ill-being. J Happiness Stud Interdisciplinary Forum Subjective Well-Being 7:397–404

Diener E, Clifton D (2002) Life satisfaction and religiosity in broad probability samples. Psychol Inquiry 13:206–209

Diener E, Emmons RA, Larsen RJ, Griffin S (1985) The satisfaction with life scale. J Pers Assess 49:71–75

Diener E, Ng W, Harter J, Arora R (2010) Wealth and happiness across the world: material prosperity predicts life evaluation, whereas psychosocial prosperity predicts positive feeling. J Pers Soc Psychol 99:52–61

Diener E, Tay L, Myers DG (2011) The religion paradox: if religion makes people happy, why are so many dropping out? J Pers Soc Psychol 101:1278–1290

Dill LJ (2017) "Wearing my spiritual jacket": the role of spirituality as a coping mechanism among African American Youth. Health Educ Behav 44(5):696–704

Dimitrova R, Aydinli-Karakulak A (2016) Acculturation orientations mediate the link between religious identity and adjustment of Turkish-Bulgarian and Turkish-German adolescents. Springer Plus 5:1024

Dorahy MJ, Lewis CA, Schumaker JF, Akuamoah-Boateng R, Duze MC, Sibiya TE (2000) Depression and life satisfaction among Australian, Ghanaian, Nigerian, Northern Irish, and Swazi University students. J Soc Behav Pers 15(4):569–580

Dorais LJ (2007) Faith, hope and identity: religion and the Vietnamese refugees. Refugee Surv Q 26(2):57–68

Echterhoff G, Hellmann JH, Back MD, Kärtner J, Morina N, Hertel G (2020) Psychological antecedents of refugee integration (PARI). Perspect Psychol Sci 15(4):856–879

Edinger-Schons LM (2019) Oneness beliefs and their effect on life satisfaction. Psychol Relig Spiritual. https://doi.org/10.1037/rel0000259

Eisenmann C, Klein C, Swhajor-Biesemann A, Drexelius U, Keller B, Streib H (2016) Dimensions of "spirituality": the semantics of subjective definitions. In: Streib H, Hood RW Jr (eds) Semantics and psychology of spirituality. Springer International, Cham, Switzerland, pp 125–152

Ellison CG, Henderson AK (2011) Religion and mental health: through the lens of the stress process. In: Blasi A (ed) Toward a sociological theory of religion and health. Brill, Leiden, pp 11–44

Eltaiba N (2014) Counseling with Muslim refugees: building rapport. J Soc Work Pract Psychother Approaches Health, Welfare Commun 28(4):397–403

Emerson SD, Mâsse LC, Ark TK, Schonert-Reichl KA, Guhn M (2018) A population-based analysis of life satisfaction and social support among children of diverse backgrounds in British Columbia, Canada. Qual Life Res 27(10):2595–2607

Emmons RA (2000) Is spirituality an intelligence? Motivation, cognition, and the psychology of ultimate concern. Int J Psychol Religion 10(1):3–26

Esses VM, Hamilton LK, Gaucher D (2017) The global refugee crisis: empirical evidence and policy implications for improving public attitudes and facilitating refugee resettlement. Soc Issues Policy Rev 11(1):78–123

Fennig M (2020) Cultural adaptations of evidence-based mental health interventions for refugees: implications for clinical social work. Br J Soc Work:bcaa024. https://doi.org/10.1093/bjsw/bcaa024

Garssen B, Visser A, Pool G (2020) Does spirituality or religion positively affect mental health? Meta-analysis of longitudinal studies. Int J Psychol Religion. https://doi.org/10.1080/10508619.2020.17295701-17

Gebauer JE, Sedikides C, Neberich W (2012) Religiosity, social self-esteem, and psychological adjustment: on the cross-cultural specificity of the psychological benefits of religiosity. Psychol Sci 23(2):158–160

George M, Ellison V (2015) Incorporating spirituality into social work practice with migrants. Br J Soc Work 45(6):1717–1733

Gladden J (2012) The coping skills of East African refugees: a literature review. Refugee Surv Q 31(3):177–196

Goodkind JR, Bybee D, Hess JM, Amer S, Ndayisenga M, Greene RN, Choe R, Isakson B, Baca B, Pannah M (2020) Randomized controlled trial of a multilevel intervention to address social determinants of refugee mental health. Am J Community Psychol 65:272–289

Goodwin-Gill GS (2014) The international law of refugee protection. In: Fiddian-Qasmiyeh E, Loescher G, Long K, Sigona N (eds) The Oxford handbook of refugee and forced migration studies, pp 36–47

Graham C, Crown S (2014) Religion and well-being around the world: social purpose, social time, or social insurance? Int J Wellbeing 4(1):1–27

Grant L, Oman D (2018) International and global perspectives on spirituality, religion, and public health. In: Oman D (ed) Why religion and spirituality matter for public health. Springer International, Cham, Switzerland, pp 447–462

Gull F, Dawood S (2013) Religiosity and subjective well-being amongst institutionalized elderly in Pakistan. Health Promot Perspect 3:124–128

Guo Y (2018) The influence of academic autonomous motivation on learning engagement and life satisfaction in adolescents: the mediating role of basic psychological needs satisfaction. J Educ Learn 7(4):254–261

Habib DG, Donald C, Hutchinson G (2018) Religion and life satisfaction: a correlational study of undergraduate students in Trinidad. J Relig Health 57(4):1567–1580

Hakim NH, Molina LE, Branscombe NR (2017) How discrimination shapes social identification processes and well-being among Arab Americans. Soc Psychologic Personal Sci 9:328–337

Harrop E, Addis S, Elliott E, Williams G (2006) Resilience, coping and salutogenic approaches to maintaining and generating health: a review. Cardiff University, Cardiff

Hashemi N, Marzban M, Sebar B, Harris N (2019) Religious identity and psychological well-being among Middle-Eastern migrants in Australia: the mediating role of perceived social support, social connectedness, and perceived discrimination. Psychol Relig Spiritual. https://doi.org/10.1037/rel0000287

Hayward RD, Elliott M (2014) Cross-national analysis of the influence of cultural norms and government restrictions on the relationship between religion and well-being. Rev Religious Res 56:23–43

Hermann CP (2007) The degree to which spiritual needs of patients near the end of life are met. Oncol Nurs Forum 34(1):70–78

Hodge DR (2015) Spiritual assessment in social work and mental health practice. Columbia University Press, New York, NY

Hodge DR (2018) Administering spiritual assessments with refugees: an overview of conceptually distinct assessment options. J Refugee Stud:fey054. https://doi.org/10.1093/jrs/fey054

Hodge DR (2019) Spiritual assessment with refugees and other migrant populations: a necessary foundation for successful clinical practice. J Religion Spirituality Soc Work Soc Thought 38(2):121–139

Horstmann A, Jung JH (2015) Introduction: refugees and religion. In: Horstman A (ed) Building Noah's ark for migrants, refugees, and religious communities. Palgrave Macmillan, New York, NY, pp 1–20

Ikizler AS, Szymanski DM (2018) Discrimination, religious and cultural factors, and Middle Eastern/Arab Americans' psychological distress. J Clin Psychol 74(7):1219–1233

Jasperse M, Ward C, Jose PE (2011) Identity, perceived religious discrimination, and psychological well-being in Muslim immigrant women. Appl Psychol 61(2):250–271

Jenks RJ (2020) A comparison of religiosity and life satisfaction among seven different religious groups. Adv Soc Sci Cult 2(2) https://doi.org/10.22158/assc.v2n2p1

Jin B, Kim J (2017) Grit, basic needs satisfaction, and subjective well-being. J Individ Differ 38(1):29–35

Johnstone B, Yoon DP, Cohen D, Schopp LH, McCormack G, Campbell J, Smith M (2012) Relationships among spirituality, religious practices, personality factors, and health for five different faith traditions. J Relig Health 51:1017–1041

Karaman MA, Ricard RJ (2016) Meeting the mental health needs of Syrian refugees in Turkey. Prof Couns 6(4):318

Kim-Prieto C, Miller L (2018) Intersection of religion and subjective well-being. In: Diener E, Oishi S, Tay L (eds) Handbook of well-being. DEF Publisher, Salt Lake City, UT, pp 1–9

Koenig HG (2012) Religion, spirituality, and health: the research and clinical implications. ISRN Psychiatry:1–33

Krause U, Schmidt H (2020) Refugees as actors? Critical reflections on global refugee policies on self-reliance and resilience. J Refugee Stud 33(1):22–41

Lancaster BL, Palframan JT (2009) Coping with major life events: the role of spirituality and self-transformation. Mental Health Religion Cult 12(3):257–276

Laubmeier KK, Zakowski SG, Bair JP (2004) The role of spirituality in the psychological adjustment to cancer: a test of the transactional model of stress and coping. Int J Behav Med 11(1):48–55

Lim C (2015) Religion and subjective well-being across religious traditions: evidence from 1.3 million Americans. J Sci Stud Religion 54(4):684–701

Lim C, Putnam RD (2010) Religion, social networks, and life satisfaction. Am Sociol Rev 75(6):914–933

Lin CY, Saffari M, Koenig HG, Pakpour AH (2018) Effects of religiosity and religious coping on medication adherence and quality of life among people with epilepsy. Epilepsy Behav 78:45–51

Linley PA, Joseph S (2011) Meaning in life and posttraumatic growth. J Loss Trauma 16(2):150–159

Long KN, Gregg RJ, Vander Weele TJ, Oman D, Laird LD (2019) Boundary crossing: meaningfully engaging religious traditions and religious institutions in public health. Religions 10(7):412. https://doi.org/10.3390/rel10070412

Lun VM, Bond MH (2013) Examining the relation of religion and spirituality to subjective well-being across national cultures. Psychol Relig Spiritual 5:304–315

Maier K, Surzykiewicz J (2020) Mediated association between spirituality and life satisfaction in chronically ill undergraduate students. Psychol Relig Spiritual 12(3):311–323

Mallett R, Hagen-Zanker J (2018) Forced migration trajectories: an analysis of journey- and decision-making among Eritrean and Syrian arrivals to Europe. Migration Develop 7:341–351

Markova V, Sandal GM, Guribye E (2020) What do immigrants from various cultures think is the best way to cope with depression? Introducing the cross-cultural coping inventory. Front Psychol. https://doi.org/10.3389/fpsyg.2020.01599

Marques SC, Lopez SJ, Mitchell J (2013) The role of hope, spirituality and religious practice in adolescents' life satisfaction: longitudinal findings. J Happiness Stud Interdisciplinary Forum Subjective Well-Being 14(1):251–261

Maslow AH (1943) A theory of human motivation. Psychol Rev 50:370–396

McSherry W (2010) Spiritual assessment: definition, categorisation and features. In: McSherry W, Ross L (eds) Spiritual assessment in healthcare practice. M&K Publishing, Cumbria, CA, pp 57–78

Muruthi BA, Young SS, Chou J, Janes E, Ibrahim M (2020) "We pray as a family": the role of religion for resettled Karen refugees. J Family Issues. https://doi.org/10.1177/0192513X20911068

Naja WJ, Aoun MP, El Khoury EL, Abdallah FJB, Haddad RS (2016) Prevalence of depression in Syrian refugees and the influence of religiosity. Compr Psychiatry 68:78–85

Narayanasamy A (2010) Recognising spiritual needs. In: McSherry W, Ross L (eds) Spiritual assessment in healthcare practice. M&K Publishing, Cumbria, CA, pp 37–55

Neimeyer RA, Burke LA (2014) Loss, grief, and spiritual struggle: the quest for meaning in bereavement. Religion Brain Behav 5(2):131–138

Nejat N, Whitehead L, Crowe M (2017) The use of spirituality and religiosity in coping with colorectal cancer. Contemp Nurse 51(1):48–59

Nesterko Y, Jäckle D, Friedrich M, Holzapfel L, Glaesmer H (2020) Health care needs among recently arrived refugees in Germany: a cross-sectional, epidemiological study. Int J Public Health 65(6):811–821

Newman DB, Graham J (2018) Religion and well-being. Handbook of well-being. DEF Publishers, Salt Lake City, UT

Oishi S, Diener E (2014) Residents of poor nations have a greater sense of meaning in life than residents of wealthy nations. Psychol Sci 25(2):422–430

Oishi S, Diener EF, Lucas RE, Suh EM (1999) Cross-cultural variations in predictors of life satisfaction: perspectives from needs and values. Pers Soc Psychol Bull 25(8):980–990

Okulicz-Kozaryn A (2010) Religiosity and life satisfaction across nations. Mental Health Religion Cult 13(2):155–169

Oman D (2018) Clinical practice, religion, and spirituality. In: Oman D (ed) Why religion and spirituality matter for public health. Springer International, Cham, Switzerland, pp 245–260

Omata N (2017) The myth of self-reliance. Economic lives inside a Liberian refugee camp. Berghahn, Oxford, New York

Pandya SP (2018) Spirituality for mental health and well-being of adult refugees in Europe. J Immigr Minor Health 20(6):1396–1403

Pargament KI (1997) The psychology of religion and coping: theory, research, practice. Guilford Press

Pargament KI (2009) The spiritual dimension of coping: theoretical and practical considerations. In: de Souza M, Francis LJ, O'Higgins-Norman J, Scott D (eds) International handbook of education for spirituality, care and wellbeing. Springer, Dordrecht, pp 209–230

Posselt M, Eaton H, Ferguson M, Keegan D, Procter N (2018) Enablers of psychological well-being for refugees and asylum seekers living in transitional countries: a systematic review. Health Soc Care Community 27(4):808–823. https://doi.org/10.1111/hsc.12680

Pulla V, Woods J (2016) The Lhotsampa in Australia: their spirituality for coping and resilience. Soc Cult South Asia 2(1):59–78

Renner A, Hoffmann R, Nagl M, Roehr S, Jung F, Grochtdreis T, König HH, Riedel-Heller S, Kersting A (2020) Syrian refugees in Germany: perspectives on mental health and coping strategies. J Psychosom Res 129:109906

Roh S, Lee YS, Lee JH, Martin JI (2014) Typology of religiosity/spirituality in relation to perceived health, depression, and life satisfaction among older Korean immigrants. Aging Ment Health 18(4):444–453

Ryan RM, Deci EL (2000) The darker and brighter sides of human existence: basic psychological needs as a unifying concept. Psychol Inquiry 11(4):319–338

Ryan RM, Deci EL (2017) Self-determination theory: basic psychological needs in motivation, development, and wellness. Guilford Publications

Ryan RM, Ryan WS, Di Domenico SI, Deci EL (2019) The nature and the conditions of human autonomy and flourishing: self-determination theory and basic psychological needs. In: Ryan RM (ed) The Oxford handbook of human motivation, 2nd edn. https://doi.org/10.1093/oxfordhb/9780190666453.013.6

Sabouni F (2019) Exploring the psychosocial needs of Syrian refugees in the UK: accounts of community service providers. Dissertation, University of Manchester

Safak-Ayvazoglu A, Kunuroglu F (2019) Acculturation experiences and psychological well-being of Syrian refugees attending universities in Turkey: a qualitative study. J Div Higher Educ. https://doi.org/10.1037/dhe0000148

Sanchez M, Dillon F, Ruffin B, De La Rosa M (2012) The influence of religious coping on the acculturative stress of recent Latino immigrants. J Ethn Cult Divers Soc Work 21(3):171–194

Schick M, Morina N, Mistridis P, Schnyder U, Bryant RA, Nickerson A (2018) Changes in post-migration living difficulties predict treatment outcome in traumatized refugees. Front Psych 9:476. https://doi.org/10.3389/fpsyt.2018.00476

Schouler-Ocak M, Wintrob R, Moussaoui D, Villasenor Bayardo SJ, Zhao XD, Kastrup MC (2016) Background paper on the needs of migrant, refugee and asylum seeker patients around the globe. Int J Cult Ment Health 9(3):216–232

Shaw SA, Peacock L, Ali LM, Pillai V, Husain A (2019) Religious coping and challenges among displaced Muslim female refugees. Affilia 34(4):518–534

Shoeb M, Weinstein HM, Halpern J (2007) Living in religious time and space: Iraqi refugees in Dearborn, Michigan. J Refugee Stud 20(3):441–460

Silove D, Ventevogel P, Rees S (2017) The contemporary refugee crisis: an overview of mental health challenges. World Psychiatry 16:130–139

Snodgrass JG, Most DE, Upadhyay C (2017) Religious ritual is good medicine for indigenous Indian conservation refugees. Curr Anthropol 58(2) https://www.journals.uchicago.edu/doi/abs/10.1086/691212

Spatrisano J, Robinson RV, Eldridge GD, Rosich RM (2020) Conceptualizing refugee resilience across multiple contexts. In: Güngör D, Strohmeier D (eds) Contextualizing immigrant and refugee resilience. Springer, Cham, pp 163–182

Stuart J, Ward C, Robinson L (2016) The influence of family climate on stress and adaptation of Muslim immigrant young adults in two Western countries. Int Perspect Psychol Res Pract Consult 5:1–17

Tay L, Diener E (2011) Needs and subjective well-being around the world. J Pers Soc Psychol 101:354–365

Tempany M (2009) What research tells us about the mental health and psychosocial wellbeing of Sudanese refugees: a literature review. Transcult Psychiatry 46(2):300–315

Tippens JA (2017) Urban Congolese refugees in Kenya: the contingencies of coping and resilience in a context marked by structural vulnerability. Qual Health Res 27(7):1090–1103

Unanue W, Gómez ME, Cortez D, Oyanedel JC, Mendiburo-Seguel A (2017) Revisiting the link between job satisfaction and life satisfaction: the role of basic psychological needs. Front Psychol. https://doi.org/10.3389/fpsyg.2017.00680

VanderWeele TJ (2017) Religious communities and human flourishing. Curr Dir Psychol Sci 26:476–481

Veenhoven R (2015) The overall satisfaction with life: subjective approaches. In: Glatzer W, Camfield L, Møller V, Rojas M (eds) International handbooks of quality-of-life. Global handbook of quality of life: exploration of well-being of nations and continents. Springer, Dordrecht, pp 207–238

Villani D, Sorgente A, Iannello P, Antonietti A (2019) The role of spirituality and religiosity in subjective well-being of individuals with different religious status. Front Psychol. https://doi.org/10.3389/fpsyg.2019.01525

Weinstein N, Khabbaz F, Legate N (2016) Enhancing need satisfaction to reduce psychological distress in Syrian refugees. J Consult Clin Psychol 84(7):645–650

von Werthern M, Robjant K, Chui Z, Schon R, Ottisova L, Mason C, Katona C (2018) The impact of immigration detention on mental health: a systematic review. BMC Psychiatry 18(1):1–19

Wilkinson J, Santoro N, Major J (2017) Sudanese refugee youth and educational success: the role of church and youth group in supporting cultural and academic adjustment and schooling achievement. Int J Intercult Relat 60:210–219

Woods J, Pulla V (2016) Spirituality, coping, and resilience of the Lhotsampa. In: Pulla V (ed) The Lhotsampa people of Bhutan. Palgrave Macmillan, New York, pp 95–119

Zbidat A, Georgiadou E, Borho A, Erim Y (2020) The perceptions of trauma, complaints, somatization, and coping strategies among Syrian refugees in Germany. A qualitative study of an at-risk population. Int J Environ Res Public Health 17(3):693. https://doi.org/10.3390/ijerph17030693

Çetin M (2019) Effects of religious participation on social inclusion and existential well-being levels of Muslim refugees and immigrants in Turkey. Int J Psychol Religion 29(2):64–76

PART V

Findings in Different Populations: Healthy Populations

CHAPTER 25

Spiritual Needs of Parents with Health-Affected Children

Arndt Büssing and Olga Riklikienė

Background

Most studies indicate a positive impact of spirituality on people's health and illness. A connection between spirituality and health manifests at different stages of persons' life and disease, that is, in terms of mortality, coping and compliance, and the course of recovery from acute and chronic diseases (Tabei et al. 2016).

Even if the need to study the spiritual dimension in humans (linking it to the state of health) has arisen a long time ago, investigating the spiritual aspects of a person is a scientifically difficult approach because of the

A. Büssing (✉)
Professorship Quality of Life, Spirituality and Coping, Faculty of Health, Witten/Herdecke University, Herdecke, Germany

IUNCTUS—Competence Center for Christian Spirituality, Philosophical-Theological University of Münster, Münster, Germany
e-mail: arndt.buessing@uni-wh.de

O. Riklikienė
Faculty of Nursing, Medical Academy, Lithuanian University of Health Sciences, Kaunas, Lithuania

A. Büssing (ed.), *Spiritual Needs in Research and Practice*,
https://doi.org/10.1007/978-3-030-70139-0_25

proximity of these aspects to the realm of religion, on the one hand, and the lack of reliable instruments to measure the different aspects of the multidimensional "spirituality" construct, on the other hand. Nevertheless, researchers have been concerned about the lack of evidence on mental health components of an individual as it is gradually becoming evident that the subjective assessment of an individual's spiritual vision, beliefs and spiritual needs becomes an important source of information about his or her health status.

Responding to patients' spiritual needs is considered to be an essential element of high-quality care. Nurses are formal caregivers and their own spiritual well-being is likely to affect the quality of the care they can deliver and the way in which they can meet spiritual needs of the patients (Jahandideh et al. 2018). Parents or other family members also play active roles in the care process as informal caregivers. Their faith, religiosity and spirituality are important factors that reflect their participation in the child's care and healing process, influence effective coping strategies and the overall quality of life. By knowing parents' spiritual concerns, nurses and other health professionals would be able to address them much better during the care process to help the family to achieve security and confidence, find or regain a purpose in life and give meaning to holistic care.

In the following, we will discuss data from mothers of sick newborns and preterm infants from Germany, mothers of children with Down syndrome[1] as a contrasting group from Germany, and mothers of neurologically ill children from Lithuania with a different cultural background. Mothers are the focus of this chapter because they have a very intensive emotional relation to their children and are in most cases responsible for their care and education, and often also have an additional job and/or have to manage the household. This multiple burden often leads to feelings of being overwhelmed and coming to the limits. What are their specific spiritual needs and how do these relate to perceived burden and life satisfaction?

Mothers of Sick Newborn or Premature Infants

Most young mothers may expect that they will deliver a healthy baby and they can start a happy family life. However, in some cases mothers have a sick newborn or a premature infant. While in most cases the prognosis of their child might be good, it is in few cases either unclear or even bad. In

[1] We would like to emphasize that we do not assume that these children are necessarily "sick".

these unexpected situations, they are confronted with the requirement that their child has to stay in hospital for surveillance or treatment. Although mothers will get the necessary medical information by the hospital staff, they nevertheless have to cope with their fears and worries, their insecurities about the future course of treatment and deal with a sick child at home later on.

A further aggravating factor is that the family will be separated as in most cases the mother is attending her child in hospital *throughout*, while her partner and other children will be possibly at home and eventually coming for visits to support her. Moreover, often mothers of sick children or premature infants are afraid to handle the "fragile" child resulting in distancing behaviors. This insecurity is a further stressor for the mothers (Brandon et al. 2011), and may persist for several years and can disturb bonding with the child (Shaw et al. 2013; Schappin et al. 2013). Mothers of preterm infants were found to be more stressed compared to other mothers, as they experience phases of anxiety and insecurity, grief and depressive states (Shaw et al. 2013; Cho et al. 2008; Shah et al. 2011), which all are indicators of posttraumatic stress disorders. Thus, although the child is at the center of the medical treatment, also its mother requires further support—from the hospital team, their partner, family and friends. They have to find their own strategies to cope with their fears and the unclear situation, and several rely on their faith as a resource of hope and meaning finding (Corrine et al. 1992; Jesse et al. 2007; Caldeira and Hall 2012; Crowther and Hall 2015). A Danish study group has found that a birth with complications may result in existential and spiritual needs and considerations (Prinds et al. 2014a, b, 2016), a fact that would underline that mothers of sick or health-affected children also require psychological and/or pastoral support. In most cases, their specific spiritual needs are unknown to the hospital team as these are not in all cases seen as a part of the professional tasks.

To analyze what spiritual needs were of relevance to mothers of sick newborns or premature infants and how these relate to stress perception and perceived impairment of life concerns, we analyzed data of 125 mothers with a mean age of 31 ± 5 years (Büssing et al. 2017). Among them, 33% had premature infants without complications, 15% had premature infants with some complications (newborn infections, respiratory distress syndrome, hyperbilirubinemia, adaptation disturbance, etc.), 33% were sick newborns with good prognosis (new-born infection, hyperbilirubinemia, hypoglycemia, skin abscess, respiratory distress syndrome, adaptation disturbance, small for age, etc.) and 19% had children with severe health impairments and unclear or even poor prognosis (sepsis, systemic inflammatory response syndrome, asphyxia, pneumonia, pneumothorax, ventricular septum defects, spina bifida, hydrocephalus, cramps, etc.) (Büssing et al. 2017). Most of these mothers were informed that the health impairment of their child is only temporary, and they were assured by the hospital staff that they need not worry about their child's prognosis. Only 10% of mothers felt inadequately informed and 12% were unsure about it. Nevertheless, despite the fact that the majority of mothers had the required information and social support resources to rely on, and despite the fact that their life satisfaction scores are very high (BMLSS-10: 81.6 ± 13.1), mothers perceived an impairment of their daily life concerns and felt "under pressure".

In these mothers, Religious needs (0.64 ± 0.80) and Existential needs (0.37 ± 0.50) scored low, while Inner Peace needs (1.47 ± 0.86) and Giving/Generativity needs (0.92 ± 0.77) were of moderate relevance (Büssing et al. 2017). Their SpNQ-20 mean score, ranging from 0 to 3, was rather low (0.78 ± 0.51) (Fig. 25.1). For them, the need to talk with someone about their fears and worries (N2: 2.12 ± 1.02), turning to

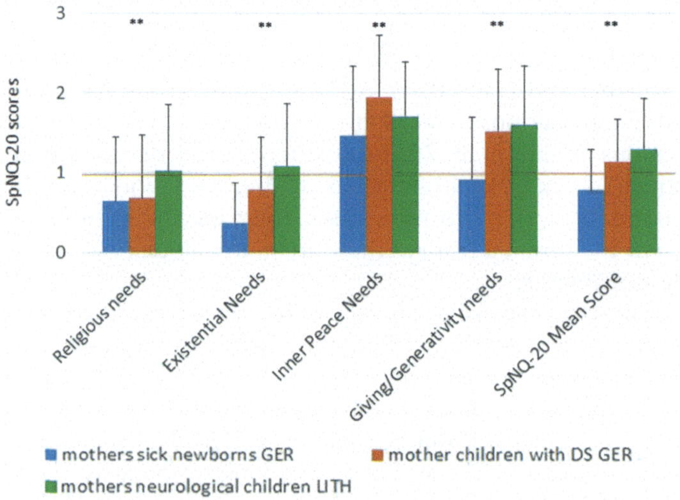

Fig. 25.1 Comparison of spiritual needs among the three samples of mothers from Germany (GER) and Lithuania (LITH). (** p<0.001 (ANOVA))

someone in a loving attitude (N13: 2.30 ± 0.99) and feeling connected with the family (N25: 2.55 ± 0.90) were of outstanding relevance, while talking with someone about the possibility of life after death (N12: 0.11 ± 0.46) or about the meaning in life (N11: 0.23 ± 0.72) was irrelevant.

When their child's prognosis was unclear or even poor or when they did not have the knowledge that their child's symptoms are only temporary, then their perceived daily life impairment and their feelings of being under pressure, on the one hand, and feelings of grief and emotional tiredness, on the other hand, were higher compared to the other mothers of this group. However, the indicators of burden and stress were not significantly related to their spiritual needs (as measured with the SpNQ-20) or to their spiritual well-being (as measured with the FACIT-Sp). The only significant differences were found for *Religious* needs, which were higher in mothers of children with unclear or poor prognosis ($F = 8.6$, $p < 0.004$) (Büssing et al. 2017). Praying (for help) and turning to a more powerful instance (God) that may help in this difficult situation are thus strategies to cope with this insecurity and helplessness.

Mothers' stress perception (Cohen's Perceived Stress Scale) was nevertheless moderately related to their *Inner Peace* needs ($r = 0.34$). This means, the need for peaceful conditions was triggered because of perceived stressors in their daily life concerns, and supporting them may have a beneficial effect. Further weak associations were found between grief and *Inner Peace* needs ($r = 0.23$), despair and *Religious* needs ($r = 0.20$), and between perceived daily life affections and *Inner Peace* needs ($r = 0.25$) and *Religious* needs ($r = 0.26$). This would underline that the need for inner peace is also a matter of negative mood states, particularly grief that is strongly related to stress perception ($r = 0.55$). None of the four spiritual needs domains were significantly related to mothers' life satisfaction, to satisfaction with partner or hospital team support, to a depressive intention to escape from the burdening situation or to having friends to talk with. However, having people to help them was moderately positively related to *Religious* needs ($r = 0.32$) and to the Faith domain of spiritual well-being ($r = 0.40$), indicating that both resources are activated because one has access to them also in difficult times.

The finding that *Religious* needs and *Existential* needs scored low in this group of mothers (which includes 21% of women without religious affiliations) does not mean they are irrelevant. In fact, 36% had strong to very strong needs to pray (particularly those mothers who were more stressed because of an unclear or poor prognosis of their child's health situation) and to find any "meaning in illness and/or suffering" (Büssing et al. 2017). However, the intensity of these spiritual needs was not clearly related to the severity of prognosis. Also in the Danish study among mothers with preterm children and timely newborns, praying did not differ between both groups (Prinds et al. 2016).

Thus, although mothers were principally informed about the prognosis of their child and although they were very satisfied with the support of the hospital staff and their partner, they nevertheless experienced stress and restrictions in their daily life concerns, and expressed specific spiritual needs, particularly *Inner Peace* needs. These needs can be explained best by their stress perception (Beta = 0.373; T = 4.27; $p < 0.0001$) and additionally by the week of gestation (Beta = 0.196; T = 2.24; $p = 0.027$). These two predictors would explain only 16% of the *Inner Peace* needs variance, while negative mood states were not among the significant predictors. This means, other relevant predictors remain to be identified.

Mothers' unmet spiritual needs should be supported by the hospital staff to provide hope, hold and orientation during the hospital stay. Information delivery is a matter of course, and continuing talks about their fears and worries and their difficulties to face the unexpected situation is essential. Supporting mothers in this ways may help them to adjust to the new and difficult situation—and maybe to promote the bonding to their child.

Spiritual Needs of Mothers of Children with Down Syndrome

Next, we analyzed mothers of children with Down syndrome who are reported to be exposed to higher stress compared to other mothers (Bodenmann et al. 2008). Parental care for a child with Down syndrome may be related to challenges in its upbringing and care, and often leads to personal restrictions in work, leisure and social contacts. The child's acceptance can be difficult for parents, and parents can experience fears of the future for their children (Roach et al. 1999; Lessenberry and Rehfeldt 2004).

Persons with Down syndrome have a chromosomal disorder that is often associated with intellectual impairment (ranging from mild to moderate) and with a higher risk for different diseases, that is, heart defects, digestive disorders, hypothyroidism, or leukemia. Particularly younger mothers may argue that their child is "special", but not "sick" (Büssing et al. 2019), to find ways of accepting and loving their child as it is. However, it is unclear why some parents get along well when they have a child with special needs, and others do not (Raina et al. 2005).

Research has highlighted that parents' stress is greater for the parent who is the primary caregiver (Saloviita et al. 2003). Stress is indeed a predictor of the reduced well-being of mothers caring for children with autism (Davis and Kiang 2020). A child with special needs can thus be a potential "stressor" (like any other child, too), primarily for the mother as the primary caregiver (Olsson and Hwang 2001, 2003; Raina et al. 2005; Bourke et al. 2008; Gabriel et al. 2008). Some parents described processes of positive transformation as they changed their view of their child from a burden to a blessing or to part of God's plan (Landsman 2009; Michie and Skinner 2010). However, most of the research has focused on mothers' quality of life, while there are only a few studies that analyze the relevance of mothers' spirituality as a resource or on which spiritual needs they would express. In fact, it was suggested that spirituality can play a key role in supporting these mothers (Kaye and Raghavan 2002).

Gallagher et al. (2015) conducted a study on parents of children with a variety of developmental disabilities (autism, Smith-Magenis syndrome, Down syndrome, Cornelia de Lange syndrome, etc.) and measured spirituality, depression and social support, with spirituality characterized separately from religious practice. The results revealed that social support was inversely related to depression, while higher levels of spirituality were positively related and predictive of increased depression among parents; spirituality was also higher in parents with less social support. Here, their spiritual convictions (as measured with Beliefs and Values Scale) might be triggered because of their burdening situation and are thus positively associated with their depression scores. The follow-up qualitative study with the same mothers confirmed that spirituality serves for them as a mechanism to obtain release from stress, as a source of support, and as a last resort (Gallagher et al. 2015).

Enrolling 203 mothers (mean age 44 ± 7 years) of children with Down syndrome, it was assessed which spiritual needs were of relevance to them and how these relate to their self-perceived burden and how they expected securing and supplying for their child's future (Büssing et al. 2019). The mean age of their children was 9 ± 7 years, and most were living with them in the family. Among the mothers, 42% see the future of their child as secured, 31% are undecided and 26% do not see them as secured. Similar proportions were found for the statement whether they consider their child as cared for in the future. Unfortunately, older mothers were not participating and their views might be different from those of younger mothers. Enrolled mothers' life satisfaction was rather moderate (BMLSS-10: 67.8 ± 18.9) and much lower as compared to mothers of sick newborn or premature infants ($p < 0.0001$, Mann-Whitney-U test). They were moderately stressed, felt moderately under pressure and impaired in their daily life concerns; 18% felt strongly under pressure and 7% very strongly, while 16% felt strongly impaired in their life concerns and 3% very strongly (Büssing et al. 2019).

Religious needs (0.68 ± 0.79) and *Existential* needs (0.79 ± 0.65) scored low in these women, while *Inner Peace* needs (1.95 ± 0.77) and *Giving/Generativity* needs (1.52 ± 0.74) were of stronger relevance (Büssing et al. 2019). Their SpNQ-20 mean score, ranging from 0 to 3, was higher (1.14 ± 0.53) compared to the mothers with the newborns (Fig. 25.1). With the exception of *Religious* needs, all spiritual needs factors were significantly higher in mothers of children with Down syndrome compared to younger mothers with sick newborn or premature infants ($p < 0.0001$, Mann-Whitney-U test). Whether the mothers of children with Down syndrome had a religious affiliation or not, their perception of burden and stress was similar (stress perception and feelings of being under pressure were in trend only higher in nonreligious persons).

The spiritual needs that were of particular importance were to feel connected with the family (N25: 2.33 ± 0.95), to dwell at a place of quietness and peace (N: 2.27 ± 0.91), to plunge into beauty of nature (N6: 2.09 ± 0.99), passing own life experiences to others (N26: 1.97 ± 0.92) and finding inner peace (N8: 1.86 ± 1.11). Thus, mothers of children with Down syndrome have, particularly, needs for emotional retreat and peaceful quietness, on the one hand, and emotional support (talking with others and being connected with the family), on the other hand.

Particularly *Existential* needs and *Inner Peace* needs were moderately to strongly related to mothers' perceived burden (stress perception, feelings of being under pressure and daily life affections), negative mood states (grief, hopelessness, emotional tiredness) and low life satisfaction (Büssing et al. 2019). *Religious* needs were not at all associated with burden indicators, and weakly only with grief and hopelessness. Mothers' expectation that the future of their child is secured and that their child is cared for in the future was moderately negatively related to *Inner Peace* needs, and weakly to *Existential* needs, but neither with *Religious* needs nor with *Giving/Generativity* needs.

Thus, compared to the group of (younger) mothers with sick or premature newborns, women caring for their child with Down syndrome seem to be more impaired in their life concerns and have a significantly lower life satisfaction. Mothers of children with Down syndrome had low satisfaction particularly with their own health situation and with themselves in general. A relevant proportion felt significantly impaired and under pressure - and these require specific support and relief. The strong correlation between grief and hopelessness and mothers' *Existential* needs would indicate that these needs are triggered by negative mood states and may result in reflection processes about their own and their child's life. Detailed analyses revealed that their grief was best related to the need of talking with someone about the question of meaning in life (N11: $r = 0.42$) and to find meaning in illness and/or suffering (N10: $r = 0.37$); further also hopelessness was best related to both needs (N11: $r = 0.47$; N10: $r = 0.43$). Again, adequate support will include persons who are able to listen and to respond to their communication needs. These needs may be the hint that someone should see their problems and is willing to respond, and this may facilitate letting go of their worries.

Spiritual Needs of Parents Taking Care of Their Neurologically Ill Children from Lithuania

Lithuania is a post-communist country with a Christian background but different cultural socialization compared to Germany. To contribute to the scientific evidence on parents' spiritual needs while caring for sick children, both mothers and fathers of neurologically ill children with chronic conditions were recruited at the Children Neurology Department of University Hospital's Pediatric Centre in the capital city.

The spiritual needs, as measured with the SpNQ both in its 27-item Lithuanian version (Riklikienė et al. 2019a, b) and its 20-item SpNQ-20 version (Büssing et al. 2018), satisfaction with life, as measured with the 10-item Brief Multidimensional Life Satisfaction Scale (BMLSS-10) (Büssing et al. 2009), and spiritual well-being, as measured with John Fisher's SHALOM questionnaire in its Lithuanian version (Riklikiene et al. 2018), were analyzed in 176 parents (response rate 98%) during the period from April 2018 to July 2019. Parents responded to the questionnaires during their stay in hospital. However, more mothers ($n = 150$) than fathers ($n = 21$) responded; their mean age was 37 ± 7 [26–64] years and those of 30–39 years composed the largest group (59%). Because of this gender disbalance, the primary focus of the following analyses will be on mothers. Two-thirds of parents were urban residents and half of respondents had higher education degree. In relation to family structure, 69% lived in marriage, 13% were divorced and all others were either single or lived with a partner. The average duration of their child's chronic condition and care was 4.0 ± 3.7 years, with the longest duration of 18 years; 48% of parents took care of their sick child for 3–6 years and 8% less than 1 year. Their child's main health problem was epilepsy, while other children were hospitalized because of cerebral palsy disease or developmental disabilities. In relation to religiousness, 72% of parents declared being religious (93% Christians, 62% of them Roman Catholics).

Mothers' life satisfaction was slightly reduced (68.2 ± 14.9); 11% had scores <50, indicating severe restrictions. Their spiritual needs (SpNQ-20) were higher compared to German mothers, particularly *Religious* needs (1.02 ± 0.83) and *Existential* needs (1.08 ± 0.78), while *Inner Peace* needs (1.70 ± 0.68) and *Giving/Generativity* needs (1.60 ± 0.73) were in a similar range (Fig. 25.1). Lithuanian mothers' SpNQ-20 mean score was 1.29 ± 0.63. With the exception of *Religious* needs (which were significantly lower in men; $p = 0.006$, Mann-Whitney-U test), their parents' spiritual needs were not significantly different between mothers and fathers.

The most important needs for these parents were to be connected with the family (N25: 91%), to be complete and safe (N24: 85%) and to be re-involved into the family life (N25: 85%). As the largest proportion of respondents were women it is expected that they stayed with a sick child and took care of other children by being supported by other family members. When the physiological need of parents to solve the health problems of their child is satisfied in the health care institution, the next step is to assure safety and completeness by receiving quality health care.

Further relevant unmet needs of parents were to plunge into beauty of nature (N6: 1.90 ± 0.91), to dwell at a place of quietness (N7: 1.69 ± 1.01), finding inner peace (N8: 1.89 ± 0.9) and to be assured that life was meaningful and of value (N27: 1.78 ± 1.02). Feelings connected to nature and value of nature activities have been shown to be beneficial to well-being (Lumber et al. 2017). The connectedness with nature is stimulated by the contact, emotion, meaning, compassion and beauty that people feel and wish to constantly experience. Possibly nature is a place where parents can find inner peace and a breathing space during crisis.

Lithuanian society is highly religious, and thus for mothers of sick children with chronic neurological diseases faith-related activities were of importance too, particularly praying for oneself (N20: 1.49 ± 1.06) and turning to a higher presence (i.e., God) (N23: 1.33 ± 1.12). It is known that more women than men actively participate in religious ceremonies and that they perceive the protective effect of weekly religious attendance of the same magnitude as the other health behaviors (e.g., smoking, physical activity, alcohol consumption) (Strawbridge et al. 2000). Mothers also reported higher needs to turn to others in a loving attitude and to keep contact with the family by participating in its life compared with the few fathers.

The health and life perspectives of parents' children were not necessarily critical. Consequently, for parents it is essential to accept the situation by adapting to the illness of their child, learning how to live with it and how to manage the symptoms or deteriorations. In this situation, parents may have the need to reflect back on life (N4: 1.16 ± 0.97) and to talk with others about their fears and worries (N2: 1.33 ± 1.03), while their need to talk with someone about the possibility of life after death (N12: 0.55 ± 0.87) was rather low.

With respect to the partner status (married, single, divorced), there were no significant differences for mothers' spiritual needs, while there were some weak differences with respect to the educational status. Those with a lower educational status had somewhat higher *Existential* needs ($F = 2.7$, $p = 0.031$) and *Religious* needs ($F = 2.6$, $p = 0.041$) compared to those with a higher status. For parents with basic level of education, it was more important to dissolve open aspects of their life, to find meaning in illness and /or suffering, to discuss life after death and to give solace to someone or be forgiven. One cannot exclude the possibility that persons with higher educational level have more possibilities to understand the complexity of their own and their child's situation, to have other strategies to cope with the burden and thus to reduce worries and doubts, and to remain more psychologically resistant compared to those with lower level of education.

How do these needs in this specific sample relate to mothers' life satisfaction and to their spiritual well-being? Mothers' spiritual needs showed only marginal negative correlation with respect to *Existential* needs ($r = -0.18$, $p = 0.024$) and *Inner Peace* needs ($r = -0.17$, $p=0.036$), a nonsignificant (positive) with *Giving/Generativity* needs ($r = 0.13$), and no association with *Religious* needs ($r = 0.03$). Instead, their life satisfaction was moderately related to their spiritual well-being as an ideal, particularly to the Personal (r = 0.38), Communal (r = 0.34) and Transcendental (r = 0.34) aspects, while for the lived experience of spiritual well-being only the Personal aspect showed a moderate association with life satisfaction (r = 0.41).

With respect to mothers' spiritual needs, the Transcendental aspect of spiritual well-being as a lived experience was strongly positively related to their *Religious* needs (r = 0.59), which is consistent from a theoretical point of view, and moderately with *Existential* needs (r = 0.30) and *Giving/Generativity* needs (r = 0.31). The Communal aspect of their spiritual well-being as a lived experience (r = 0.30) and also the Environmental aspect (r = 0.38) were moderately related only to *Giving/Generativity* needs, while the Personal aspect was weakly only related to *Giving/Generativity* needs (r = 0.28). It is thus striking that mothers' *Giving/Generativity* needs were related so often with the different aspects of spiritual well-being, particularly the Environmental aspect that involves connection with nature, awe at a breathtaking view, oneness with nature, harmony with the environment, and sense of 'magic' in the environment. Here, the need of giving solace to someone (N15) was related best with the lived experience of Environmental spiritual well-being (r = 0.35).

How well people cope with their illness or with the illness of their child depends on their internal relationship with themselves, with others around them, the natural and social environment, and God or the belief in a "higher being". In these four areas of relationships, namely, with Self, Others, Environment/Nature, and/or the Transcendent, a person's spiritual well-being might be represented (Fisher 2012). Next, the interconnectedness of body–mind–spirit leads individuals toward a state of mature spirituality, where they are at peace with themselves and the world around (Chan et al. 2006). It is evident that spiritual needs are not simply expressed as an indicator of low spiritual well-being; instead, these resources can be activated when the ideal and the lived experience are not matching. A person's spiritual well-being is, of course, linked to (mental) health and survival factors, such as quality of life, hope, coping with pain, spiritual practices, end of life interventions and similar, and it is also related to happiness and life satisfaction (Riklikienė et al. 2020). However, the causal relationships remain to be clarified, and further, how spiritual well-being could be facilitated. Whether this would indeed reduce a person's specific spiritual needs remains to be shown. It might be that some spiritual needs are permanent ("desires") and cannot be satisfied or fulfilled at all.

Conclusions

Here three groups of mothers from two culturally different contexts were analyzed. These groups differed significantly with respect to their life satisfaction ($p < 0.0001$, ANOVA) and their spiritual needs (Fig. 25.1). Young mothers with sick newborns/preterm infants had the highest life satisfaction and the lowest spiritual needs. Most of them had the knowledge and expectations that their child's health affection is only temporary and that the prognosis is good. In contrast, mothers of children with Down syndrome (DS) had significantly lower life satisfaction and higher spiritual needs. They have to live with the fact that their child has a chromosomal disorder that cannot be treated in terms of healing, that their child may have special needs that require more intensive care and support, and that it has higher risks for several relevant diseases. As a consequence, they may worry about their child's health and social perspectives and—depending on their own age—who and how their child will be cared for in the future. Also mothers of children with neurological diseases have to live with the fact that—depending on the underlying condition—their child will have to live with it. Their life satisfaction was moderately reduced, too, and their spiritual needs were the highest compared to both groups of mothers from Germany. Particularly their *Religious* needs and their *Existential* needs were high, while their *Inner Peace* needs and *Giving/Generativity* needs were similarly high compared to mothers with children with Down syndrome (Fig. 25.1).

All of these mothers require specific support, with respect to (1) an often more intensive care for their child with special needs and an often unclear future situation, (2) the challenge to manage these complex conditions alone as the "responsible" mother, and (3) their feelings of being overwhelmed by the different additional tasks of daily life and care of other children in the family. It was striking that particularly *Inner Peace* needs were of high relevance to all of them, indicating that they need time-out breaks in a peaceful surrounding, which they probably will not find during their daily routine. Also *Giving/Generativity* needs were of relevance, indicating that they need peer support groups to talk to about their situation and to help each other, and of being affirmed that all efforts are worth it and that their life is (nevertheless) meaningful.

Often mothers of children with chronic diseases and persisting disorders may feel "guilty" and "consumed" by the exhausting care of their child whose situation in several cases will not become better. This may result in phases of depression and reduced quality of life, as it was shown for mothers of children with Down syndrome and children with epilepsy (Swanepoel and Haw 2018; Senses Dinc et al. 2019; Reilly et al. 2018; Koc et al. 2019). Whether and how addressing their spiritual needs will help them to cope with the difficult situation is the question for further investigations. The knowledge that others are aware of their situation and are available for relieving talks, and offer their help and support, will have a positive effect but may not change their situation.

Acknowledgments We are grateful to Silke Broghammer-Escher, Sophia Hippen und Julia Eichhorn for recruiting the sample of mothers in Germany.

References

Bodenmann G, Gabriel B, Zender N (2008) Stress und Coping bei Eltern von einem Kind mit einem Down-Syndrom. Die Überprüfung eines theoretischen Modells Zeitschrift für Familienforschung 20:80–95

Bourke J, Ricciardo B, Bebbington A, Aiberti K, Jacoby P, Dyke P, Msall M, Bower C, Leonard H (2008) Physical and mental health in mothers of children with Down syndrome. J Pediatr 153:320–326

Brandon DH, Tully KP, Silva SG, Malcolm WF, Murtha AP, Turner BS, Holditch-Davis D (2011) Emotional responses of mothers of late-preterm and term infants. J Obstet Gynecol Neonatal Nurs 3:719–731

Büssing A, Fischer J, Haller A, Heusser P, Ostermann T, Matthiessen PF (2009) Validation of the brief multidimensional life satisfaction Scale in patients with chronic diseases. Eur J Med Res 14:171–177

Büssing A, Wassermann U, Hvidt NC, Längler A, Thiel M (2017) Spiritual needs of mothers with sick new born or premature infants. Woman and Birth 31:e89–e98

Büssing A, Recchia DR, Koenig H, Baumann K, Frick E (2018) Factor structure of the Spiritual Needs Questionnaire (SpNQ) in persons with chronic diseases, elderly and healthy individuals. Religions 9:13. https://doi.org/10.3390/rel9010013

Büssing A, Hippen S, Eichhorn J, Baumann K (2019) Spirituelle Bedürfnisse und Belastungserleben von Müttern mit Kindern mit Down-Syndrom. Spiritual Care 8:263–273

Caldeira S, Hall J (2012) Spiritual leadership and spiritual care in neonatology. J Nurs Manag 20:1069–1075

Chan CL, Ng SM, Ho RT, Chow AY (2006) East meets West: applying Eastern spirituality in clinical practice. J Clin Nurs 15:822–832

Cho J, Holditch-Davis D, Miles MS (2008) Effects of maternal depressive symptoms and infant gender on the interaction between mothers and their medically at-risk infants. J Obstet Gynecol Neonatal Nurs 37:58–70

Corrine L, Bailey V, Valentin M (1992) The unheard voices of women: spiritual interventions in maternal-child-health, insight into the client's spiritual life can yield strategies for overcoming crisis. MCN Am J Matern Child Nurs 17:141–145

Crowther S, Hall J (2015) Spirituality and spiritual care in and around childbirth. Women Birth 28:173–178

Davis R, Kiang L (2020) Parental stress and religious coping by mothers of children with autism. Psychol Relig Spiritual 12:137–148

Fisher JW (2012) The Importance of Relating with God for Spiritual Well-Being. In: Fowler MC, Weiss M, Hochheimer JL (eds) Spirituality: New Reflections on Theory, Praxis & Pedagogy. InterDisciplinary Press, Oxford, pp 147–161.

Gabriel B, Zeender N, Bodenmann G (2008) Stress und Coping bei Eltern von einem Kind mit einem Down-Syndrom: die Überprüfung eines theoretischen Modells. Zeitschrift für Familienforschung 20:80–95

Gallagher S, Phillips A, Lee H, Carroll D (2015) The association between spirituality and depression in parents caring for children with developmental disabilities: social support and/or last resort. J Relig Health 54:358–370

Jahandideh S, Zare A, Kendall E, Jahandideh M (2018) Nurses' spiritual well-being and patients' spiritual care in Iran. COJ Nursing & Healthcare 1(3). https://doi.org/10.31031/cojnh.2018.01.000514

Jesse DE, Schoneboom C, Blanchared A (2007) The effect of faith or spirituality in pregnancy: a Conten analysis. J Holist Nurs 25:151–158

Kaye J, Raghavan SK (2002) Spirituality in disability and illness. J Relig Health 41:231–242

Koc G, Bek S, Vurucu S, Gokcil Z, Odabasi Z (2019) Maternal and paternal quality of life in children with epilepsy: who is affected more? Epilepsy Behav 92:184–190

Landsman GH (2009) Reconstructing motherhood and disability in the age of 'perfect' babies. Routledge, New York

Lessenberry BM, Rehfeldt RA (2004) Evaluating stress levels of parents of children with disabilities. Counc Except Child 70:231–244

Lumber R, Richardson M, Sheffield D (2017) Beyond knowing nature: contact, emotion, compassion, meaning, and beauty are pathways to nature connection. PLoS One 12:e0177186. https://doi.org/10.1371/journal.pone.0177186

Michie M, Skinner D (2010) Narrating disability, narrating religious practice: reconciliation and Fragile-X syndrome. Intellect Dev Disabil 48:99–111

Olsson MB, Hwang CP (2001) Depression in mothers and fathers of children with intellectual disability. J Intellect Disabil Res 45:535–543

Olsson MB, Hwang PC (2003) Influence of macrostructure of society on the life situation of families with a child with intellectual disability: Sweden as an example. J Intellect Disabil Res 47:328–341

Prinds C, Hvidt NC, Mogensen O, Buus N (2014a) Making existential meaning in transition to motherhood—a scoping review. Midwifery 30:733–741

Prinds C, Hvidtjorn D, Mogensen O, Skytthe A, Hvidt NC (2014b) Existential meaning among first-time full-term and preterm mothers: a questionnaire study. J Perinat Neonatal Nurs 28:271–279

Prinds C, Hvidtjørn D, Skytthe A, Mogensen O, Hvidt NC (2016) Prayer and meditation among Danish first time mothers—a questionnaire study. BMC Pregnancy Childbirth 16:8. https://doi.org/10.1186/s12884-016-0802-6

Raina P, O'Donnell M, Rosenbaum P, Brehaut J, Walter SD, Russell D, Swinton M, Zhu B, Wood E (2005) The health and well-being of caregivers of children with cerebral palsy. Pediatrics 115:626–636

Reilly C, Atkinson P, Memon A, Jones C, Dabydeen L, Das KB, Gillberg C, Neville BGR, Scott RC (2018) Symptoms of depression, anxiety, and stress in parents of young children with epilepsy: a case controlled population-based study. Epilepsy Behav 80:177–183

Riklikiene O, Kaseliene S, Fisher J (2018) Translation and validation of spiritual well-being questionnaire SHALOM in Lithuanian language, culture and health care practice. Religions 9:156. https://doi.org/10.3390/rel9050156

Riklikienė O, Spirgienė L, Kaselienė S, Luneckaitė Ž, Tomkevičiūtė J, Büssing A (2019a) Translation, cultural, and clinical validation of the Lithuanian version of the spiritual needs questionnaire among hospitalized cancer patients. Medicina (Kaunas, Lithuania) 55:738. https://doi.org/10.3390/medicina55110738

Riklikienė O, Spirgienė L, Kaselienė S (2019b) Association of religiosity and spirituality with the perception of cancer patients' spiritual wellbeing and spiritual needs. Nurse Education, Research, & Practice 9:19–25

Riklikienė O, Kaselienė S, Spirgienė L, Karosas L, Fisher JW (2020) Spiritual wellbeing of cancer patients: what health-related factors matter? Journal of Religion and Health, Advance online publication. https://doi.org/10.1007/s10943-020-01053-0

Roach MA, Orsmond GI, Barratt MS (1999) Mothers and fathers of children with Down syndrome: parental stress and involvement in childcare. Am J Ment Retard 104:422–436

Saloviita T, Itälinna M, Leinonen E (2003) Explaining the parental stress of fathers and mothers caring for a child with intellectual disability: a Double ABCX Model. J Intellect Disabil Res 47:300–312

Schappin R, Wijnroks L, Venema MM, Jongmans MJ (2013) Rethinking stress in parents of preterm infants: a meta-analysis. PLoS One 8:e54992

Senses Dinc G, Cop E, Tos T, Sari E, Senel S (2019) Mothers of 0-3-year-old children with Down syndrome: effects on quality of life. Pediatr Int 61:865–871

Shah PE, Clements M, Poehlmann J (2011) Maternal resolution of grief after preterm birth: implications for infant attachment security. Pediatrics 127:284–292

Shaw RJ, Bernhard RS, Storfer- Isser A, Rhine W, Horwitz SM (2013) Parental coping in the neonatal intensive care unit. J Clin Psychol Med Settings 20:135–142

Strawbridge WJ, Cohen RD, Shema SJ (2000) Comparative strength of association between religious attendance and survival. Int J Psychiatry Med 30:299–308

Swanepoel M, Haw T (2018) A pilot study evaluating depression in mothers with children diagnosed with Down syndrome in state health care. J Intellect Disabil Res 62:952–961

Tabei SZ, Zarei N, Joulaei H (2016) The impact of spirituality on health. Shiraz E-Med J 17:e39053. https://doi.org/10.17795/semj39053

CHAPTER 26

Spiritual Needs of Elderly

Arndt Büssing, Renata Spalek, Norbert Gerard Pikuła, Eckhard Frick, and Janusz Surzykiewicz

Introduction

In 2019, 20% of the European population was aged 65 years and over. This percentage is higher in Italy (23%) and Germany (22%) compared to Poland (18%) (Eurostat 2019). Currently, the population of the elderly (65 years and over) is increasing in these countries. This constant increase of the elderly within a society will have important consequences not only for the

A. Büssing (✉)
Professorship Quality of Life, Spirituality and Coping, Faculty of Health, Witten/Herdecke University, Herdecke, Germany

IUNCTUS—Competence Center for Christian Spirituality, Philosophical-Theological University of Münster, Münster, Germany
e-mail: Arndt.buessing@uni-wh.de

R. Spalek
Rehabilitation Unit, 'Mons. L. Novarese' Hospital, Moncrivello, Vercelli, Italy

Department of Geriatrics, Neurosciences and Orthopedics, Center for Geriatric Medicine, Institute of Internal Medicine and Geriatrics, Catholic University of the Sacred Hearts, Rome, Italy
e-mail: renata.spalek@unicatt.it

A. Büssing (ed.), *Spiritual Needs in Research and Practice*,
https://doi.org/10.1007/978-3-030-70139-0_26

health insurance system, but also for health care in general and the ways to live as an older person with reduced vitality and health conditions and lower abilities to participate in social life. Research draws on disengagement, reengagement, and activity theory to show how religion and spirituality can be integrated in the care of older adults. It is crucial that the elderly find new ways to build community, find spiritual and cultural interests, and continue to work for as long as they can render service, even if limited.

The psychosocial model of mental health postulates that well-being in late life is significantly influenced by external factors such as social resources, income and negative life events. Recently, the gerontological literature is drawing attention to the influential role of existential factors such as religiosity, spirituality and personal meaning in terms of psychological well-being of older adults. It has been suggested to gerontologically explore spirituality as an independent component of "successful aging" in different cultural contexts (Crowther et al. 2002; Fassino et al. 2002; MacKinlay 2017; Janhsen et al. 2019). Holistic health care requires the health professional to focus on the person's dignity, culture, values, beliefs and rights that intersect with spiritual needs (Goh et al. 2014; Erichsen and Büssing 2013; Man-Ging et al. 2015; Jackson et al. 2016; Łukasik et al. 2018a; Straßner et al. 2019).

With respect to 'successful aging', a person's spirituality among other significant components explains relevant aspects, even by chronical illness conditions (Young et al. 2009; Papadopoulos 2020). Spirituality or

N. G. Pikuła
Chair of Social Pedagogy, Faculty of Social Sciences, Pedagogical University, Krakow, Poland
e-mail: norbertpikula@gmail.com

E. Frick
Research Unit Spiritual Care, Clinic and Policlinic for Psychosomatic Medicine and Psychotherapy, Klinikum rechts der Isar, Technical University of Munich, Munich, Germany
e-mail: eckhard.frick@tum.de

J. Surzykiewicz
Faculty of Philosophy and Education, Katholische Universität Eichstätt-Ingolstadt, Eichstätt, Germany

Faculty of Education, Cardinal Stefan Wyszynski University in Warsaw, Warsaw, Poland
e-mail: Janusz.Surzykiewicz@ku.de

religious commitment, a complex and multidimensional part of human experience, has a positive impact on health outcomes and the well-being of older adults (McFadden 1999; Berkman et al. 2011; Noronha 2015; Tomás et al. 2016; Villani et al. 2019).

It is an observation in different countries that the number of elderly with unmet care and support needs is increasing. A scoping review by Abdi et al. (2019) identified three main categories which require special attention: (1) social activities and relationships; (2) psychological health; (3) mobility, self-care and domestic life. Maintaining independence was seen as crucial. However, in several cases elder persons have to live in protected housing areas (i.e., retirement homes, assisted accommodation, nursing homes) where basic needs of support and security are provided. Here, they may experience phases or even states of depression because of perceived physical affections and limitations, loneliness and lack of social support (Jongenelis et al. 2004). However, also those elderly living in their own apartments/houses are often lonely and depressed; living a distance away from family and friends and low satisfaction with living accommodation and finances are risk factors (Wilson et al. 2007). Both groups may suffer from a decline of reliable social networks and thus experience loneliness and depressive phases or even states. A decline of physical fitness and often also mental capabilities may aggravate these problems. Further problems of elderly are related to the fact that they miss social recognition. In the late 1980s it was stated that "older persons have significant needs that cannot be met by psychotherapy, social work, or other disciplines," particularly because they "often feel useless and without dignity," on the one hand, and have to struggle with "thoughts of dying," on the other hand (Shea 1986). One systematic review identified 94 articles or reports that have documented the unmet needs of patients with cancer during their illness experience (Harrison et al. 2009).

Referring to Alderfer's ERG model (Alderfer 1972), which includes the dimensions Existence (i.e., physiological and safety needs), Relatedness (i.e., belongingness and external esteem needs) and Growth (i.e., self-actualization and internal esteem needs), one can assume that elderly's Existence dimension becomes more and more insecure, while their Development potential is increasingly restricted (because no one cares for their views and creativity potentials), and thus their Relatedness needs (with respect to friends and family) will be more important in order to compensate for the other needs. These relatedness needs may either refer to concrete persons or also to God as an external source to address one's prayers for shelter, protection, anger, hope and gratitude. Faith/religion as a resource is investigated in several studies. It seems that in the elderly, the level of spirituality is quite stable at higher age (Forlenza and Vallada 2018; Bailly et al. 2018). This may mean that the elderly already have found meaning in their life and can rely on their faith as a stable resource. Older adults' spirituality was further related to higher levels of social support and flexibility (Bailly et al. 2018).

Though meaning in life tends to increase with age (Reker 2005), Erikson's theory of adult development suggests some normative struggle around the choice of generativity versus stagnation in old age (Slater 2003). When older people access senior aged, they are typically facing substantial health and lifestyle related changes, particularly when autonomy and potentials for self-sufficiency are educed. Then, maintaining a quality of life becames more relevant - with a focus on dignity, human rights and social, physical and emotional care provided by others (WHO 2002). However, aging is part of individual development over the life span. Therefore, one may expect that over the life span not only physiological and social needs but also other needs will increase, that is, the need for security, need for self-realization, relationship and also spiritual and religious needs. They might overlap depending on age and individual stage of development, situation or social circumstances. In its role as an important predictor of well-being, spirituality has also been included in psychological approaches to the 'good life' (Cowlishaw et al. 2013; Steger 2012; Van Dierendonck 2012; Van Dierendonck and Mohan 2006; Łukasik et al. 2018b), particularly in those studies that address the fulfillment of basic psychological needs (van Dierendonck 2012; Tomás et al. 2016; Fabiś 2015; Molesztak 2015).

Existential or spiritual concerns are especially important for older people and those faced with their own fragility and mortality (Bruce et al. 2011). However, one may assume that persons lacking this resource would indeed also lack social support and social networks. When the elderly experience phases of depression, one may suggest that religiosity could be a relevant buffer. However, a meta-analysis by Smith et al. (2003) found a marginal inverse correlation between religiousness and depressive symptoms only, while, however, this association was somewhat stronger when persons were experiencing stressful life events. In the elderly from Korea, Jung et al. (2017) found that depression, well-being and suicidal ideation did not significantly differ between those with a religious affiliation and others lacking it. However, the effects of the mood states were moderated by participants' religious engagement (Jung et al. 2017). Another study from Korea found that depressive states and quality of life were not related to religiosity/spirituality in Buddhists, but in Protestants and Catholics (Moon and Kim 2013). Thus, whether or not the elderly could benefit from their religion is dependent on different factors, including own religious engagement, but also on support and cohesion of an available religious community.

A systematic review by Agli et al. (2015) analyzed the effects of spirituality/religion in older persons with dementia and found that religious involvement and maintaining social interactions reduced or stabilized their cognitive disorders, helped them to cope in terms of disease acceptance coping strategies to help accept their disease, to maintain hope and relationships and hope and to find meaning in life that would improve their quality of life. Although some of these associations should be seen with caution and may depend on the indicators of spirituality, it is nevertheless striking that older persons who have a vital spiritual practice and can rely on it as a resource, may benefit from it particularly in old age.

In the following, we intend to describe which spiritual needs were of relevance for elderly living in retirement homes, assisted living homes or nursing homes, and what may trigger these. For that purpose, we will discuss findings from studies among the elderly from Germany, Poland and Italy, which are different with respect to their cultural and religious backgrounds.

Spiritual Needs of the Elderly living in Germany

Germany is regarded as a rather secular country with two main Christian denominations, Protestant and Catholics, and an increasing group of (younger) persons who are nonreligious. The interest in institutional religiosity is constantly decreasing, and this refers to both churches in Germany. This decline is not exclusively due to demographic factors, but more due to permanent leaves of Church members and exits and fewer entries and lower Baptisms (Peters et al. 2019). Those who have left their church stated that they are "indifferent" to the church, that one "does not need religion for life" and that the church is fundamentally "untrustworthy," as a 2014 study of the Protestant Church in Germany stated (Evangelische Kirche in Deutschland 2014).

In the general population, 53% are never or seldom attending religious services, and 57% are seldom or never praying, while 60% nevertheless believe in God (Pew Research Center 2018). With respect to praying as an indicator of religiosity, in 2012, 17% were praying on a daily basis, 8% once a week, 17% less often and 39% not at all (Infratest Dimap 2012). In a larger study among young adults from Germany (age 18 ± 2 years), 73% would not regard themselves as religious, and thus they had no interest in religious issues, but interest in existential issues and a conscious dealing with others and the environment (Büssing et al. 2016). In persons with chronic diseases (mean age 55 ± 14 years), 47% regarded themselves as not religious, despite their Christian denomination); 27% were praying regularly, 24% often, 33% seldom and 16% never (data taken from: Büssing et al. 2012).

To further analyze whether and which spiritual needs are prevalent among the elderly, data of 345 elderly (77% women and 24% men; mean age 84 ± 7 [53–100] years) living in retirement homes were descried and discussed. They were recruited in three regions of Germany, the North (29%) (Erichsen and Büssing 2013), South (63%) (Man-Ging et al. 2015; Mayr et al. unpublished) and West (9%) (Büssing et al. unpublished). Most had a Christian affiliation (87%), 2% had other religious affiliations and 11% none. Among them, 69% had access to their family, 31% not. Half were living in an old people's home, 17% in assisted living, 29% in a nursing home and 4% other. With respect to their self-care abilities, 26% cared for themselves completely alone, 38% mostly and 36% required help from other persons.

In these persons, *Inner Peace* needs were of strongest relevance, followed by *Giving/Generativity* needs and *Religious* needs, while *Existential* needs scored lowest (Fig. 26.1). The different regions of Germany have a differential cultural and religious background. The North (Schleswig-Holstein) is primarily Protestant, the South (Bavaria) Catholic and the West (North-Rhine Westphalia) a mix of both Christian confessions. While the life satisfaction is similar in the elderly from these three regions (BMLSS-9: 68.1 ± 13.5; $F = 0.8$, n.s.), their spiritual needs differed. The main differences were found for *Religious* needs that scored high in the South (1.34 ± 0.87) and the West (1.07 ± 0.95) but low in the North (0.54 ± 0.58) ($F = 33.8$, $p<0.0001$) and for *Existential* needs, which scores low in all regions, and lowest in the North ($F = 7.2$, $p = 0.001$). For *Inner Peace* needs and *Giving/Generativity* needs, there were no regional differences. Further, gender-related differences were found only for *Religious* needs that scored higher in women than in men ($F = 4.9$, $p = 0.027$). With respect to the self-care abilities, there were significant

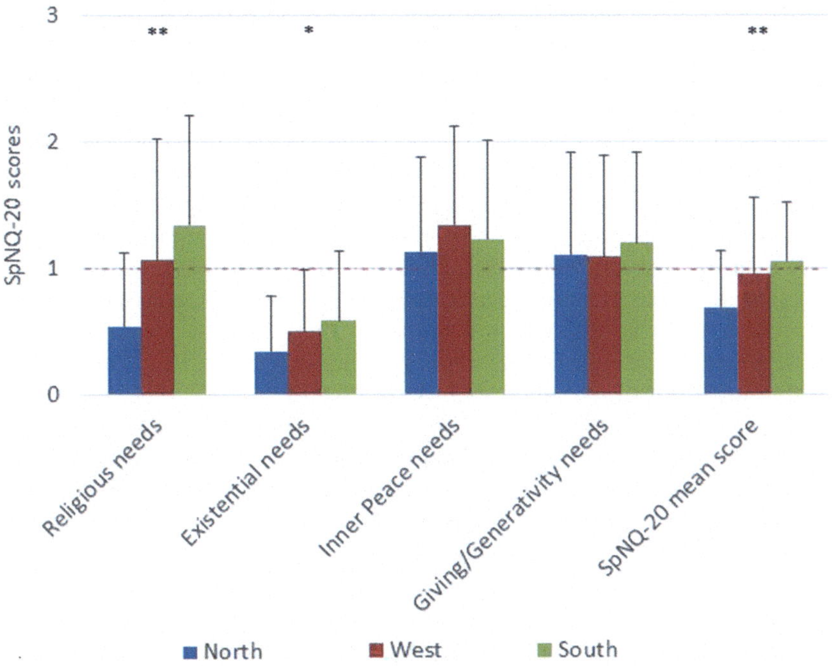

Fig. 26.1 Spiritual needs in the elderly (n=345) from different regions in Germany: South (n=213), North (n=100), West (n=32). ** $p < 0.0001$; *$p < 0.05$ (ANOVA)

differences only for *Religious* needs ($F = 3.4$, $p = 0.034$), which were lowest in the elderly who were completely independent of the help of others (0.92 ± 0.91) compared to mostly independent persons (1.23 ± 0.87), and to those who require the help of others (1.05 ± 0.85). This dependency is also related with significantly higher perceived affections of daily life activities ($F = 77.7$, $p < 0.0001$) and reduced life satisfaction ($F = 17.4$, $p < 0.0001$).

The following spiritual needs were of higher importance for the enrolled elderly persons: To plunge into beauty of nature (N6: 2.21 ± 1.04), to be connected with the family (N25: 1.72 ± 1.32) and to pray (N26: 1.72 ± 1.25), and to reflect back on life (N4: 1.68 ± 1.16). However, need to clarify open aspects (N5: 0.48 ± 0.95) or to forgive someone from a distinct period of life (N16: 0.38 ± 0.83) or to be forgiven (N17: 0.27 ± 0.69) were not of relevance. It seems they have found some forms of "inner peace" and distance from their "previous" phases of life. Indeed, need for inner peace scored rather low (N8: 0.94 ± 1.20).

Interestingly, most other needs of these elderly persons scored quite low. It might also be that several have downregulated their expectations towards life and thus their needs, too. Some stated that they of course would like to pass their life experiences to others, but that their children and grandchildren have to interest (Erichsen and Büssing 2013). Talking about fears and worries (N2: 0.73 ± 1.08), about meaning in life (N11: 0.69 ± 1.03) or about the possibility of life after death (N12: 0.59 ± 0.99) were less relevant. It would seem they do not have these needs—either because no one is available for them or they are not too interested. However, that someone of the religious community (i.e., the pastor) cares for them was not of relevance (N3: 0.40 ± 0.81).

The aforementioned higher scoring spiritual needs have in common that they refer to a multidimensional involvement (connection with others, with God and nature) and to a reflection on life—because the future may not hold too many surprises anymore. During the talks with the elderly from North Germany, several of their comments indicated emotional tiredness and often resignation that no one has interest in their views and concerns (Erichsen and Büssing 2013), or that their partner has died a long time ago and old friends are not able to come to visit or have passed away too. Therefore, it is worth analyzing whether and how negative mood states are related to their spiritual needs. In fact, grief was moderately positively related with *Existential* needs ($r = 0.35$) and weakly with *Inner Peace* needs ($r = 0.26$). Hopelessness was weakly related to *Existential* needs ($r = 0.24$), while emotional tiredness was weakly related to *Existential* needs ($r = 0.25$) and *Religious* needs ($r = 0.24$). Further, reduced life satisfaction (BMLSS-9) was moderately related to *Existential* needs ($r = -0.35$). Thus, the *Existential* needs were related to elderly's negative mood states and reduced life satisfaction. Detailed analyses revealed that particularly the need to clarify open aspects of life (N5) was related to their grief ($r = 0.31$) and hopelessness ($r = 0.25$), but less relevantly their need to talk with somebody about meaning in life or afterlife ideas or to forgive or to be forgiven. Life satisfaction (which is strongly negatively related to grief and moderately negatively to hopelessness) was best related to elderly's needs to find some meaning in life (N10: $r = -0.30$) and to clarify open aspects of life (N5: $r = -0.26$). In an attempt to analyze the best predictors of these *Existential* needs, reduced life satisfaction (Beta = -0.25, $T = -4.2$, $p < 0.001$) was identified as the best predictor (alone explaining 13% of variance), with further weak effects of grief, age and region (which would explain a further 6% of *Existential* needs variance). Self-care abilities, perceived impairment of daily life activities, hopelessness and emotional tiredness were no significant predictors in this regression model. Thus, there are some other, not yet defined, predictors why elderly would express *Existential* needs. In contrast to propositions on the relation of spirituality and aging, the spiritual task of aging for the elderly in Germany does not so much seem as a shift from finding single to ultimate meaning, but could be seen as two parallel processes combining the cultural and biographic imprint of the aging person. While for the elderly the search for meaning itself becomes a higher priority with aging, it is nevertheless in a particular way catalyzed in relation to the experiences of the many years lived and the related sociocultural imprinting. At the same time opportunities for meaningful participation are therefore aligned by experiences of acceptance, purpose of life in later life, age and interaction with a larger social–cultural context. Age-related changes are also responsible for transformation and building of that performative dimension of spirituality (Janhsen et al. 2019).

Spiritual Needs of the Elderly in Poland

Poland is geographically a direct neighbor of Germany, and still has a vital Catholic faith tradition. Most Polish people, particularly the older generation, belong to the Roman Catholic Church. The population of believers in the Roman Catholic Church is 88% of the total population (Religious denominations in Poland 2019). Being a Catholic in Poland is been seen as identical with being a Pole, as a stereotype says. It can be assumed that among a number of sociocultural determinants, the Polish attachment to Christianity and especially to Catholicism is connected with the history of Poland, where for many decades the country was divided by different countries with different confessional roots of Orthodoxy or Protestantism, while Catholicism was a peculiar force that identified the majority of Poles in the fight for national identity. Probably also in the new history the resistance against Nazism during the occupation as well as the post-war struggle with atheistic communism led to the consolidation of beliefs around Christianity and the Catholic Church. This may have to do with the identity-generating role the Catholic Church has played in the majority of the Polish population. Nevertheless, as observed in different Western European countries, also in Poland there are changes related to secularization and a distancing from the religious sphere in its institutional aspects.

There is an obvious decline of regular religious practices, and a rather modest share of believers subjectively assessing themselves as highly religious (Zarzycka 2008; Mariański 2013; Marody and Mandes 2012; Stachowska 2019; Garbowski 2020). There is a relatively stable level of declarations expressing faith and firm belief in Poland. This is confirmed by the 2018 data of the Centre for Public Opinion Research (Centrum Badania Opinii Społecznej, CBOS) that states 49% of respondents participated regularly in liturgy. Irregularly 38% of the respondents participated in this form of activity and 13% of Poles declared passivity in this respect (Boguszewski 2018).

This kind of stabile tendency of Polish religiousness over the last years has been seen from research conducted by the Central Statistical Office (GUS), according to which the level of self-declaration of faith in 2018 among different age groups in Poland was 81%, of which 11% of the respondents identified themselves as deeply believing. A similar percentage of respondents (11%) described themselves as undecided/seeking, 6% were religiously indifferent and 3% nonbelievers (Religious life in Poland. Results of the Social Cohesion Survey 2018). At the same time, there is a greater share of auto-identification indicating deep faith among the elderly, as in 2018 there were 29% of them in the oldest age group (75 years and more). Among the 65–74-year-old cohort, the share of deep faith was 16%, and among people aged 55–64 years, it was 13%. In contrast, among the youngest people aged 16–24 years, only 5% identified as deep faith believers (Religious life in Poland. Results of the Social Cohesion Survey 2018). In addition, a higher percentage of people identifying themselves as nonbelievers, indifferent, and indecisive was observed in younger age groups (Religious life in Poland. Results of the Social Cohesion Survey 2018).

Because of these age-related differences, praying was much higher in older persons from Poland compared to younger ones. In 2018, 7% of all enrolled persons prayed daily and 35% almost daily, while 8% of the respondents did not pray. In the age group of 75 years and more, 24% prayed daily and 51% almost daily, while among the 65–74-year-olds, 11% pray several times a day and 49% daily or almost daily (Results of the Social Cohesion Survey 2015 and 2018).

Polish religiosity is strongly Church-oriented, with a focus on the Church's sacraments and spirituality, strict dogmatic attitudes and ideologies. Nevertheless, during the course of life, personal experiences as well as social changes such as individualization, pluralization, liberalization, and globalization with its decrease of the monopoly of religious institutions has led to a subjectification and critical reflection of these adopted value and belief systems as well as the role of religious institutions with regard to their personal spirituality. Despite this, religiosity is still an important element for older adults in Poland. For many, religious faith is a source of support in times of illness. Spiritual perspectives enable some patients to find meaning even in the difficult experience of a chronic disease and they should therefore be supported to utilize their religious resources. Spiritual care is an important key to the spiritual needs of the chronically and terminally sick. In order to develop this field in Poland, recognition is needed about what exactly is helpful for the patients.

To analyze which spiritual needs were of relevance for Polish elderly, a group of 292 persons (63% women, 37% men, with a mean age of 74 ± 8 [50–92] years) was analyzed. They were recruited in the area of Warsaw and Krakow. Among them, 94% were Catholics; 53% were living in retirement homes, 31% in special care homes, 9% in assisted living home and 8% other. Of these, 61% were completely caring for themselves, 26% were depending on others' help in part and 13% only with the help of others. The life satisfaction (BMLSS-9: 69.1 ± 19.1) differed significantly between these self-care abilities groups ($F = 5.3$, $p = 0.006$) and was highest in those who are independent of the help of others.

With respect to their spiritual needs, *Religious* needs and *Inner Peace* needs scored high, *Giving/Generativity* needs the highest and *Existential* needs the lowest (Fig. 26.2). The SpNQ-20 mean scores was 1.10 ± 0.65. In all cases, women had significantly higher spiritual needs than men (data not shown). The spiritual needs that scored highest were: to be connected with the family (N25: 2.05 ± 1.18); followed by: to participate at a religious service (N21: 1.75 ± 1.19), to turn to a higher presence (God) (N23: 1.52 ± 1.28) and to pray (N20: 1.48 ± 1.26). Thus, for Polish elderly, the topic of connectedness (with family and God) was most relevant. Interestingly, participating in a religious service (Sunday service in church) was much more relevant than praying, indicating that the sacramental and congregational (public) aspects of religiosity are more vital in Polish religiosity than the private aspects. Talking about fears and worries were of some relevance (N2: 1.05 ± 1.07), while talks about meaning in life were less relevant (N11: 0.83 ± 1.10), and least relevant, talks about the possibility of life after death (N12: 0.45 ± 0.85). The more specific the talks, the stronger the need. However, that someone of the religious

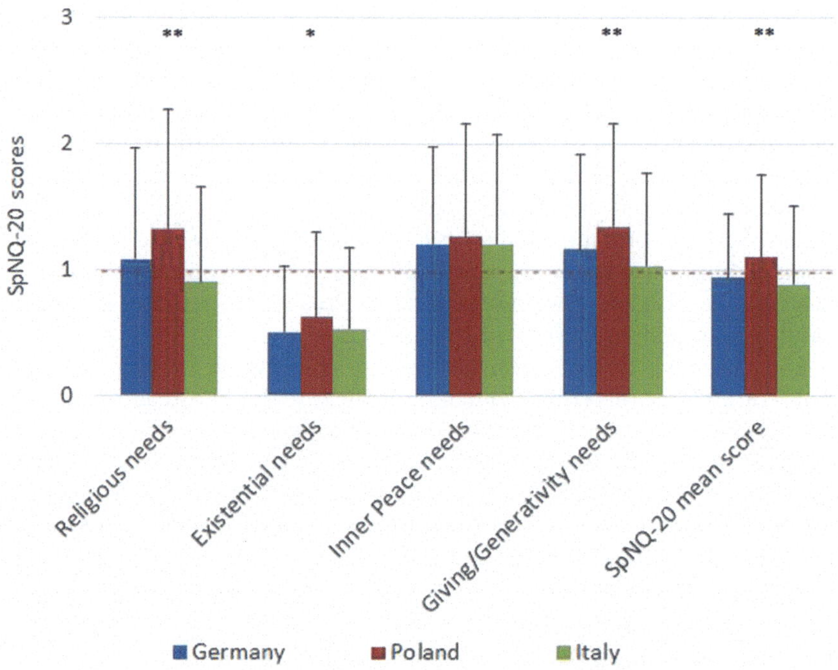

Fig. 26.2 Spiritual needs in the elderly from Germany (n = 345), Poland (n = 292) and Italy (n = 164). ** $p < 0.0001$; *$p < 0.05$ (ANOVA)

community (i.e., the pastor) cares for them was not of relevance (N3: 0.41 ± 0.86).

What are the triggers of the respective needs? With the exception of *Giving/Generativity* needs, all spiritual needs were significantly higher in elderly who were depending on the help of others (data not shown). As these "dependent" persons have significantly lower life satisfaction, lower well-being and higher depressive intentions to escape from their situation, it is conceivable that they will express higher needs than the independent persons because of their perceived restrictions in life.

Correlation analyses indeed revealed that *Religious* needs were moderately related to their reliance in God's help (RGH: $r = 0.49$), and weakly to their intention to escape from their situation (Escape: $r = 0.24$), while they were not significantly related to their life satisfaction, well-being or loneliness. These *Religious* needs are thus more an indicator of their religiosity rather than triggered by low well-being. Regression analyses revealed that their *Religious* needs were best predicted by reliance on God's help (indicating that God is perceived as a source of hope, hold and help), female gender and perceived daily life affections, which together would explain 33% of variance. Their *Existential* needs were weakly to moderately related to low life satisfaction (BMLSS-9: r = -0.30), perceived daily life affections (VAS: r = 0.27) and loneliness (UCLA: r = 0.26). Here, the best predictors were low self-care abilities, low life satisfaction, daily life affections, reliance on God's help and female gender, explaining altogether 26% of variance. *Inner Peace* needs were moderately related to loneliness (r = 0.32) and perceived daily life affections (r = 0.31). Best predictors were perceived daily life affections, reliance on God's help, low well-being and female gender, which would explain 20% of variance. *Giving/Generativity* needs showed weak correlations only with the intention to escape from the life situation (r = 0.22) and with their reliance on God's help (r = 0.23), and were explained with weak predictive power (R^2 = 0.16) by female gender and escape. Thus, one may see a differential pattern of related stressors and variables that may be associated with specific spiritual needs or trigger them, among them are perceived daily life affections, reduced quality of life and reliance on God's help as a resource as relevant predictors. Reliance on God's help was moderately high in the Polish sample (RGH: 64.9 ± 33.8), but with large variance; 19% had scores <40 indicating disinterest in this resource, and 61% scores >60 indicating stronger reliance on God's help; the others were rather indifferent. Thus, this resource was of relevance for most Polish elderly.

Spiritual Needs of the Elderly in Italy

Similar to other Western European countries, also in Catholic Italy the number of people who attend religious services (39% seldom or never) and pray is decreasing (39% seldom or never), while for 73% God was nevertheless seen as important (Pew Research Center 2018).

The Italian sample consisted of 164 persons (54% women and 46% men; mean age 71 ± 8 [57–91] years) from the North Italian region Piedmont. Most were Catholics (92%) and 8% had no religious affiliation. Among them, 20% were living in a retirement home, 48% in rehabilitation center and 32% in other resorts or at home. With respect to their self-care abilities, 57% cared for themselves completely alone, 30% mostly and 13% required help from other persons. Their life satisfaction was high (BMLSS-9: 72.0 ± 19.1).

Their *Religious* needs and *Existential* needs scored rather low and their *Inner Peace* and *Giving/Generativity* needs scored higher (Fig. 26.2). The SpNQ-20 mean scores were 0.88 ± 0.63. Women had significantly higher scores for *Religious* needs ($F = 8.1$, $p = 0.005$) and *Giving/Generativity* needs ($F = 14.2$, $p < 0.001$), but not for the other needs. All spiritual needs scored significantly higher in persons depending on the help of others (data not shown).

Of highest relevance for Italian older persons was to be connected with the family (N25: 2.09 ± 1.19), to turn to someone in a loving attitude (N13: 1.46 ± 1.10), and to plunge in the beauty of nature (N6: 1.46 ± 1.31). Turn to a higher presence (God) (N23: 1.33 ± 1.22) and to participate at a religious ceremony (Sunday service) (N21: 1.30 ± 1.07) was of stronger relevance than own praying (N20: 0.85 ± 1.09). That someone from the religious community (i.e., the pastor) cares was least relevant (N3: 0.22 ± 0.65), too.

How are these spiritual needs related to well-being and loneliness? Surprisingly, *Religious* needs were only weakly related to their reliance on God's help ($r = 0.25$), but moderately with daily life affections ($r = 0.44$). Regression analyses indicated that the best predictors of *Religious* needs were their self-care abilities, female gender, perceived health affections and reliance on God's help; these four variables would explain 38% of variance. Here, daily life affections were the strongest predictor. *Existential* needs were moderately related to the intention to escape from their situation/illness ($r = 0.47$), low life satisfaction ($r = -0.46$), loneliness ($r = 0.36$) and perceived daily life affections ($r = 0.32$). Regression analyses showed that self-care abilities were the best predictors (explaining alone 23% of variance), followed by low life satisfaction, reliance on God's help and female gender. These four variables would explain altogether 37% of variance. *Inner Peace* needs were moderately negatively related to life satisfaction ($r = -0.40$), loneliness ($r = 0.36$) and low well-being ($r = -0.33$). Here, daily life affections were the best predictor (explaining 16% of variance), followed by reliance on God's help and low well-being. These three variables would explain 26% of variance. *Giving/Generativity* needs was best and moderately related to low perceived daily life affections ($r = 0.37$). Regression analyses indicated that female gender was a significant predictor and daily life affections, which both would only explain 17%, indicating that other relevant predictors remain to be identified. In Italian elderly, perceived daily life affections were of strong relevance (which could be explained by the fact that a large proportion were from rehabilitation centers) and reliance on God's help. This is of interest because its mean score was rather low in the Italian sample (RGH: 52.3 ± 33.8), but with large variance; 27% had scores <40 indicating disinterest in this source, and 45% scored >60 indicating stronger reliance on God's help; the others were rather indifferent. Thus, this resource was of some relevance for a larger proportion of elderly from the Piedmont region.

Comparison of Needs between the Different Samples

Religious needs (p = 0.002; Mann-Whitney-U test) and *Giving/ Generativity* needs (p = 0.004) and the SpNQ-20 mean score (p = 0.003) were significantly higher in Polish elderly compared to those from Germany, while their *Existential* needs and their *Inner Peace* needs did not significantly differ. This cannot be solely explained by gender or age differences as more and older women were prevalent in the German sample. Also their life satisfaction was similar, while their perceived daily life affections were lower in Polish elderly (p < 0.0001). It seems that particularly the centrality of their religiosity and cultural aspects would explain these differences. This could be substantiated by the fact that *Religious* needs in the elderly from the predominantly Catholic South of Germany (Bavaria) have similar intensity compared to the Catholic Polish elderly, while the elderly particularly from the Protestant North of Germany (Schleswig-Holstein) scored low on *Religious* needs. In that area of Germany the public religiosity is practiced much more cautiously than in the South of Germany.

How do these data compare to that of older persons from the Piedmont region in North Italy? Reliance on God's help scored lower in the Italian sample compared to the Polish sample, but this difference was not significant. Nevertheless, as shown in Fig. 26.2, particularly *Religious* needs and *Giving/Generativity* needs differed significantly in these three samples. Polish and Italian elderly were identified as Catholics; however, the *Religious* needs from Polish elderly were significantly higher than in Italian elderly (p < 0.0001; Mann-Whitney-U test); also German and Polish elderly (p = 0.002) differed significantly, while the difference between German and Italian elderly was significant in trend only (p = 0.051). Because of a higher proportion of person living in rehabilitation units in the Italian sample, one could argue that their perceptions of daily life impairment and life satisfaction might be lower, but this presumption was not true, as life satisfaction in the Italian sample was similar compared to

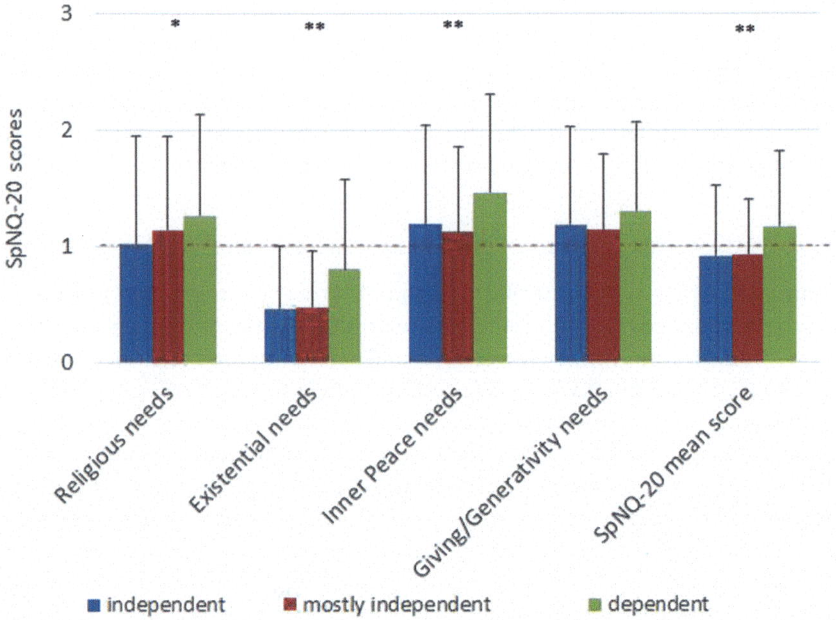

Fig. 26.3 Spiritual needs in the elderly from Germany, Poland and Italy (n = 766) differentiated for their self-care abilities. ** $p < 0.0001$; *$p < 0.05$ (ANOVA)

the other samples ($F = 2.9$, $p = 0.0657$), while perceived daily life affection was highest in German elderly ($F = 3.5$, $p = 0.032$), which are the oldest compared to the others ($F = 229.0$, $p < 0.0001$).

With respect to their self-care abilities, the elderly from Germany represented the highest proportion of persons who are depending on the help of others compared to the Polish and Italian elderly (36% vs. 13% vs. 13% $p < 0.001$; Chi^2 test). As shown in Fig. 26.3, the higher the dependence on the help of others, the higher their *Religious* needs, *Existential* needs and *Inner Peace* needs are in the combined data set from the three samples. *Giving/Generativity* needs did not significantly differ with respect to these "independence" indicators. This could indicate that this dependency on others would result in more spiritual needs because the respective persons would lack "something", that is, independence, vitality, health. However, comparing independent and dependent people reveals that the effect size is weak for *Religious* needs (Cohen's $d = 0.27$) and for *Inner Peace* needs (Cohen's $d = 0.32$), moderate for *Existential* needs (Cohen's $d = 0.55$), and irrelevant for *Giving/Generativity* needs (Cohen's d =

0.13). Here, *Existential* needs may show the strongest effect, but the intensity of these needs is nevertheless rather low.

Regression analyses in this combined data set with the independent variables self-care abilities, perceived daily life affections, life satisfaction, age and gender showed that older persons' spiritual needs cannot be sufficiently explained by these variables alone. Although these show relevant effects in the respective German, Polish and Italian samples, they nevertheless explain in most cases less that 5% of the variance. The best prediction model was found for *Existential* needs, which are explained by reduced life satisfaction, self-care abilities and female gender, but would altogether explain only 19% of variance. These findings would again underline that other influences are of relevance, too, to explain why they express the respective spiritual needs. Among these could be negative mood states and cultural/religious influences as discussed above.

Assessment and Support of Elderly's Spiritual Needs

To support the spiritual needs of the elderly in particular, a spiritual support plan is required. First, unmet spiritual needs have to be identified, and then the spiritual care team has to consent who could address which need. Such a spiritual care team may involve nurses, social workers, psychologists, therapists, pastoral workers, parish nurses, family members, etc. The different professions have their specific points of view and diverse professional skills that they could bring into such intervention processes, whether they see themselves as a religious/spiritual person or not. For nurses it was stated that long-term care residents thought that these could support their spirituality and could facilitate visits with religious personnel, showing kindness, having adequate time to listen to them, and showing respect for their needs (Wallace and O'Shea 2007). It is interesting that these topics were also ascribed to assumed "nonprofessionals" in terms of spirituality instead to trained pastoral workers. In fact, the personnel of retirement and nursing homes have constant contacts with the elderly and can notice when mood states change, when vitality decreases, and when the residents or patients withdraw from others. Also the cleaning staff should be part of the team because they are in most cases available for short talks. Nevertheless, to provide adequate spiritual care, professional training is required with necessary time resources and empathy.

Spiritual assessment in the elderly is a crucial topic. So far, two approaches are recommended, an initial spiritual screening and in-depth spiritual assessments (Fitchett 2012; McSherry and Ross 2010). These are in most cases face-to-face interviews. However, not all are trained to do this and may feel uncomfortable to talk about such "private" things or will argue that the necessary time is lacking. To assist a standardized assessment that includes various psychosocial, existential and spiritual needs, the extended SpNQ may be an option. Handing out the questionnaire to the residents enables a certain respect for the possible discomfort during the answering, as the residents can fill it out by themselves and in a self-chosen environment, without being observed and thus influenced by people waiting to take the questionnaire back. However, several older persons have reading impairments or even disabilities and may apply for the option of an assisted interview. Here, a trusted person is reading the items loud and enters the answers according to the reactions and comments of the older person. This allows directly reacting to someone that is either emotionally moved or unclear about specific things. These direct reactions were often very moving, for example when older persons stated that so far no one has asked them about their spiritual needs and valued this interest in their concerns (Erichsen and Büssing 2013). The interviewer has thus the chance to directly respond and initiate in-depth discussions when this is wanted.

For some persons with reduced vitality and limited attention abilities, the extended instrument with its 27 items (and free text options) might be too burdening, and thus the 8-item "Spiritual Needs Screener" might be an option (see Appendix). This short instrument uses three *Inner Peace* needs items (N2—talk with others about your fears and worries; N7—dwell at a place of quietness and peace; N8—find inner peace), two *Existential* needs items (N11—talk with someone about the question of meaning in life; N17—be forgiven) and three *Religious* needs items (N20—pray for yourself; N21—participate in a religious ceremony (i.e., Sunday service); N23—turn to a higher presence). This Spiritual Needs Screener is not intended as a research instrument, but as a practical tool for the direct encounter with the elderly by palliative care providers, parish nurses, etc., and to facilitate communication about their needs. Its internal consistency was acceptable in the German sample (Cronbach's alpha = 0.71) and the Polish sample (Cronbach's alpha = 0.79) and good in the North Italian sample (Cronbach's alpha = 0.84) and it can thus be applied as an easy to handle starter to communicate.

Practical Consequences

Spiritual needs and persons' intention to satisfy these seem to be a basic motivation in life. Such needs are the expression of what is necessary to sustain and to develop as a person during the different phases of life. These emphasize the necessity to be fulfilled or satisfied—although this is not always possible. What is considered as indispensable, however, depends on the respective level of development of a culture and society.

How can unmet spiritual needs of the elderly be supported when several may feel weak, unwanted and unnecessary and thus withdraw from others, becoming depressive and isolated, and resist talking about their needs? Of course, many elderly people may have a strong will to be involved in social processes and may have a good fitness and vitality, while others may be mentally weak, experience losses and require constant medication because of health affections, etc. The term "elderly" refers to a very heterogeneous group, and thus their abilities, preferences and needs will be heterogeneous, too.

Connectedness and involvement are relevant topics as described above. Connection was also identified by older persons from Australia as an important aspect of spirituality (Harrington et al. 2019). However, even in their faith tradition they may feel isolated and not involved anymore as an active person who has something to give, instead of being a passive recipient. Further, when family members are not (or seldom only) available, who could provide the required spiritual and social support? The data show that the interest that someone from their religious community cares (the pastor for example) was rather limited. Maybe we have to reconsider what older persons' "community" is or could be, and what "connection" may mean to them. Their connection needs may have a horizontal direction (i.e., friends, families, others) and also a vertical direction (i.e., God). When the contact with the family is restricted and friends are not available, and when they already know all their housemates' stories, it is not surprisingly that their connection needs may be either high (when they still wait for someone who cares for them) or even low (when they do not expect any longer that someone may have interest in their concerns). The analysis of their spiritual needs revealed that they have both, needs for inspirational talks with others and also to generatively give their time, affect, experience and company. It seems that not just any talks are of relevance to the elderly enrolled in our studies, but specific ones. The more specifc these talks could be (i.e., about their fears and worries), the stronger the need was articulated. Here, constant presence is important to build trusting relationships with reliable relations who are easily available. As was advised by Jackson et al. (2016), this requires "spending time, being present, active listening, and passive responses and would see the practitioner contributing to the person's life not only in conversation but in practical and in physical ways". Here, the organizations running the residential homes are in charge of encouraging the personnel to address and support their residents' spiritual needs too. This requires commissioning, structures, time resources, and spiritual care trained personnel. However, one cannot ignore the fact that several people are reluctant to talk about such "private" things such as hope, fears or faith. The first step should come from the "externals", as some elderly stated (Erichsen and Büssing 2013), because several have withdrawn from others in fear of disinterest in their concerns. This is clearly a self-induced emotional withdrawal because of their fear of not being relevant and interesting anymore.

To address their pronounced *Giving/Generativity* needs and their wish to talk about their life experiences and to be seen as "experts of life" who could guide the next generation, why not start creativity projects? Younger persons or students of arts (i.e., painting, sculpturing) or creative writing instructors could be invited to discuss and organize creativity projects and exhibitions in the respective housing facilities, thereby underlining that they still have the motivation to exchange ideas with others, to learn new things, and become creative and active again—instead of waiting in withdrawal. The individual creative outputs of such projects could also be seen as a spiritual "legacy" and presented as temporary exhibitions or permanent installations (in the public areas of the retirement or communal areas or even exhibition halls, in the parish, in the town hall, etc.) and made visible and "tangible" to others. This would help the elderly to experience feelings of pride, self-worth, and social recognition and involvement. An intergenerational project that involves preschool children and a retirement community by Eggers and Hensley (2004) raised older persons' "sense of relatedness to others and hope for the future" and thereby increasing their positive affect, well-being and spirituality. These findings link to the *Giving/Generativity* needs that were found to be of relevance for the elderly from all three samples. Guiding the next generation will further provide a sense of meaning and underline that they are still relevant and needed. This refers to Erikson's psychosocial development stage "Generativity" (Erikson 1974). He stated that during this phase persons should put aside thoughts of death and instead turn to "the only happiness that is lasting: to increase, by whatever is yours to give, the goodwill and higher order in your sector of the world". This has a clear "spiritual" dimension as it points beyond one's own life toward the Sacred.

With respect to their *Religious* issues, public prayers (with others) were less relevant for the elderly analyzed herein than private prayers. Nevertheless, ritualized forms of prayers can be helpful as they provide a reliable structure most will know and recognize, while also inspirational spiritual texts, poems and prayers to contemplate are of relevance. Particularly, the more religious elderly from Poland and Italy stated needs to participate in a religious ceremony (meaning the Sunday service to receive the sacraments). Apart from recognizable rituals (to connect to their past) and a familiar service schedule (with inspirational readings of the scriptures, receiving the Sacrament of communion, and the blessing to connect to the Sacred), which help to connect to the Sacred, participating in a religious service means to be involved in a religious community, which may give support and hope. Spiritual rituals provide recognizable patterns and symbols that the elderly may be familiar with (Jackson et al. 2016). When these are essential to them, the elderly can thus easily connect with their own history (remembering themselves as a child, an adult, and an old person) and, depending on the faith tradition, with the Transcendent. This can also be seen as part of a reminiscence process that would contribute to "developing a greater sense of meaning in older age and a sense of resilience rather than fear" (Jackson et al. 2016). Such meetings, as with a group of persons with similar faith traditions in a carefully prepared surrounding, could also invite them to talk about important points in their life, about their life experiences, etc., and would further foster cohesion among the elderly. These narratives may allow them to remember what may have been hidden and forgotten, and are thus a chance to reconcile with their own life story and their religious tradition. This is also an option for the spiritual care providers to understand which aspects of spirituality are central to them, what may provide hold, hope and meaning, and how they could be supported.

Unmet *Inner Peace* needs were a further central point, particularly the experience of nature and the need to "dissolve" in nature and the intent to become part of a "paradisiacal state" where everything is right and peaceful (remembering one's own childhood days), resulting in states of inner peace and congruence with life. It might be that these needs are rather constant desires than needs that can be met and that will finally disappear. Nevertheless, where could these times and places be to reconnect to the Sacred and the Beauty in life that seem to be lost? The topic of healing architecture is currently a developing area of interest in health care research to increase a person's sense of well-being (Fricke et al. 2019; Núñez-González et al. 2020). Meanwhile one could consider guided trips in beautiful gardens or woods in the neighborhood, or virtual walks for those who are incapable of leaving their areas. It is also possible to bring nature into public and private rooms, either as flowers, budding branches and leaves, or even large pictures that refer to the different seasons. This would also draw their attention to the changes in nature and their surroundings. Also helpful are diaries to write down what has moved them during the day, where they stopped in times of wondering awe (Büssing et al. 2014) and what made them grateful, which persons they remembered from their past and what they would like to tell them, etc. As a consequence of such a reflection process, the elderly may more easily remember the "good" things in their life and can consult this diary in difficult times, and further, these reflections help to connect to their life and other persons (whether they are available or not). Again, this can be part of a reminiscence process to generate states of peacefulness and well-being.

With respect to conventional care and support, there are several hindrances that interfere with older persons' needs: (1) lack of professional advice on self-care strategies; (2) poor communication and coordination of services; and (3) lack of information on services such as care pathways, as identified by Abdi et al. 2019. The same might be true for their unmet spiritual care. Therefore, spiritual care models and support services have to be developed that take the needs of older people seriously and support them adequately.

Conclusions

We have analyzed three samples of older persons from three culturally different countries and found both, similarities in specific unmet spiritual needs and significant differences that refer particularly to *Religious* needs and *Existential* needs. The underlying causes are probably multifactorial and involve cultural and religious differences, on the one hand, and negative mood states, feelings of loneliness and perceived daily life affections (and thus low self-care abilities and independence), on the other hand. Loss of connectedness and involvement were identified as crucial, and thus support concepts could start with these topics. If what is missing is expressed as a need and if elderly′ mobility and fitness are limited, then it should be made available where older persons life. As there is evidence that "many services and care delivery models are still not based on the needs of older adults" (Abdi et al. 2019), creative support projects should be encouraged. These should be suited to facilitating elderly's social participation and inclusion, on the one hand, and their independence and generative giving abilities, on the other hand, which would help to maintain feelings of meaningfulness and psychosocial and spiritual well-being.

Acknowledgements Thanks to Nora Beata Erichsen, Jülyet Öven Uslucan and Beta Mayr for their help in recruiting our participants in Germany, and to Karzyna Jagielska and Joanna M. Łukasik in Poland, and to Marco Calabrese in Italy.

References

Abdi S, Spann A, Borilovic J, de Witte L, Hawley M (2019) Understanding the care and support needs of older people: a scoping review and categorisation using the WHO international classification of functioning, disability and health framework (ICF). BMC Geriatr 19:195. https://doi.org/10.1186/s12877-019-1189-9

Agli O, Bailly N, Ferrand C (2015) Spirituality and religion in older adults with dementia: a systematic review. Int Psychogeriatr 27(5):715–725

Alderfer CP (1972) Existence, Relatedness, and Growth. Human Needs in Organizational Settings. Free Press, New York

Bailly N, Martinent G, Ferrand C, Agli O, Giraudeau C, Gana K, Roussiau N (2018) Spirituality, social support, and flexibility among older adults: a five-year longitudinal study. Int Psychogeriatr 30(12):1745–1752

Boguszewski R (2018) *Religijność Polaków i ocena sytuacji Kościoła katolickiego.* Komunikat z badań CBOS, 147. Centrum Badania Opinii Społecznej, Warszawa

Berkman LF, Ertel KA, Glymour MM (2011) Aging and social intervention: Life course perspectives. In: Binstock RH, George LK (eds) Handbook of aging and the social sciences, 7th edn. Elsevier Academic, San Diego, CA, pp 337–351

Bruce A, Schreiber R, Petrovskaya O, Boston P (2011) Longing for ground in a ground(less) world: A qualitative inquiry of existential suffering. BMC Nursing 10(1):1–9. https://doi.org/10.1186/1472-6955-10-2

Büssing A, Reiser F, Michalsen A, Zahn A, Baumann K (2012) Engagement of Patients With Chronic Diseases in Spiritual and Secular Forms of Practice: Results with the Shortened SpREUK-P SF17 Questionnaire. Integrative Medicine: A Clinician's Journal 2012 11(1):28–38

Büssing A, Wirth AG, Reiser F, Zahn A, Humbroich K, Gerbershagen K, Schimrigk S, Haupts S, Hvidt NC, Baumann K (2014) Experience of gratitude, awe and beauty in life among patients with multiple sclerosis and psychiatric disorders.

Health Qual Life Outcomes 12(63) http://www.hqlo.com/content/12/1/63
Büssing A, Recchia DR, Surzykiewicz J, Baumann K (2016) Ausdrucksformen der Spiritualität bei Schülern und jungen Erwachsenen. Spiritual Care 5:261–272
Cowlishaw S, Niele S, Teshuva K, Browning C, Kendig H (2013) Rowe and Kahns' model of successful aging revisited: Positive spirituality, the forgotten factor. Gerontologist 33(7):1243–1262
Crowther MR, Parker MW, Achenbaum WA, Larimore WL, Koenig HG (2002) Rowe and Kahn's model of successful aging revisited: Positive spirituality—The forgotten factor. Gerontologist 42(5):613–620
Eggers S, Hensley SJ (2004) Empowering Spirituality and Generativity through Intergenerational Connections. J Relig Spiritual Aging 51:161–175
Erichsen NB, Büssing A (2013) Spiritual Needs of Elderly living in Retirement / Nursing Homes. Evidence-based Complementary and Alternative Medicine Article ID913247. https://doi.org/10.1155/2013/913247
Erikson EH (1974) Dimensions of a new identity. Norton, New York
Eurostat (2019) https://ec.europa.eu/eurostat/statistics-explained/index.php?title=File:Population_age_structure_by_major_age_groups,_2009_and_2019_(%25_of_the_total_population).png. Accessed 20 August 2020
Evangelische Kirche in Deutschland (2014) Engagement und Indifferenz Kirchenmitgliedschaft als soziale Praxis. V. EKD-Erhebung über Kirchenmitgliedschaft https://www.ekd.de/ekd_de/ds_doc/ekd_v_kmu 2014.pdf. Accessed 22 August 2020
Fabiś A (2015) Rozwój duchowy jako atrybut dojrzałości w starości. *EXLIBRIS Biblioteka Gerontologii Społecznej* 1(9):11–18
Fassino S, Leombruni P, Daga GA, Brustolin A, Rovera GG, Fabris F (2002) Quality of life in dependent older adults living at home. Arch Gerontol Geriatr 35(1):9–20
Fitchett G (2012) Next steps for spiritual assessment in healthcare. In: Cobb M, Pulchaski C, Bruce R (eds) Oxford textbook of spirituality in healthcare. Oxford University Press, Oxford, pp 298–303
Fricke OP, Halswick D, Längler A, Martin DD (2019) Healing Architecture for Sick Kids. Z Kinder Jugendpsychiatr Psychother 47(1):27–33
Forlenza OV, Vallada H (2018) Spirituality, health and well-being in the elderly. Int Psychogeriatr 30(12):1741–1742
Goh AM, Eagleton T, Kelleher R, Yastrubetskaya O, Taylor M, Chiu EAM, Trauer HB, Lautenschlager NT (2014) Pastoral care in old age psychiatry: Addressing the spiritual needs of inpatients in an acute aged mental health unit. Asia Pac Psychiatry 6(2):127–134
Garbowski C (2020) Catholicism in the New Poland: A Religion and Society in Transition. Occasional Papers on Religion in Eastern Europe 40(5):6. https://digitalcommons.georgefox.edu/ree/vol40/iss5/6

Harrington A, Williamson V, Goodwin-Smith I (2019) Understanding the Diverse Forms of Spiritual Expression of Older People in Residential Aged Care in Australia. J Relig Health 58:1561–1572

Harrison JD, Young JM, Price MA, Butow PN, Solomon MJ (2009) What are the unmet supportive care needs of people with cancer? A systematic review. Support Care Cancer 17(8):1117–1128

Infratest DIMAP (2012) http://www.livenet.de/news/international/263371-jeder_zweite_amerikaner_betet_fuer_sich_und_seine_familie.html. Accessed 20 August 2020

Jackson D, Doyle C, Capon C, Pringle E (2016) Spirituality, spiritual need, and spiritual care in aged care: What the literature says. J Relig Spiritual Aging 28:281–295

Janhsen A, Golla H, Mantell P, Woopen C (2019) Transforming spirituality through aging: coping and distress in the search for meaning in very old age. J Relig Spiritual Aging. https://doi.org/10.1080/15528030.2019.1676362

Jongenelis K, Pot AM, Eisses AMH, Beekman ATF, Kluiter H, Ribbe MW (2004) Prevalence and risk indicators of depression in elderly nursing home patients: the AGED study. J Affect Disord 83:135–142

Jung J, Roh D, Moon YS, Kim DH (2017) The Moderating Effect of Religion on the Relationship Between Depression and Suicidal Ideation in the Elderly. J Nerv Ment Dis 205(8):605–610

Łukasik J, Pikuła N, Jagielska K (2018a) Senior citizens' existential needs and education for the meaning of life. Pedagogy 6(90):805–816

Łukasik JM, Jagielska K, Pikuła NG (2018b) Spirituality/religiosity of man from the perspective of quality of life - a review of Polish research in social studies. Journal of Rare Cardiovascular Disease 8(3):259–265

Man-Ging CI, Öven Uslucan J, Fegg M, Frick E, Büssing A (2015) Reporting Spiritual Needs of Older Adults Living in Bavarian Residential and Nursing Homes. Journal of Mental Health, Religion and Spirituality 18(10):809–821

Mariański J (2013) Kościół katolicki w Polsce w przestrzeni życia publicznego. Wydawnictwo Adam Marszałek, Torun

Marody M, Mandes S (2012) Przemiany polskiej religijności. In: Jasińska-Kania WA (ed) Wartości i zmiany. Przemiany postaw Polaków w jednoczącej się Europie. Scholar; Warzawa, Warszawa, pp 191–206

McFadden SH (1999) Religion, personality, and aging: A life span perspective. J Pers 67(6):1081–1104. https://doi.org/10.1111/1467-6494.00083

MacKinlay E (2017) The spiritual dimension of ageing. Jessica Kingsley Publishers, London, UK

McSherry W, Ross L (2010) Spiritual assessment in healthcare practice. M&K Publishing, Cumbria, UK

Molesztak A (2015) Duchowość a zadowolenie z życia seniorów. *EXLIBRIS Biblioteka Gerontologii Społecznej* 1(9):133–146

Moon YS, Kim DH (2013) Association between religiosity/spirituality and quality of life or depression among living-alone elderly in a South Korean city. Asia Pac Psychiatry 5(4):293–300

Noronha KJ (2015) Impact of religion and spirituality on older adulthood. J Relig Spiritual Aging 27(1):16–33

Núñez-González S, Delgado-Ron JA, Gault C, Lara-Vinueza A, Calle-Celi D, Porreca R, Simancas-Racines D (2020) Overview of "Systematic Reviews" of the Built Environment's Effects on Mental Health. J Environ Public Health 2020:9523127

Papadopoulos D (2020) The Role of Well-Being, Spirituality, and Religiosity for Successful Aging in Late Life: A Brief Review. Advances in Aging Research 9(2):98467. https://doi.org/10.4236/aar.2020.92003

Peters F, Ilg W, Gutmann D (2019) Demografischer Wandel und nachlassende Kirchenzugehörigkeit: Ergebnisse aus der Mitgliederprojektion der evangelischen und katholischen Kirche in Deutschland und ihre Folgen für die Religionspädagogik. Zeitschrift für Pädagogik und Theologie 71:196–207

Pew Research Center (2018) Being Christian in Western Europe: Religious practice and belief. https://www.pewforum.org/2018/05/29/religious-practice-and-belief/ Accessed 28 August 2020

Reker GT (2005) Meaning in life of young, middle-aged, and older adults: Factorial validity, age, and gender invariance of the Personal Meaning Index (PMI). Personal Individ Differ 38(1):71–85

Religious life in Poland. Results of the Social Cohesion Survey (Życie religijne w Polsce. Wyniki badania spójności społecznej 2018) (2018). Informacje sygnalne, GUS: https://stat.gov.pl/obszary-tematyczne/inne-opracowania/wyznania-religijne/zycie-religijne-w-polsce-wyniki-badania-spojnosci-spolecznej-2018,8,1.html. Accessed 20 August 2020

Shea G (1986) Meeting the pastoral care needs of an aging population. Health Prog 67:36–68

Slater CL (2003) Generativity versus stagnation: An elaboration of Erikson's adult stage of human development. Journal of Adult Development 10(1):53–65

Smith TB, McCullough ME, Poll J (2003) Religiousness and depression: evidence for a main effect and the moderating influence of stressful life events. Psychol Bull 129(4):614–636

Stachowska E (2019) Światowe dni młodzieży w Krakowie w perspektywie socjologii religii. Nomos, Kraków

Steger MF (2012) Experiencing meaning in life: Optimal functioning at the nexus of spirituality, psychopathology, and well-being. In: Wong PTP (ed) The human quest for meaning. Routledge, New York, pp 165–184

Straßner C, Frick E, Stotz-Ingenlath G, Buhlinger-Göpfarth N, Szecsenyi J, Krisam J, Schallhorn F, Valentini J, Stolz R, Joos S (2019) Holistic care program for elderly patients to integrate spiritual needs, social activity, and self-care into disease management in primary care (HoPES3): study protocol for a cluster-randomized trial. Trials 20(1):364. https://doi.org/10.1186/s13063-019-3435-z

Tomás JM, Sancho P, Galiana L, Oliver A (2016) A double test on the importance of spirituality, the "forgotten factor", in successful aging. Social Indicators Research 127(3):1377–1389

Young Y, Frick KD, Phelan EA (2009) Can successful aging and chronic illness coexist in the same individual? A multidimensional concept of successful aging. J Am Med Dir Assoc 10(2):87–92

Van Dierendonck D (2012) Spirituality as an essential determinant for the good life, its importance relative to self-determinant psychological needs. Journal of Happiness Studies 13(4):685–700

Van Dierendonck D, Mohan K (2006) Some thoughts on spirituality and eudaemonic well-being. Mental Health, Religion and Culture 9:227–238

Villani D, Sorgente A, Iannello P, Antonietti A (2019) The Role of Spirituality and Religiosity in Subjective Well-Being of Individuals With Different Religious Status. Front Psychol 10:1525. https://doi.org/10.3389/fpsyg.2019.01525

Wallace M, O'Shea E (2007) Perceptions of spirituality and spiritual care among older nursing home residents at the end of life. Holist Nurs Pract 21(6):285–291

World Health Organization (2002) Active ageing: A policy framework (No. WHO/NMH/NPH/02.8). World Health Organization. https://www.who.int/ageing/publications/active_ageing/en. Accessed 20 August 2020

Wilson K, Mottram P, Sixsmith A (2007) Depressive symptoms in the very old living alone: prevalence, incidence and risk factors. Int J Geriatr Psychiatry 22:361–366

Zarzycka B (2008) Tradition or charisma—Religiosity in Poland. In: Stiftung B (ed) What the World Believes: Analysis and Commentary on the Religion Monitor. Bertelsmann-Stiftung, Gütersloh, pp 26–29

CHAPTER 27

Spiritual Needs of Patients' Relatives

Arndt Büssing, Charlotte Wapler, Christoph Dodt, Andreas Beivers, Kristin Härtl, and Eckhard Frick

Introduction

The therapeutic strategy of emergency room(s) is necessarily patient-centered. Relatives who accompany patients to the Emergency Room may be separated from the patient in acute treatment moments, for example, during cardiopulmonary resuscitation (Johnson 2017). In other moments, however, maybe for hours, families and friends share the patient's waiting (Bournes and Mitchell 2002; Forsgärde et al. 2016; Hsiao et al. 2017; Barreto et al. 2019; Cetin-Sahin et al. 2019; Hassankhani et al. 2019;

A. Büssing
Professorship Quality of Life, Spirituality and Coping, Faculty of Health, Witten/Herdecke University, Herdecke, Germany

IUNCTUS—Competence Center for Christian Spirituality, Philosophical-Theological University of Münster, Münster, Germany
e-mail: Arndt.buessing@uni-wh.de

C. Wapler • E. Frick (✉)
Research Unit Spiritual Care, Clinic and Policlinic for Psychosomatic Medicine and Psychotherapy, Klinikum rechts der Isar, Technical University of Münster, Munich, Germany
e-mail: eckhard.frick@tum.de

A. Büssing (ed.), *Spiritual Needs in Research and Practice*,
https://doi.org/10.1007/978-3-030-70139-0_27

Ocak and Avsarogullari 2019), especially when the patient is classified as "non-urgent" or "less urgent" than others in the triage process (Coughlan and Corry 2007; Dahlen et al. 2012; Elmqvist et al. 2012; Forsgärde et al. 2016; Larsson et al. 2017; Hassankhani et al. 2019; Rantala et al. 2019).

Frequently, relatives seek a balance between keeping a calm posture and expressing their suffering from uncertainty, anxiety, unmet needs (Barreto et al. 2017). They are considered as information sources, carriers, translators, co-carers or even as interpreters of the patient's needs, for example, vigorously shouting: "Me First, Others Later" (Hassankhani et al. 2019), identifying themselves with the patient's needs. The relatives' own needs, conversely, are rarely noticed and still less frequently studied.

Consequently, relatives may wait for the patients and their needs to be addressed, or they may accompany the patients' waiting. In both situations, they experience a strange mixture of emergency (lack of time) and dull, maybe boring monotony, interrupted by more or less accidental events and encounters with health professionals and other visitors of the emergency room: "a vigilant attentiveness surfacing amid an ambiguous turbulent lull as contentment emerges with uplifting engagements", as stated by Bournes and Mitchell (2002: 66). This ambiguity of turbulence and stillness creates a permanent distress of accompanying relatives or, in other words, their unmet need for inner peace.

Previous studies investigated some of the largely overlooked needs of relatives as a part of their "emotional roller-coaster" (Linnarsson et al. 2010) and their powerlessness (Forsgärde et al. 2016). The (cognitive) need for information and explanation and for instrumental support is often a need for contact (Coughlan and Corry 2007; Rantala et al. 2019), for a momentary relief from the caregiving situation (Rantala et al. 2019). A South-African study (Botes and Langley 2016) found (using the Critical Care Family Needs Inventory) the families' need for "meaning" more important than for "communication" and "support". Other studies using

C. Dodt
Clinic for Emergency Medicine, Clinic Bogenhausen, Munich, Germany
e-mail: Christoph.Dodt@muenchen-klinik.de

A. Beivers • K. Härtl
Hochschule Fresenius, Munich, Germany
e-mail: beivers@hs-fresenius.de; kristin.haertl@hs-fresenius.de

the same instrument found "hope" (Linnarsson et al. 2010) or "communication" (Hsiao et al. 2017) as the most important need of relatives in the emergency situation.

There is no generally admitted definition about which relatives' needs have to be named "spiritual". Frequently, spirituality is restricted to End of Life Care (Hennessy et al. 2020). However, a recent Delphi-process states that relatives' spiritual needs are not limited to the palliative situation:

> *"Spirituality is a dynamic and intrinsic way in which we seek meaning, purpose, and transcendence. […] Spiritual distress is the overwhelming sense of unrelieved suffering that happens when a person's sense of meaning, purpose, connection, hope, or identity becomes acutely more vulnerable or is challenged. […] Spiritual distress is a normal response to physical, emotional, and psychological suffering or loss. Critical illness and ICU care introduce many stressors for family members. Spiritual distress in this setting is often underrecognized. Family members may experience spiritual distress at any time during a patient's stay in the ICU, not only at the end of life"* (Roze des Ordons et al. 2020).

Jones et al. (2019) surveyed individuals suffering from spinal cord injury together with one caring relative. In both parts of these dyads they found strong links between spiritual resources and resilience.

The spiritual needs of relatives in an Emergency Room have not yet been assessed in German-speaking countries. We approached these persons while waiting for the patient or waiting with the patient. The following data have been collected during a study about spiritual needs of patients attended in an Emergency Room of a municipal hospital (Frick et al. 2020). Using the SpNQ, this chapter addresses the following research questions:

1. How do the relatives rate their own spiritual needs?
2. Are there differences between the patients' and their relatives' spiritual needs?
3. Are the relatives' spiritual needs related to patient-related indicators or to own attitudes and behaviors?

Description of the Sample of Patients' Relatives

We analyzed data of 97 relatives from patients at a hospital´s emergency room. There were 60% women and 40% men; their mean age was 54 ± 25 [13-92] years. Among them, 42% were partner of the patient, 16% parent or brother/sister of the patient, 23% child of the patient, 20% attending friend or other relative—68% were Christians, 9% Muslim and other, and 23% had no religious affiliation.

Patients were treated as internal (27%), surgical (37%), urological (8%) or general medicine (28%) patients; 52% were treated as out-patients and 48% were hospitalized as in-patients.

Patients' Emergency Severity Index was 2 in 18% (which means that the patient's risk is high and he or she should be treated rapidly), while it was 3 in 57%, 4 in 22% and 5 in 3% (both are lower risk stages); patients´ mean ESI score was 3.1 ± 0.7.

Relatives' Spiritual Needs

As shown in Table 27.1, relatives' main needs were to "plunge into beauty of nature" (N6), which means to escape from the situation to a peaceful place in nature, and nevertheless to turn to someone "in a loving attitude" (N13) and to "give solace to someone"(N15), probably the sick patient. Further, they had the need to be "connected with the family" (N25), which can give further backing support for both the relative and the patient, and the need to "have good friends who support you" (N31). Nevertheless, two generative needs scored high, too: "pass own life experiences to others" (N26) and to "be assured that your life was meaningful and of value" (N27). It might be that the unclear situation with the patient in the emergency unit caused them to think about their life and their spiritual legacy.

As one may assume that relatives waiting in the Emergency Room will be mentally focused on the patient's situation, existential needs might be high. In fact, the need to reflect back on life (N4) was somewhat higher, but not the items that would address the next steps of such reflection processes, probably because the diagnosis and treatment options might be at that early time unclear, for example, talk with someone about the question of meaning in life (N11) or about the possibility of life after death (N12), or to find meaning in illness and/or suffering (N10). Interestingly, among the religious needs, praying for themselves (N20) was much higher than

Table 27.1 Expression of spiritual needs in relatives and patients

Item ID and topic	*Agreement score Relatives [Mean ± SD]*	*Agreement score Patients [Mean ± SD]* [b]
Number	97	379
Religious needs score	0.70 ± 0.83	0.73 ± 0.84
N18 pray with someone	0.43 ± 0.93	0.49 ± 0.97
N19 someone prays for you	0.71 ± 1.14	0.65 ± 1.06
N20 pray for yourself	1.01 ± 1.22	1.08 ± 1.24
N21 participate at a religious ceremony (i.e., Sunday service)	0.85 ± 1.10	0.84 ± 1.09
N22 read religious/spiritual books	0.37 ± 0.80	0.48 ± 0.93
N23 turn to a higher presence (i.e., God, Allah)	0.85 ± 1.10	0.85 ± 1.15
N3[a] that someone of your religious community (i.e., pastor) cares for you	0.25 ± 0.74	-
Existential needs score	0.71 ± 0.61	0.67 ± 0.61
N4[a] reflect back on your life	1.03 ± 1.20	1.09 ± 1.15
N5 dissolve/clarify open aspects of your life	0.75 ± 1.09	0.69 ± 1.07
N10 find meaning in illness and/or suffering	0.45 ± 0.96	0.39 ± 0.81
N11 talk with someone about the question of meaning in life	0.58 ± 0.98	0.73 ± 1.05
N12 talk with someone about the possibility of life after death	0.72 ± 1.09	0.73 ± 1.05
N16 forgive someone from a distinct period of your life	0.79 ± 1.11	0.69 ± 1.06
N17 be forgiven	0.92 ± 1.09	0.78 ± 1.09
Inner Peace needs score	1.49 ± 0.74	1.49 ± 0.74
N6 plunge into beauty of nature	2.39 ± 0.91	2.31 ± 1.03
N7 dwell at a place of quietness and peace	1.35 ± 1.25	1.48 ± 1.24
N8 find inner peace	1.07 ± 1.14	1.21 ± 1.20
N2 talk with others about your fears and worries	1.12 ± 1.18	0.94 ± 1.14
Giving/Generativity needs score	1.71 ± 0.76	1.59 ± 0.73
N14 give away something of yourself	1.51 ± 1.16	1.56 ± 1.19
N15 give solace to someone	1.79 ± 1.12	1.52 ± 1.19
N13[a] turn to someone in a loving attitude	1.99 ± 1.09	-
N26 pass own life experiences to others	1.79 ± 1.14	1.73 ± 1.10
N27 be assured that your life was meaningful and of value	1.74 ± 1.13	1.55 ± 1.21
SpNQ-20 Mean Score	1.06 ± 0.55	1.04 ± 0.54
Support needs	-	-
N25[a] feel connected with family	2.39 ± 1.03	2.52 ± 0.87
N30[a] receive more support from your family	0.89 ± 1.17	0.84 ± 1.18
N31[a] have good friends who support you	1.68 ± 1.29	-

[a]informative items not used for the factor calculation;
[b]data from Frick et al. (2020)

praying with someone (N18). Reading inspirational religious/spiritual books (N22) was irrelevant to them, while participating at a religious ceremony (N21) was at least of some relevance. Also a visit of a chaplain (N3) was less relevant to them, probably because they do not assume that the situation is so dramatic that sacramental help is needed.

Women had significantly higher *Religious* needs ($F = 7.4$, $p = 0.008$), *Existential* needs ($F = 7.5$, $p = 0.007$), *Inner Peace* needs ($F = 13.8$, $p < 0.001$), and *Giving/Generativity* needs ($F = 9.3$, $p = 0.003$). Womens′ SpNQ-20 Mean Score was significantly higher, too (1.24 ± 0.57 vs. 0.80 ± 0.42; $F = 16.6$, $p < 0.0001$). There were no statistically significant differences between the age groups, neither for the subscales ($F < 2.1$; $p < 0.10$) nor for the SpNQ-20 Mean Score ($F = 1.9$; n.s.). The relational status (i.e., partner, parents, etc.) had no significant effect on the needs ($F < 1.4$; n.s.).

Religious needs were lowest in nonreligious persons compared to Christians or Muslims (0.27 ± 0.59 vs. 0.86 ± 0.84 vs. 0.61 ± 0.84; $F = 4.7$, $p = 0.011$), while for the other needs no significant religion-associated differences were found ($F < 0.8$, n.s.).

Discussion of Findings

Concerning the research questions formulated in this chapter's introduction, we can state a preponderance of the SpNQ subscale *Inner Peace*, especially of the item N6 "plunge into beauty of nature". This finding represents a strong contrast with the stressful situation in the Emergency Room, urging the relatives to seek a balance between keeping a calm posture and expressing their suffering from uncertainty, anxiety, unmet needs (Barreto et al. 2017). Such needs for inner peace may be interpreted as a desire for such a balance or as a coping attitude (denying that they are enclosed in a waiting room or emergency unit with artificial light and sticky atmosphere). What about the patients' situation and its influence on their relatives' spiritual needs; are these needs related to patient-related indicators or to own attitudes and behaviors?

With respect to the medical profession patients were treated in (i.e., internal, surgical), there were no significant differences for the subscales of their relatives ($F = 2.6$, $p < 0.10$). However, whether the patients were treated as out-patients or as in-patients had a significant influence on relatives' *Inner Peace* needs, which were higher in an out-patient situation

(1.72 ± 0.74 vs. 1.34 ± 0.73; $F = 4.4$, $p = 0.040$), but not on the other needs ($F < 1.8$; n.s.).

Patients´ Emergency Severity Index (ESI) was not significantly related to their relatives' spiritual needs ($r < 0.20$; n.s.). Lower ESI means higher risk (which is also related to patients´ duration of hospital stay: $r = -0.42$, $p < 0.0001$). This duration of stay at the hospital as an in-patient was weakly and inversely related with relatives' *Inner Peace* needs ($r = -0.26$, $p = 0.034$). Detailed analyses revealed that their "need for inner peace" (N8) during the initial diagnostic measures was best related to the patients' hospitalization time ($r = -0.27$, $p = 0.025$), followed by the need to "dwell at a place of quietness and peace" (N7: $r = -0.26$, $p = 0.031$), while talk "about fears and worries" (N2: $r = -0.18$) or the need to escape "into beauty of nature" (N6: $r = 0.06$) were not significantly related. The inverse association is worth mentioning because it means that the longer patients were hospitalized, the lower are the *Inner Peace* needs and vice versa at the beginning of hospitalization. Consequently, patients' symptom severity perceived either consciously or subconsciously by their relatives during their emergency room attendance may be considered as an indicator of hospitalization time. Given that uncertainty is more important when hospitalization starts, relatives' fear and consequently their *Inner Peace* needs may increase. However, our sample encompasses relatives of patients suffering from symptoms of moderate severity; that is, less frequently facing End of Life situations than other patients' relatives. Consequently, satisfying *Inner peace* needs is more important than other spiritual needs, especially those clearly related to transcendence.

A further important finding is that the spiritual needs of relatives are not significantly different from the patients´ needs (Table 27.1): Neither the SpNQ subscales scores nor the single items differ significantly (Mann-Whitney-U), with the exception, however, of item N15 ($p = 0.048$). One explanation could be that patients and relatives might have a similar religious history (when they are direct partners within a family) and thus their attitudes and practices might be similar too. This can at least be underlined by similar scores for praying needs, attendance of religious ceremonies, reading religious/spiritual books, and need to relate to a higher presence (God). A further explanation could be that both are in a similar phase of early insecurity about the implications of patients´ symptoms and illness. During the later course of being ill, patients' needs could change, depending on the implications of disease. However, the spiritual needs of patients' relatives investigated herein may be experienced by all persons suffering from significant stressors, either due to disease, insecurity or hopelessness, etc. This note could be true, too, because a similar pattern of spiritual needs was also observed in stressed young mothers with sick newborn or premature infants (Büssing et al. 2017), mothers of children with Down syndrome (Büssing et al. 2019), stressed soldiers (Büssing and Recchia 2016), and elderly living in retirements homes (Erichsen and Büssing 2013; Man-Ging et al. 2015).

Conclusions

Patients and relatives alike experience a situation of uncertainty while enclosed in an emergency room, which is a transitional space either toward hospitalization in an ICU or in an ordinary ward or discharge toward home or death. Unfavorable outcomes are possible and even physically close and visible when regarding more urgent patients and their relatives.

Maintaining hope and a spiritual ground shared with the patient seems to be an important strategy of the relatives studied in this chapter.

Including and respecting the relatives in communication, information and decision-making processes can be a first support for their spiritual relationship with the patient.

References

Barreto MS, Garcia-Vivar C, JLGd S, Maciel DGS, Matsuda LM, Marcon SS (2019) Meanings attributed by family and patients to family presence in emergency rooms. Rev Bras Enferm 72:1684–1691

Barreto MS, Marcon SS, Garcia-Vivar C (2017) Patterns of behaviour in families of critically ill patients in the emergency room: a focused ethnography. J Adv Nurs 73:633–642

Botes ML, Langley G (2016) The needs of families accompanying injured patients into the emergency department in a tertiary hospital in Gauteng. Curationis 39:1–7

Bournes DA, Mitchell GJ (2002) Waiting: the experience of persons in a critical care waiting room. Res Nurs Health 25:58–67

Büssing A, Recchia DR (2016) Spiritual and Non-spiritual Needs Among German Soldiers and their Relation to Stress Perception, PTDS Symptoms, and Life Satisfaction – Results from a Structural Equation Modeling Approach. J Relig Health 55:747–764

Büssing A, Wassermann U, Hvidt NC, Längler A, Thiel M (2017) Spiritual needs of mothers with sick new born or premature infants. Woman and Birth 31:e89–e98

Büssing A, Hippen S, Eichhorn J, Baumann K (2019) Spirituelle Bedürfnisse und Belastungserleben von Müttern mit Kindern mit Down-Syndrom. Spiritual Care 8:263–273

Cetin-Sahin D, Ducharme F, McCusker J, Veillette N, Cossette S, Vu TM et al. (2019) Experiences of an emergency department visit among older adults and their families: Qualitative findings from a mixed-methods study. Journal of Patient Experience:2374373519837238

Coughlan M, Corry M (2007) The experiences of patients and relatives/significant others of overcrowding in accident and emergency in Ireland: A qualitative descriptive study. Accid Emerg Nurs 15:201–209

Dahlen I, Westin L, Adolfsson A (2012) Experience of being a low priority patient during waiting time at an emergency department. Psychol Res Behav Manag 5:1–9

Elmqvist C, Fridlund B, Ekebergh M (2012) On a hidden game board: the patient's first encounter with emergency care at the emergency department. J Clin Nurs 21:2609–2616

Erichsen NB, Büssing A (2013) Spiritual Needs of Elderly living in Retirement / Nursing Homes. Evidence-based Complementary and Alternative Medicine Article ID913247. https://doi.org/10.1155/2013/913247

Forsgärde E-S, From Attebring M, Elmqvist C (2016) Powerlessness: Dissatisfied patients' and relatives' experience of their emergency department visit. Int Emerg Nurs 25:32–36

Frick E, Büssing A, Rodrigues Recchia D, Härtl K, Beivers A, Wapler C, Dodt C (2020) Spirituelle Bedürfnisse von Patienten eines Notfallzentrums. Medizinische Klinik Intensivmedizin und Notfallmedizin 115. https://doi.org/10.1007/s00063-00020-00653-00068

Hassankhani H, Soheili A, Vahdati SS, Amin Mozaffari F, Wolf LA, Wiseman T (2019) "Me First, Others Later". A focused ethnography of ongoing cultural features of waiting in an Iranian emergency department. Int Emerg Nurs 47:100804

Hennessy N, Neenan K, Brady V, Sullivan M, Eustace-Cooke J, Timmins F (2020) End of life in acute hospital setting-A systematic review of families' experience of spiritual care. J Clin Nurs 29:1041–1052

Hsiao P-R, Redley B, Hsiao Y-C, Lin C-C, Han C-Y, Lin H-R (2017) Family needs of critically ill patients in the emergency department. Int Emerg Nurs 30:3–8

Johnson C (2017) A literature review examining the barriers to the implementation of family witnessed resuscitation in the Emergency Department. Int Emerg Nurs 30:31–35

Jones KF, Simpson G, Briggs L, Dorsett P, Anderson M (2019) A study of whether individual and dyadic relations between spirituality and resilience contribute to psychological adjustment among individuals with spinal cord injuries and their family members. Clin Rehabil 33:1503–1514

Larsson G, Holmén A, Ziegert K (2017) Early prehospital assessment of non-urgent patients and outcomes at the appropriate level of care: A prospective exploratory study. Int Emerg Nurs 32:45–49

Linnarsson JR, Bubini J, Perseius K-I (2010) Review: a meta-synthesis of qualitative research into needs and experiences of significant others to critically ill or injured patients. J Clin Nurs 19:3102–3111

Man-Ging CI, Öven Uslucan J, Fegg M, Frick E, Büssing A (2015) Reporting Spiritual Needs of Older Adults Living in Bavarian Residential and Nursing Homes. Journal of Mental Health, Religion and Spirituality 18:809–821

Ocak U, Avsarogullari L (2019) Expectations and needs of relatives of critically ill patients in the emergency department. Hong Kong Journal of Emergency Medicine 26:328–335

Rantala A, Ekwall A, Forsberg A (2019) Significant others' perceptions of being taken seriously by the Swedish Ambulance Service when the patient is assessed as nonurgent. Scand J Caring Sci. https://doi.org/10.1111/scs.12811

Roze des Ordons AL, Sinclair S, Sinuff T, Grindrod-Millar K, Stelfox HT (2020) Development of a clinical guide for identifying spiritual distress in family members of patients in the intensive care unit. J Palliat Med 23:171–178

PART VI

Relevance of Addressing Spiritual Needs for Clinical Support

CHAPTER 28

Spiritual Needs, Hopes and Resources: A Chaplain's Mantra

Anne Vandenhoeck

Introduction

It is a chaplain's job and vocation to address spiritual needs of patients, families and even staff. But spiritual needs are inevitably linked to spiritual resources and hopes that people have. Consider it a chaplain's mantra: we listen to spiritual needs, hopes and resources. And of course we address them. Observing or listening to spiritual needs is only the beginning of spiritual care. This chapter aims to make the point that spiritual needs are only part of the story. Focusing solely on spiritual needs creates the risk of a power imbalance where a patient has a need and we, as health care professionals, need to provide a solution for that need. This kind of thinking could endorse a sort of paternalism in health care that many would like to avoid. Focusing in addition to spiritual resources provides the space for patients to own their meaning-making processes. Working with the hopes patients have adds tremendously to their meaning-making processes.

A. Vandenhoeck (✉)
Faculty of Theology and Religious Studies, Catholic University Leuven, Leuven, Belgium
e-mail: anna.vandenhoeck@kuleuven.be

A. Büssing (ed.), *Spiritual Needs in Research and Practice*,
https://doi.org/10.1007/978-3-030-70139-0_28

This chapter also starts from the distinction between generalist and specialist spiritual care. Generalist spiritual care can be integrated into the practice of every health care professional. Specialist spiritual care is the task of chaplains or spiritual care professionals. Both types of spiritual care are at the top of their game when combined in an interdisciplinary take on whole-person care. Generalist spiritual care is enriched by specialist spiritual care and vice versa. Applied to spiritual needs, a spiritual needs questionnaire can be used by both generalist and specialist spiritual caregivers. But both parties will do different things with them, each from their own professional perspective. Chaplains are the only health care professionals who have the opportunity to address spiritual needs of patients and family members with every visit. It is part of their approach and professionalism. Evidence shows that involving chaplains for specialist spiritual care impacts the well-being of patients and their overall satisfaction with the care they receive (Iler et al. 2001).

In many health care facilities, chaplains are teaching other health care professionals to discern and address spiritual needs. They encounter the barriers that health care professionals feel regarding spiritual care. In this chapter, we talk about different strategies to support health care professionals to overcome those hurdles.

Spiritual Needs, Hopes and Resources

Back in the days when I worked as a chaplain in a hospital, I visited a young woman with severe Diabetes mellitus type 1 (a "juvenile" form of diabetes in which the hormone insulin producing cells are destroyed). Her life had been completely dominated by her disease for years. She needed to be hospitalized several times a year. Patients like her were eligible for (in those days sometimes experimental) treatments for this severe form of diabetes: internal insulin pump, external inhalation pump, islet cell transplantations, etc. One of the treatments actually worked for her and gave her the opportunity to start living again: studying, working, having relationships, in fact a realm of possibilities. But she had been locked up, dependent and isolated for so long. She had difficulties imagining all these new possibilities. She told me she needed to do something to help her over the threshold. Could I help? She was good in drawing and she loved it. So I asked her to draw how she felt. She drew a bird cage. The little door was open but the bird was still inside. We did a ritual in the chapel, using the drawing, reading a psalm, lighting a candle, praying for her and blessing her. It touched the spiritual resources she had and it strengthened her. It enabled her to make the click and to start imagining a different future.

This case shows that the patient's spiritual needs go together with her spiritual resources. Does everyone have the right resources for their spiritual needs? Probably not. But chaplains look for them, wondering what the reasons are for people to keep living. Those reasons are meaning-makers and can turn into resources. They are as important to integrate into spiritual care as spiritual needs. Often they help giving patients ownership over their meaning-making processes. Contemporary mental health practices confirm the fundamental link between needs and resources in their recovery-oriented care paradigm. Recovery is perceived as a process in which someone learns to live with a disorder, using his or her resources and the resources that are offered by mental health providers (Davidson et al. 2006). Spiritual care by chaplains has a lot in common with the mental health paradigm regarding working with the potential of the patient. Chaplains do listen for spiritual needs but at the same time look for resources that can support meaning-making processes in patients.

Arthur Lucas, the former head of the spiritual care service at BJC Health in Saint Louis, distilled out of the case studies of his chaplains a model: the Discipline for Pastoral Care Giving (VandeCreek & Lucas 2001). It begins with the notion that every chaplain starts with listening to the patient's story and in particular to the spiritual needs, hopes and resources. The model commences, thus, with the concept of the patient's spiritual needs. The connection with the medical care model is most evident in the starting point of the discipline. The traditional care model sees the patient as an individual with needs. The health care professional detects the needs and then meets them as much as possible. This problem-solving thinking, one of the foundations of traditional medical health care, sees the patient as a collection of needs and the care provider as a collection of solutions (De Jong & Berg 2015). Spiritual care addresses spiritual needs but also works with patient's resources and hopes. Hope is essential in the spirituality of people. Without future stories, without a future time dimension integrated in the present, life has no meaning (Lester 1995). For chaplains it is essential to understand the future stories patients have in order to understand their losses today. If you truly aim to understand the person in front of you, you need to know what he or she is hoping for (Yalom 1980). Needs and resources have no perspective and perhaps no meaning without hope. From listening to spiritual needs, hopes and resources, chaplains start to think of an outcome that would be beneficial for the patient. But it needs to be a shared desired outcome. If the patient goes another route, the chaplain changes gears. In order to get to a shared desired outcome, a plan and interventions are needed. An example: A young couple has a stillborn baby. Their spiritual need is to give the baby a name. They want to recognize the baby as a human being and as theirs. The chaplain checks some possible interventions: do they want a ritual, a prayer, a naming ceremony? The couple decides on a naming ceremony. The outcome of the chaplain's visit is that the baby was recognized and honored as a human being and as a child of her parents, thus meeting the need of the parents.

Spiritual needs are often, but not always, linked to experiencing loss of meaning. In order to find, receive, experience meaning in life, a person needs connectedness with self, others, nature and the sacred. When suffering comes in, changes occur in the purposes and goals that a person has. But spiritual needs can also come forth from within the experience of deep meaningfulness. When a person works on his or her own spirituality and deepens the awareness of being connected, the spiritual need for a greater awareness or a deepened connection can arise.

Spiritual needs, hopes and resources are the foundation to build spiritual care on. They inspire the content of spiritual care. Chaplains tap into the resources and hopes that patients have. They often meet the spiritual needs of patients well, make their stay easier and help them connect with their resources (Flannelly et al. 2009).

Spiritual Care Meets Spiritual Needs

When I started to work in the spiritual care team of a university hospital in the 1990s, one of the older team members expressed there were differences in spiritual care for patient populations. The differences had to do with the pathology that the patients were treated for. He did not know the term spiritual needs at that time and used pathology-linked characteristics to describe what he instinctively knew after so many years of chaplaincy on different units. For example he said: "Most patients on the cardiac floors have been living life to the fullest in one way or another, that is why they are there. Often they are in for a life changing shock to their system. What they need from you is assistance in rearranging their priorities and reassurance they will be ok." Of course, this is only valid for part of the patients with cardiac problems and of course this is very unnuanced, but it shows that even before we started doing research on spiritual needs, chaplains already knew, through reflection on their experiences, that specific pathologies are linked to specific spiritual needs. Today's research only confirms that initial reflection on the practice. One of the first researches on spiritual needs that came to my attention categorized specific spiritual needs for palliative care patients (Hermann 2001).

A significant part of today's research on spiritual needs is not done by chaplains themselves nor by researchers in the field of chaplaincy. Despite chaplains being those health care professionals that consistently work with spiritual needs. The advantage of others researching spiritual needs is that spiritual care becomes more of an interdisciplinary concern. One of the disadvantages is that research regularly fails to take the difference between generalist and specialist spiritual care into consideration. Even to the point where research discussions do not mention any form of possible interventions by chaplains. Research done by chaplains should focus among others on the impact of addressing spiritual needs of patients and family members, on the impact of teaching spiritual needs to other health care professionals and on improving tools to discern spiritual needs. One of the important questions today for chaplains is if they meet the spiritual needs of patients and family members. Who better to ask then patients and family members themselves? Today we have two forms of research regarding chaplaincy that tries to answer the question if chaplains meet spiritual needs from the perspective of patients: patient satisfaction questionnaires and outcome-oriented research. We refer to three important researches in that regard (ACPE et al. n.y.).

Patient satisfaction surveys in the United States are used, among others, to indicate the overall satisfaction of patients with the spiritual care they received. Some research based on patient satisfaction lists show patients' opinions regarding their spiritual needs being addressed. In Mount Sinai hospital, New York, 9000 patients participated in a satisfaction survey (Marin et al. 2015). Those who were visited by a chaplain gave higher ratings to all satisfaction items including having their spiritual and emotional needs addressed.

A 2010 survey in the United States provides evidence that patients want the assistance of chaplains regarding their spiritual needs (Piderman et al. 2010). Some numbers regarding explicit religious needs: 78% of patients want chaplains to remind them of God's care and presence, 62% of patients want chaplains to pray or read scriptures or sacred texts. Some numbers regarding broader spiritual needs: 71% of patients want chaplains to offer support to their family and friends, 69% of patients want chaplains to be with them during times of particular anxiety or uncertainty. In this research, the desired interventions of chaplains meet the spiritual and religious needs of patients. It seems more than likely that if this survey were to be conducted in other parts of the world, the spiritual needs and the desired interventions of chaplains based on them would be expressed differently. Religion and spirituality are embedded and expressed culturally. In Western Europe, for example, chaplains work in secularized societies where people have grown further away from religious traditions (detraditionalization). Broader spiritual needs dominate religious needs when listening to patients and families. Because of their training and experience, chaplains learn to discern those broader spiritual needs. Often spiritual needs are expressed through relational meaning or lack thereof. When religious languages are seldom used, people look for other languages to express their spirituality and spiritual needs. For example, Marc Desmet, a palliative care physician described "euthanasia talk" as a way for patients to describe severe loss of meaning (Desmet 2015). It doesn't mean that those patients will all request euthanasia but talking about ending life through euthanasia becomes a way to express spiritual pain. Chaplains thus need to be vigilant for new ways to express spirituality and spiritual needs.

Patient Reported Outcome Measures (PROMS) are an important tool in health care to integrate patients′ feedback on treatments, state of illness, quality of life, etc. The Scottish PROMS for spiritual care give patients the opportunity to voice how spiritual care by a chaplain impacted them (Snowden et al. 2018). Did the chaplain meet their spiritual needs? Items like "I was listened to," "I was able to talk about what was on my mind," "My situation was understood," "My faith/beliefs were valued" were to be evaluated by patients after a visit from a chaplain. "I was able to talk about what was on my mind" was validated the highest by the participating patients. Clearly, chaplaincy is meeting the spiritual needs of patients by giving them space to talk about what really is on their mind that day, that visit.

Chaplains Teach Others about Spiritual Needs

Chaplains, as specialist spiritual caregivers, are teaching across disciplines how to discern and meet spiritual needs. They do that formally and informally. They teach during introduction sessions of new health care staff, they have sessions in training programs of hospitals and nursing homes; they are invited to train staff on various occasions. More likely than not, the topics of spiritual screening and spiritual needs will be integrated in teachings. How, to what extent and where chaplains are involved in training programs depends on the health care institutions and on the initiatives of the spiritual care services themselves. Informal teaching happens in day-to-day communication between chaplains and other staff. Often the language that chaplains use to chart communicates to others what the spiritual needs are for that particular patient or family. Interdisciplinary team meetings are another way chaplains use to communicate about their perspectives on patients and families, which include their spiritual needs.

In teaching about spiritual needs, chaplains encounter barriers that health care professionals are experiencing regarding generalist spiritual care. Although researchers and educators stress the importance of listening to spiritual needs and the impact meeting them has on health and well-being of patients, the practice still shows a lack of attention for spiritual needs. Research that gives a voice to patients and family caregivers highlights that spiritual distress and spiritual needs are present but they remain unmet (Selman et al. 2017). According to the literature review by Rogiers, Steegen and Vandenhoeck, barriers to spiritual care can be classified in three categories (Rogiers et al. 2019). A first category contains environmental factors. Examples are an uneasiness to speak about spirituality in a secularized culture, feeling anxious in the face of existential questions and most of all the experience of lack of time to respond to spiritual needs. A second category refers to missing aspects of professionalism. Examples are a lack of skills to recognize spiritual needs, having no tools to address spiritual needs, seeing spiritual care as the exclusive domain of chaplains. The last category contains personal factors. Examples are a lack of spiritual self-awareness, the reluctance to integrate generalist spiritual care, and fear of emotions associated with spiritual needs.

To remedy this, Rogiers, Steegen and Vandenhoeck consider three strategies that are best applied together for an optimal result (Rogiers et al. 2019). The first strategy refers to the best possible care culture to integrate spiritual care and address spiritual needs. Researchers on spiritual care stress the importance of a culture of compassionate care (van Heijst 2005) that enhances the integration of generalist (and specialist) spiritual care (Puchalski et al. 2014). Contemporary management-oriented care thus needs to be in dialogue with a perspective on care where connectedness with fellow human beings is paramount. A second strategy is to reform the way spiritual care is taught in the context of training programs in health care institutions today. It is not sufficient to teach a group of physicians and nurses on spiritual care for 2 h and then send them back to patients. After a 2-h session there is an increased attention that gradually fades away. Efficient training should correspond to the three barriers for spiritual care that health care professionals experience. The training needs to touch health care professionals personally, for example, by applying the spiritual needs questionnaire to themselves or by learning to communicate about the content of their own global meaning system. The training needs to enhance or add to professional skills, for example, by learning how to use a tool for spiritual needs and learning about the underpinnings of a tool. The training needs to be in dialogue with environmental factors, for example, through case discussions or bedside teaching by specialist spiritual caregivers. A follow-up on the training is as important. Post trainings chaplains can, for example, organize follow-up talks or check in if health care professionals integrated charting about spiritual needs. The third strategy is to integrate a course on generalist spiritual care in the education of nurses, physicians, physiotherapists and other health care professions. I am extremely fortunate to have the opportunity to teach generalist and specialist spiritual care at the Catholic University of Leuven (KU Leuven) where all students have one mandatory course on religion, meaning of life and life views. This course is given in all faculties by professors of the faculty of Theology and Religious Studies. The course needs to fit with the end goals of the educational program of every faculty. Thus, I teach generalist spiritual care to students in medicines, physiotherapy and pharmacology. My course is a mixture of theory and practice. Students and staff appreciate the combination of lived experience of spiritual care from my background as a chaplain, the research I bring in as an academic and the tools they can take from it. Those who teach spiritual care to students in medical professions have a number of competences in mind that are mostly based on active actions like observing spiritual needs, discussing them in interdisciplinary teams, charting them, addressing them. But a case can be made for the preservation of incompetence (Waaijman 2004). Incompetence refers to the lack of answers and action we all have regarding existential questions or other issues that refer to meaninglessness. Maintaining incompetence in that regard ensures that existential questions from patients that do not yet need answers, do not receive any from professional caregivers. Only in the field of spirituality can "maintaining incompetence" create space for solidarity, connectedness and endurance.

Conclusion

Spirituality cannot progress, deepen or heal meaninglessness without spiritual needs. These often come to the surface when experiencing suffering and loss of meaning. Every health care professional should be able to address those needs. The professional approach of chaplains integrates working with the spiritual needs, hopes and resources of patients and family members. As specialist spiritual caregivers, chaplains are well chosen to educate and train other health care professionals in addressing spiritual needs.

References

ACPE, APC, CASC, NACC and NESHAMA (n.d.) The impact of Professional Spiritual Care. https://www.professionalchaplains.org/Files/resources/The%20Impact%20of%20Professional%20Spiritual%20Care_PDF.pdf. Accessed 23 August 2020

Davidson L, O'Connell M, Tondora J, Styron T, Kangas K (2006) The top ten concerns about recovery encountered in mental health system transformation. Psychiatr Serv 57:640–645

Desmet M (2015) Euthanasie: Waarom niet? Pleidooi voor nuance en niet-weten. Lannoo, Tielt

Flannelly K, Oettinger M, Galek K, Braun-Storck A, Kreger R (2009) The correlates of Chaplains' effectiveness in meeting the spiritual/religious and emotional needs of patients. J Pastoral Care Counsel 63(1–2):1–16

Hermann CP (2001) Spiritual needs of dying patients. A Qualitative Study Oncology Nursing Forum 28:67–72

Iler W, Obenshain D, Camac M (2001) The impact of daily visits from chaplains on patients with chronic obstructive pulmonary disease (COPD): a pilot study. Chaplaincy Today 17:5–11

de Jong K, Berg I (2015) De kracht van oplossingen. Handboek oplossingsgericht werken, Pearson Benelux.

Lester A (1995) Hope in pastoral care and Counseling. Westminster John Knox Press, Louisville, Kentucky

Marin D, Sharma V, Sosunov E, Egorova N, Goldstein R, Handzo G (2015) Relationship between chaplain visits and patient satisfaction. J Health Care Chaplain 21:14–24

Piderman K, Marek D, Jenkins S, Johnson M, Buryska J, Shanafelt T, O'Bryan F, Hansen P, Howick P, Durland H, Lackore K, Lovejoy L, Mueller P (2010) Predicting Patients' expectations of hospital chaplains: a multisite survey. Mayo Clin Proc 85:1002–1010

Puchalski C, Vitillo R, Hull S, Reller N (2014) Improving the spiritual dimension of whole person care: reaching national and international consensus. J Palliat Med 17:642–656

Rogiers E, Steegen M, Vandenhoeck A (2019) Verpleegkundigen en eerstelijns spirituele zorg: een harmonieuze combinatie binnen de hedendaagse zorgcontext? Op zoek naar een ondersteunend (in)competentieprofiel en de bijhorende vorming. Collationes Vlaams Tijdschrift voor Theologie en Pastoraal 49(4):427–448

Selman L, Brighton L, Sinclair S, Karvinen I, Egan R, Speck P, Powell R, Deskur-Smielecka E, Glajchen M, Adler S, Puchalski C, Hunter J, Gikaara N, Hope J (2017) Patients' and caregivers' needs, experiences, preferences and research priorities in spiritual care: a focus group study across nine countries. Palliat Med 32:216–230

Snowden A, Lobb E, Schmidt S, Swing A, Logan P, Macfarlane C (2018) What's on your mind?' the only necessary question in spiritual care. Journal for the Study of Spirituality 8:19–33

VandeCreek L, Lucas AM (2001) The discipline for pastoral care giving : foundations for outcome oriented chaplaincy. J Health Care Chaplain 10 & 11:1–174

Van Heijst A (2005) Menslievende zorg. Een ethische kijk op professionaliteit. Klement, Kampen

Waaijman K (2004) Spiritualiteit in de zorg. In de interactie tussen zorgvrager en zorgverlener. In: Bouwer J (ed) Spiritualiteit en zingeving in de gezondheidszorg. Kok, Kampen

Yalom I (1980) Existential psychotherapy. Hachette Book Group, New York

CHAPTER 29

Relevance of Addressing Spiritual Needs for Clinical Support: Nursing Perspective

Linda Ross and Wilfred McSherry

Introduction

In this chapter, we seek to answer the question of whether or not it is important for nurses to address the spiritual needs of those in their care, and if so, whether this is possible in the current busy milieu of competing demands and limited resources.

But first, we clarify what is meant by 'spiritual needs' and whether addressing them falls within the remit of nursing. To do that we briefly

L. Ross (✉)
School of Care Sciences, Faculty of Life Sciences and Education,
University of South Wales, Pontypridd, UK
e-mail: linda.ross@southwales.ac.uk

W. McSherry
Department of Nursing, School of Health and Social Care,
Staffordshire University, Staffordshire, UK

University Hospitals of North Midlands NHS Trust, Stoke-on-Trent, UK

VID Specialized University, Bergen/Oslo, Norway
e-mail: W.McSherry@staffs.ac.uk

A. Büssing (ed.), *Spiritual Needs in Research and Practice*,
https://doi.org/10.1007/978-3-030-70139-0_29

discuss definitions, models and theories of nursing, and how the role of the nurse has evolved over time to adjust to the changing landscape of healthcare provision and service user need. We identify the core elements of nursing that never change and that put spiritual care firmly within the nurse's domain: advocacy and care co-ordination, holistic care and evidence-based practice.

We then move on to consider how realistic it is for nurses to provide spiritual care on top of everything else. Finally, we tackle the thorny issue of how we can prepare nurses for spiritual care drawing upon a recently completed European project that sought to establish best practice in undergraduate spiritual care education. We conclude that nurses cannot fulfill their true remit without attending to the spiritual needs of the people they care for. We offer a model to help them to do this, which need not incur extra time or resources.

Clarifying How Spirituality, Spiritual Needs and Spiritual Care are Understood

In order to answer the question of whether nurses should address the spiritual needs of those in their care, it is first necessary to clarify what is meant by 'spiritual needs'.

The issue of how spirituality is defined has been hotly debated and contested for decades with a rich diversity of definitions and understandings. In response to being asked to write a chapter on what spirituality is, in 2010 John Swinton wrote '...the more I reflect on the issue of spirituality, the less convinced I am that asking the apparently simple question—what is spirituality?—is the best way to frame the issue. The area of human experience that spirituality has come to represent is far too complicated and important to be captured in a single definition' (Swinton 2010, p. 17). Ten years on, Swinton argues that rather than asking what spirituality is, we should be asking what it does (Swinton 2020), focusing on the experience of spirituality and what it means for nursing practice and the people nurses care for. Swinton (2010) offers three approaches, or three different lenses through which spirituality might be 'experienced' (rather than defined): an approach from religion, an approach from biology and a generic approach. We briefly look at the latter two here.

Based on the work of David Hay (2006), the biological approach assumes that spirituality is present in everyone; that people are 'hard-wired for religious and spiritual experiences' and that a particular area of the brain processes these experiences. If this is true, then spirituality is relevant to all, not just people who are religious. It also may account for the body of research that demonstrates connections between spirituality, religion, and health. The biological approach links with Swinton's 'generic' approach to spirituality, which assumes a common set of spiritual needs relevant to all people, irrespective of any religious tradition. This approach means that spiritual care is for people of all faiths and none. It is this generic approach that has largely been adopted by healthcare and by nursing.

The next question that needs to be answered is, what is the common set of 'spiritual needs' that should be addressed within peoples' care? The answer to this question comes from a number of sources: consensus mapping by experts studies that have sought service users' views; concept analyses.

Consensus Mapping

In 2002, the WHO endorsed spirituality as a health-related quality of life indicator (WHOQOL-SRPB Group, 2006), encompassing aspects of the human experience including spiritual/religious/personal beliefs, connection, meaning, awe, wholeness, inner strength, peace, hope and faith. Professional bodies such as the Royal College of Nursing in the United Kingdom (RCN 2011) have adopted a similar understanding to underpin nursing practice.

In 2013, after decades of debate, international experts met to seek agreement in mapping out the spiritual territory (Puchalski et al. 2014). The resulting consensus statement has been adopted by health organizations such as the European Association of Palliative Care (EAPC, Nolan et al. 2011):

Spirituality is the dynamic dimension of human life that relates to the way persons (individual and community) experience, express and/or seek meaning, purpose and transcendence, and the way they connect to the moment, to self, to others, to nature, to the significant and/or the sacred. The spiritual field is multidimensional, containing:

1. Existential challenges (e.g. questions concerning identity, meaning, suffering and death, guilt and shame, reconciliation and forgiveness, freedom and responsibility, hope and despair, love and joy).

2. Value based considerations and attitudes (what is most important for each person, such as relations to oneself, family, friends, work, things, nature, art and culture, ethics and morals, and life itself).
3. Religious considerations and foundations (faith, beliefs and practices, the relationship with God or the ultimate'.

This understanding of spirituality is commonly referred to in nursing literature and research and it has been adopted by nurse/midwifery educators across Europe who are using it as a basis for their education programmes (McSherry et al. 2020). However, further work is needed to explore how this largely Western understanding of spirituality fits in non-Western cultures, as recent research suggests it may need to be adapted to take account of the cultural diversity and sensitivities in continents such as Asia (Deng and Liu 2020; Niu et al. 2020a, 2020b; Balthip et al. 2017).

Service User Studies

Service user studies tend to focus on two main aspects: the spiritual needs people experience and the spiritual care they desire.

Spiritual needs: A large number of studies by nurses since the 1980s have focused on exploring what spirituality means to the people they care for. The types of needs reported broadly align with the generic view of spirituality outlined above and are adequately summarized in review papers (Cockell & McSherry 2012; Pike 2011; Ross 2006; Ross & Miles 2019).

Spiritual care: The research on spiritual care suggests that it is valued but not always offered or expected (Murray et al. 2004; Selman et al. 2017). It is more likely to be offered within specialist palliative and end-of-life care settings, such as hospices or palliative care units, which adopt a holistic care model. Spiritual care seems less likely to be offered where the medical model predominates, even if people are receiving palliative or end-of-life care in those settings (Royal College of Physicians 2016). So, the care philosophy or 'ethos' of the organization (whether the focus is on cure or care), seems to be important in the provision of spiritual care.

The people providing spiritual care also seem to be important. A recent study conducted in nine countries across five continents (Selman et al. 2017) confirms the findings from previous research that the spiritual care patients and carers with life-limiting conditions welcome has more to do with *how* the nurse is rather than *what* he/she does. Patients want to be cared for by someone who is open, respectful, genuine, nonjudgmental, hopeful, honest, empathetic, kind and spiritually aware. They want to be cared for by someone who is present in the moment and puts them and their actual needs (not assumed needs) and what is important to them first, who sees spiritual care as integral to all care. In other words, spiritual care could be considered to be care that focuses on what is most important to the person at any moment in time (whether that's about a spiritual matter specifically such as hope, meaning, faith, or about a physical ailment requiring medication or treatment) and is provided by a nurse with the qualities just mentioned. This view of spiritual care resonates with Clarke's (2013) notion of all care having the potential to be spiritual; Swinton's (2010) view that it's what spiritual care does rather than what it is that is important; NHS Education Scotland's (NES) view that spiritual care is dynamic, moving 'in whatever direction need requires' (NES 2010). Such care may involve 'faith support' (prayer, rites, sacraments) or 'simply for a sensitive listener'. It will be important, however, for the nurse to get the right balance of art and science in the care he or she provides (Ross & McSherry 2010). For example, a nurse who is very good in the 'art' of nursing but is incompetent in clinical procedures (science) is an incompetent nurse and unsafe to practice; balancing the art with the science is important.

Concept Analyses

Concept analyses of 'spirituality' from many disciplines (nursing, allied health, social work, psychology, theology) and adopting different methodological approaches tend to condense the multiple aspects of spirituality mentioned above into three key elements: meaning, connection (with self, others, nature/higher power) and transcendence (Murgia et al. 2020; Tanyi 2002; Weathers 2016).

The understanding of spirituality described above, derived from expert mapping/service users/concept analyses, presents the spiritual aspects of humanity that nurses should be cognizant of in assessing, planning and providing care in partnership with patients and their loved ones. Care that seeks to foster peoples' sense of meaning and transcendence and keeps them connected with themselves, the people, things, the Ultimate that are important to them. Seen in this way, all care can be spiritual, as argued by Clarke (2013). It need not mean doing something extra, although on occasion it might. All of this assumes of course that spiritual care is part of what nurses are supposed to do.

Is Addressing Spiritual Needs Part of the Nurse's Remit?

Definitions of Nursing

One of the most seminal definitions of nursing was written by Virginia Henderson (1964, p 63):

The unique function of the nurse is to assist the individual, sick or well, in the performance of those activities contributing to health or its recovery (or to a peaceful death) that he would perform unaided if he had the necessary strength, will or knowledge; and to do this in such a way as to help him gain independence as rapidly as possible.

This definition affirms that nursing involves a reciprocal relationship between the nurse and the person(s) receiving nursing care. While the word spiritual is not used explicitly, it is implied inasmuch as a person's beliefs, values and what provides their life with meaning, purpose and fulfillment are important contributors to health and well-being.

Nursing Models and Theories

It is beyond the scope of this chapter to provide an in-depth account of all the nursing models and theories that have been developed. However, over two decades ago, Martsolf and Mickley (1998) provided a useful overview of the extent to which aspects of spirituality were found in modern nursing theories. They found that the spiritual dimension was not present in all nursing theories and models. They concluded that action was needed, stating:

Continued theoretical development in this area is essential to further understanding of the concept and to guide practice.

Since then theoretical development has continued offering a better understanding of the place that spirituality plays within nursing practice. This richer and deeper understanding is evidenced by the ever-increasing and expanding number of publications and research studies that have been undertaken in this field.

It is disappointing that, in the United Kingdom at least, many undergraduate nurse education programs give little attention to nursing models and theories. Students, therefore, miss out on important insights into the nature of the person and the role of the nurse, which these theories and models offer. Martha Raile Alligood's (2014) text *Nursing Theorists and their Work* highlights the importance of nursing theories to the development of the nursing profession and the delivery of healthcare. In a key word search of this text, the word 'spiritual' is referred to 293 times, demonstrating how the concept is now recognized within some theories of nursing.

Central themes within contemporary nursing models include 'individualized care', 'person-centered care', and 'coproduction'. McSherry (2016, p. 85) observes how the word 'care' is often prefaced by other straplines, for example, 'dignity in care' or 'compassionate care'. He suggests that these straplines may counteract 'the prevailing medical and scientific model that has infiltrated and fragmented nursing care.'

Evolving Role of the Nurse

The role of the nurse has evolved considerably over time. These changes are notable in many areas, for example, the formal education and preparation to become a registered practitioner and the scientific evidence base that has been developed underpinning the art and science of nursing. There has been a proliferation in specialist roles and titles, for example, 'Advanced Nurse Practitioner', 'Specialist Nurse', 'Nurse Consultant', which can be confusing for members of the public. Many of the myths, rituals and routines once performed by nurses have rightly been replaced with evidence-based practices that promote clinical excellence and high-quality patient care. However, one of the *dangers of such improvements* and innovation in nursing practice is that nursing may become more medically dominated, reductionist and specialized, resulting in fragmentation of care where the 'whole person' is lost sight of.

Core Elements

Although the role of the nurse has evolved considerably over time, there are core elements that never change. These include advocacy and care coordination, holistic care and evidence-based practice.

Advocacy and care coordination. Increasingly, nurses are advocating for their patients, coordinating care across sometimes complex, multi- and interdisciplinary teams and providing a 24-h, seven-day presence. It could be argued that nursing is the 'glue that holds care together', that unifies the patient and carer relationships with all other disciplines involved.

Holistic Care

Considerable emphasis has been placed upon the notion of 'holistic care' or 'holistic nursing' (Papathanasiou et al. 2013). The working definition developed by McEvoy and Duffy reads (2008, p. 418):

Holistic nursing care embraces the mind, body and spirit of the patient, in a culture that supports a therapeutic nurse/patient relationship, resulting in wholeness, harmony and healing. Holistic care is patient led and patient focused in order to provide individualised care, thereby, caring for the patient as a whole person rather than in fragmented parts.

This definition affirms the importance of seeing the individual as a 'whole' functioning unit, not as a fragmented set of systems. It has been suggested that spirituality is the thread running through the many dimensions and facets of people's lives (McSherry & Draper 1998). Similarly, the concept and importance of spirituality within many societies has often 'waxed and waned' depending upon societal influence and pressure. For example, in the United Kingdom there has been strong opposition from the National Secular Society to the use of government money to provide services to support public institutions such as the National Health Service to meet peoples′ personal, religious and spiritual beliefs (National Secular Society 2011).

The dangers of removing the spiritual dimension from care may have a detrimental impact upon the overall quality of patient care. For example, there have been some serious failings in the provision of healthcare in England (The Parliamentary and Health Service Ombudsman 2011; The Mid Staffordshire NHS Foundation Trust Public Inquiry 2013) and in Wales (Andrews & Butler 2014). It is evident, when reviewing these failings that when we lose sight of the person, this can result in a violation of dignity, depersonalization and dehumanization. Spirituality is one way of ensuring that care remains compassionate, person-centered and dignified, recognizing the value and worth of both those receiving it and those providing it.

The drive for secularization of public services may account for and explain why in the United Kingdom the Nursing and Midwifery Council (NMC) decided not to include the word 'spiritual' within its revised code of professional standards of practice and behavior for nurses (NMC 2015). Yet, this omission seems to contradict other guidance they produce for undergraduate nursing and midwifery education where spirituality has always been an integral part.

Evidence-Based Practice

Nurses must use the best available evidence to guide their practice (ICN 2012; NMC 2015). Spiritual well-being has been associated with improved coping, well-being, quality of life and reduced depression and anxiety (Balboni et al. 2017; Steinhauser et al. 2017), and unmet spiritual need has been associated with poorer quality of life (Astrow et al. 2018). Although this body of work has been criticized for lack of conceptual clarity and inconsistent methodological approaches and measurement (Clark et al. 2018; King 2014; Steinhauser et al. 2017) and further research is needed, it is currently the best available evidence. As nurses are in the business of promoting quality of life and well-being, it stands to reason that promoting spiritual well-being and reducing spiritual distress should fall within their remit.

But what interventions can they employ to promote these desirable outcomes? The answer to that is by no means clear. A recent review of seven studies identified little evidence of benefit of spiritual care (spiritual history taking, existential therapy, death-related rituals, creative therapies) within palliative care (Gijsberts et al. 2019), but these were small scale studies with methodological limitations. Whether some of these interventions were 'spiritual' is also questionable. Another review of effective spiritual interventions in heart failure in the last 5 years identified that no single intervention stood out as being effective in enhancing quality of life (Ross & Miles 2019). Interventions involving life review and mindfulness appeared ineffective, which concurs with a Cochrane review where quality of life or well-being of those patients (in their palliative phases) with or without meditation interventions did not significantly differ (Candy et al. 2012). Interventions involving talking about spiritual matters and spiritual coping may be beneficial but need further investigation. The most promising intervention wasn't an intervention as such, but rather a holistic team approach to care inclusive of spiritual assessment and follow-up (Rogers et al. 2017).

It may be that the 'compassionate presence' (Gillian et al. 2017) of team members persuaded by a holistic approach to care, is key. Further investigation is needed to delineate the active ingredient, but these findings resonate with the view of spiritual care presented above as being integral to all care and dependent on the 'way of being' or personal attributes of the caregivers rather than on specific actions. There is certainly evidence to support this. The personal spirituality of student nurses/midwives and their perception of spirituality were significant factors in self-perceived spiritual care competency in a large longitudinal multinational study discussed in more detail below; students also identified personal life events as instrumental to their learning (Ross et al. 2018). The individual's worldview, feeling of responsibility to care for the 'spirit' and experience of life events are antecedents to spiritual care identified in the concept analyses referred to above derived from empirical and theoretical literature (Murgia et al. 2020; Weathers et al. 2016). Personal attributes such as compassion, care and communication are highlighted by care providers as key to good care provision (e.g. NHS England) and emotional warmth, kindness, being spiritually aware are additional qualities highlighted by patients as important for spiritual care (Selman et al. 2017).

So, what does evidence-based spiritual care look like? Clearly further investigation is needed to answer this, but key strands highlighted by the literature include: 'compassionate presence' and personal attributes of the nurse such as spiritual awareness/well-being, compassion, emotional warmth, kindness, ability to communicate; holistic 'ethos' of the organization inclusive of spiritual care; seeing all care as spiritual rather than spiritual care as an extra; providing opportunity for people to talk about spiritual matters; fostering meaning, hope, connection, transcendence during care giving; focusing on what's most important to the person (person-centered care). This 'art' of caring must, of course, be balanced with the 'science' of caring demonstrated by competence in clinical skills.

To conclude this section, having looked at definitions and models of nursing and current evidence, it is clear that spiritual care is part of the holistic caring role of the nurse.

Preparing Nurses for Spiritual Care

It is all very well saying that nurses should be providing spiritual care but they have been saying for several decades that they feel unprepared and in need of further education (Austin et al. 2017; Egan et al. 2017; Ross 1994; RCN 2011). Part of the problem in trying to address this long-standing gap has been the lack of clarity about what is actually expected of nurses in providing spiritual care. Although there are a number of self-assessment spiritual care competency scales available (van Leeuwen et al.

2009; Frick et al. 2019[1]), there were no operational spiritual care competencies for nurses, It was also unclear how nurses might acquire spiritual caring skills or how education programs might be structured in terms of content and delivery to help nurses achieve that (McSherry et al. 2020). Some small-scale studies had tested teaching approaches, but these approaches were all different so difficult to compare and they were limited by size (all were single-centered) and methodology (Ross et al. 2014). There was a need for large multicenter robust studies to find answers to these questions.

Between 2010 and 2016, three landmark studies were conducted by a European group of nurse/midwifery academics (McSherry et al. 2020). Building on the work of van Leuuwen et al. (2009), a 54-item spiritual care competency framework for student nurses and midwives was developed from an in-depth review of the international literature and consultation with stakeholders (focus groups) and spiritual care experts (two-stage modified delphi) (Attard et al. 2019a, b). Concurrently, a cross-sectional pilot study (Ross et al. 2016) and subsequent longitudinal study involving 2,193 student nurses/midwives from 21 universities in 8 countries identified that spiritual care competency develops over students' studies, even in low-scoring students (Ross et al. 2018). The personal spirituality of students and how they perceive spirituality are key factors in self-assessed spiritual care competency. Caring for patients, personal life events and teaching/discussion are important to students in helping them develop spiritual caring skills (Ross et al. 2018).

The next step involved bringing together nurse/midwifery educators (31 from 21 European countries) and key stakeholders (e.g. Governments, professional bodies, public, students, service users) to consider this evidence and how it might be used in '***E***nhancing Nurses and Midwives Competence in ***P***roviding Spiritual Care through ***I***nnovative Education and ***C***ompassionate ***C***are' (EPICC Project funded by Erasmus+ K2). EPICC sought to address the gaps in nurse education producing important new outputs:

- Clarification on how 'spirituality' and 'spiritual care' are understood (EPICC Spiritual Care Education Standard)

[1] Spiritual Care Competence Questionnaire (SCCQ) available from https://www.spiritual-competence.net Accessed 14 September 2020

- Four spiritual care competencies (distilled from Attard et al. 2019a, b, and based on van Leeuwen et al. 2009) setting out the knowledge, skills and attitudes expected of nurses (EPICC Spiritual Care Education Standard)
- Evidence-based guidance on the content and delivery of undergraduate nurse education programs (EPICC Gold Standard Education Matrix and Standard)
- Teaching and learning activities to support student learning (EPICC Toolkit) freely available on a website (www.epicc-network.org) with opportunity for continued sharing of best practice (EPICC Network) (McSherry et al. 2020).

How Realistic Is It for Nurses to Provide Spiritual Care?

A commonly cited reason for nurses not providing spiritual care is that it takes extra time that nurses simply do not have as they strive to meet increasing demands, changing roles and often with fewer resources (Salmond & Echevarria 2017). However, if spiritual care is integral rather than additional to nursing care, as suggested in this chapter, it may not necessarily require extra time. To address this concern about time and to help nurses to provide spiritual care, we developed the Two Question Spiritual Assessment Model (2Q-SAM, Ross and McSherry 2018), which can be found in the EPICC Toolkit (www.epicc-network.org). The two questions are: 'What's most important to you? And 'How can we help? We suggest that if care is directed by these two questions, it will be person-centered, prudent, coproduced and 'spiritual' because it is responding to actual expressed and current need, focusing on what is most important and meaningful to the person at any moment—care that is dynamic and 'moves in whatever direction need requires' (NES 2010). Sometimes it may involve doing something 'extra', but it may also mean that some tasks (perceived as important by the nurse but not by the patient) are not needed. So overall it could save time, or at least ensure that time is used efficiently. Of course, peoples' situations can be complex. We address some of these complexities, such as the person who is unconscious or has difficulty in articulating their spiritual needs, in another book chapter. We also provide examples of how the model might be applied in different settings: emergency department; psychology; adolescent HIV/AIDS care in Thailand (McSherry et al. 2019).

Conclusion

It is important for nurses to be able to address the spiritual needs of the people they look after because doing so promotes well-being, which is a key aspect of their holistic caring role. One instrument that enables the assessment of spiritual needs is the Spiritual Needs Questionnaire (SpNQ)[2], which can be used both within a clinical context or as a measuring instrument in research investigations. The EPICC Project provides the first evidence-based resources to equip nurses and those who educate them for fulfilling this part of their role.

References

Alligood MR (2014) Nursing Theorists and their work (8th Edition) Elsevier St. Louis, Missouri. Available from http://docshare01.docshare.tips/files/29843/298436680.pdf. Accessed 2 September 2020

Andrews J, Butler M (2014) Trusted to Care An independent Review of the Princess of Wales Hospital and Neath Port Talbot Hospital at Abertawe Bro Morgannwg University Health Board. http://www.wales.nhs.uk/sitesplus/documents/863/1%20%28vii%29%20'Trusted%20to%20Care'%20Report.pdf. Accessed 2 September 2020

Astrow A, Kwok G, Sharma R, Fromer N, Sulmasy D (2018) Spiritual Needs and Perception of Quality of Care and Satisfaction With Care in Hematology/Medical Oncology Patients: A Multicultural Assessment. J Pain Symptom Manage 55:56–64. https://doi.org/10.1016/j.jpainsymman.2017.08.009

Attard J, Ross L, Weeks K (2019a) Developing a spiritual care competency framework for pre-registration nurses and midwives. Nurse Educ Pract 40:102604. https://doi.org/10.1016/j.nepr.2019.07.010

Attard J, Ross L, Weeks K (2019b) Design and development of a spiritual care competency framework for pre-registration nurses and midwives: a modified Delphi study. Nurse Educ Pract 39:96–104. https://doi.org/10.1016/j.nepr.2019.08.003

Austin P, MacLeod R, Siddall P, McSherry W, Egan R (2017) Spiritual Care Training is Needed for Clinical and non-Clinical Staff to Manage Patients' Spiritual Needs. Journal for the Study of Spirituality 7(1):50–53. https://doi.org/10.1080/20440243.2017.1290031

[2] Spiritual Needs Questionnaire (SpNQ) available from www.spiritualneeds.net Accessed 16 September 2020

Balboni TA, Fitchett G, Handzo GF, Johnson KS, Koenig HG, Pargament KI, Puchalski CM, Sinclair S, Taylor EJ, Steinhauser KE (2017) State of the Science of Spirituality and Palliative Care Research Part II: Screening, Assessment, and Interventions. J Pain Symptom Manage 54(3):441–453. https://doi.org/10.1016/j.jpainsymman.2017.07.029

Balthip S, McSherry W, Kittikorn N (2017) Spirituality and Dignity of Thai Adolescents Living with HIV. Religions 8:257. https://doi.org/10.3390/rel8120257

Candy B, Jones L, Varagunam M, Speck P, Tookman A, King M (2012) Spiritual and religious interventions for wellbeing of adults in the terminal phase of disease. The Cochrane Library, Wiley, London, p 5

Clark CC, Hunter J (2018) Spirituality, spiritual wellbeing, and spiritual coping in advanced heart failure. A review of the literature. J Holist Nurs 37(1):56–73

Clarke J (2013) Spiritual care in everyday nursing practice. A new approach. Palgrave Macmillan, Basingstoke

Cockell N, McSherry W (2012) Spiritual care in nursing: an overview of published international literature. J Nurs Manag 20:958–969

Deng L, Liu H (2020) Research progress in the definition, assessment tools, and practice of spiritual care. Frontiers of Nursing 7(2):81–86. https://doi.org/10.2478/FON-2020-0014

Egan R, Llewellyn R, Cox B, MacLeod R, McSherry W, Austin P (2017) New Zealand nurses' perceptions of spirituality and spiritual care: qualitative findings from a national survey. Religions 8(5):79. https://doi.org/10.3390/rel8050079

Frick E, Theiss M, Rodrigues Recchia D, Büssing A (2019) Validierung einer deutschsprachigen Skala zur Messung der Spiritual Care Kompetenz. Spiritual Care 8(2):1. https://doi.org/10.1515/spircare-2018-0066

Gillilan R, Qawi S, Weymiller A, Puchalski CM (2017) Spiritual distress and spiritual care in advanced heart failure. Heart Fail Rev 22:581–591. https://doi.org/10.1007/s10741-017-9635-2

Gijsberts M, Liefbroer A, Otten R, Olsman E (2019) Spiritual Care in Palliative Care: A Systematic Review of the Recent European Literature. Med Sci 7:25. https://doi.org/10.3390/medsci7020025

Hay D (2006) Something there: the biology of the human spirit. Darton Longman and Todd, London

Henderson V (1964) The nature of nursing. Am J Nurs 64:62–68

International Council of Nurses (2012) The ICN Code of ethics for nurses. ICN, Geneva

King M (2014) The challenge of research into religion and spirituality (Keynote 1). Journal for the Study of Spirituality 4(2):106–120

McEvoy L, Duffy A (2008) Holistic Practice – A Concept Analysis. Nurse Educ Pract 8:412–419

McSherry W, Draper P (1998) The debates emerging from the literature surrounding the concept of spirituality as applied to nursing. J Adv Nurs 27(4):683–691

McSherry W (2016) Reintegrating spirituality and dignity in nursing and health care: a relational model of practice. In: Tranvåg O, Synnes O, McSherry W (eds) Stories of Dignity within Healthcare: Research, narratives and theories, vol 6. M&K Publishing, Keswick, pp 75–96

McSherry W, Ross L, Balthip Q, Ross N, Young S (2019) Spiritual assessment in healthcare: an overview of comprehensive, sensitive approaches to spiritual assessment for use within the interdisciplinary healthcare team. In: Timmins F, Caldeira S (eds) Spirituality in Healthcare: Perspectives for Innovative Practice. Springer Nature, Switzerland

McSherry W, Ross L, Attard J, van Leeuwen R, Giske T, Kleiven T, Boughey A, and the EPICC Network (2020) Preparing undergraduate nurses and midwives for spiritual care: some developments in education over the last decade. Journal for the Study of Spirituality https://doi.org/10.1080/20440243.2020.1726053

Martsolf D, Mickley J (1998) The concept of spirituality in nursing theories: differing world-views and extent of focus. J Adv Nurs 27:294–303

Murgia C, Notarnicola I, Rocco G, Stievano A (2020) Spirituality in nursing: A concept analysis. Nurs Ethics 27(5):1327–1343. https://doi.org/10.1177/0969733020909534

Murray SA, Kendall M, Boyd K (2004) Exploring the spiritual needs of people dying of lung cancer or heart failure: a prospective qualitative interview study of patients and their carers. Palliat Med 18(1):39–45

NHS Education for Scotland (2010) Spiritual care matters. An introductory resource for all NHSScotland staff. https://www.nes.scot.nhs.uk/education-and-training/by-discipline/spiritual-care/about-spiritual-care/publications/spiritual-care-matters-an-introductory-resource-for-all-nhs-scotland-staff.aspx. Accessed 16 September 2020

National Secular Society (2011) Costing the heavens: Chaplaincy services in English NHS provider Trusts 2009/10 Available from https://www.secularism.org.uk/uploads/nss-chaplaincy-report-2011-4.pdf. Accessed 5 September 2020

Niu Y, McSherry W, Partridge M (2020a) The Perceptions of Spirituality and Spiritual Care Among People From Chinese Backgrounds Living in England: A Grounded Theory Method Journal of Transcultural Nursing https://doi.org/10.1177/2F1043659620938135

Niu Y, McSherry W, Partridge M (2020b) An understanding of spirituality and spiritual care among people from Chinese backgrounds: A grounded theory study Journal of Advanced Nursing https://doi.org/10.1111/jan.14474

Nolan S, Saltmarsh P, Leget C (2011) Spiritual care in palliative care: working towards an EAPC task force. Eur J Palliat Care 18(2):86–89

Nursing and Midwifery Council (2015) The Code. NMC, London. https://www.nmc.org.uk/standards/code

Papathanasiou I, Sklavou M, Kourkouta L (2013) Holistic nursing Care: theories and perspectives. American Journal of Nursing Science 2(1):1–5. https://doi.org/10.11648/j.ajns.20130201.11

Pike J (2011) Spirituality in nursing: a systematic review of the literature from 2006-10. Br J Nurs 20(12):743–749. https://doi.org/10.12968/bjon.2011.20.12.743

Puchalski C, Vitillo R, Hull S, Reller N (2014) Improving the spiritual dimension of whole person care: reaching national and international consensus. J Palliat Med 17(6):642–656. https://doi.org/10.1089/2Fjpm.2014.9427

Rogers JG, Patel CB, Mentz RJ, Granger B, Steinhauser K, Fiuzat M, Adams P, Speck P, Johnson K, Krishnamoorthy A, Yang H, Anstrom K, Dodson G, Taylor D, Kirchner J, Mark D, O'Connor C, Tulsky J (2017) Palliative care in heart failure: the PAL-HF randomised controlled clinical trial. J Am Coll Cardiol 70:331–341

Ross LA (1994) Spiritual aspects of nursing. J Adv Nurs 19:439–447. https://doi.org/10.1111/j.1365-2648.1994.tb01105.x

Ross LA (2006) Spiritual care in nursing: an overview of the research to date. J Clin Nurs 15(7):852–862. https://doi.org/10.1111/j.1365-2702.2006.01617.x

Ross L, Giske T, van Leeuwen R, Baldacchino D, McSherry W, Narayanasamy A, Jarvis P, Schep-Akkerman A (2016) Factors contributing to student nurses'/midwives' perceived competency in spiritual care. Nurse Educ Today 36:445–451. https://doi.org/10.1016/j.nedt.2015.10.005

Ross L, van Leeuwen R, Baldacchino D, Giske T, McSherry W, Narayanasamy A, Downes C, Jarvis P, Schep-Akkerman A (2014) Student nurses perceptions of spirituality and competence in delivering spiritual care: A European pilot study. Nurse Educ Today 34(5):697–702. https://doi.org/10.1016/j.nedt.2013.09.014

Ross L, McSherry W (2010) Considerations for the future of spiritual assessment. In: McSherry W, Ross L (eds) Spiritual assessment in healthcare practice, vol 9. M&K Publishing, Keswick, pp 161–171

Ross L, McSherry W (2018) Two questions that ensure person-centred spiritual care. Nursing Standard. https://rcni.com/nursing-standard/features/two-questions-ensure-person-centred-spiritual-care-137261. Accessed 4 October 2019

Ross L, McSherry W, Giske T, van Leeuwen R, Schep-Akkerman A, Koslander T, Hall J, Østergaard Steenfeldt V, Jarvis P (2018) Nursing and midwifery students' perceptions of spirituality, spiritual care, and spiritual care competency: a prospective, longitudinal, correlational European study. Nurse Educ Today 67:64–71. https://doi.org/10.1016/j.nedt.2018.05.002

Ross L, Miles J (2019) Spirituality in heart failure: a review of the literature from 2014-2019 to identify spiritual care needs and spiritual interventions. Curr Opin Support Palliat Care 14(1):9–18. https://doi.org/10.1097/SPC.0000000000000475

Royal College of Nursing (RCN) (2011) Spirituality Survey 2010. https://www.rcn.org.uk/professional-development/publications/pub-003861. Accessed 18 November 2019

Royal College of Physicians (2016) End of life care audit – dying in hospital: National report for England 2016. https://www.rcplondon.ac.uk/projects/outputs/end-life-care-audit-dying-hospital-national-report-england-2016. Accessed 16 October 2019

Salmond SW, Echevarria M (2017) Healthcare Transformation and Changing Roles for Nursing. Orthop Nurs 36(1):12–25. https://doi.org/10.1097/NOR.0000000000000308

Selman L, Brighton L, Sinclair S, Karvinen I, Egan R, Speck P, Powell R, Deskir-Smielecka E, Glajchen M, Adler S, Puchalski C, Hunter J, Gikaara N, Hope J (2017) Patients' and caregivers' needs, experiences, preferences and research priorities in spiritual care: a focus group study across nine countries. Palliat Med 32(1):216–230. https://doi.org/10.1177/2F0269216317734954

Steinhauser K, Fitchett G, Handzo G, Johnson K, Koenig H, Pargament K, Puchalski C, Sinclair S, Taylor E, Balboni T (2017) State of the Science of Spirituality and Palliative Care Research Part I: Definitions, Measurement, and Outcomes. J Pain Symptom Manage 54(3):428–440. https://doi.org/10.1016/j.jpainsymman.2017.07.028

Swinton J (2010) The meanings of spirituality: a multi-perspective approach to 'the spiritual'. In: McSherry W, Ross L (eds) Spiritual assessment in healthcare. M&K, Keswick

Swinton J (2020) BASS ten years on. Journal for the Study of Spirituality 10(1):6–14. https://doi.org/10.1080/20440243.2020.1728869

Tanyi R (2002) Towards clarification of the meaning of spirituality. J Adv Nurs 39(5):500–509. https://doi.org/10.1046/j.1365-2648.2002.02315.x

The Mid Staffordshire NHS Foundation Trust Public Inquiry (2013) Report of the Mid Staffordshire NHS Foundation Trust Public Inquiry https://www.gov.uk/government/publications/report-of-the-mid-staffordshire-nhs-foundation-trust-public-inquiry/ Accessed 31 October 2015

The Parliamentary and Health Service Ombudsman (2011) Care and Compassion Report of the Health Service Ombudsman on ten investigations into NHS care of older people. http://www.ombudsman.org.uk/__data/assets/pdf_file/0016/7216/Care-and-Compassion-PHSO-0114web.pdf. Accessed 31 January 2015

van Leeuwen R, Tiesinga L, Middel B, Post D, Jochemsen H (2009) The validity and reliability of an instrument to assess nursing competencies in spiritual care. J Clin Nurs 18:2857–2869
Weathers E, McCarthy G, Coffey A (2016) Concept analysis of spirituality: an evolutionary approach. Nurs Forum 51(2):79–96. https://doi.org/10.1111/nuf.12128
WHOQOL SRPB Group (2006) A cross-cultural study of spirituality, religion, and personal beliefs as components of quality of life. Soc Sci Med 62:1486–1497

CHAPTER 30

Addressing Spiritual Needs in Faith Community Nursing

Helen A. Wordsworth

Introduction

"Faith Community Nurses, (known in some countries including the United Kingdom as *Parish Nurses*), are licensed, registered nurses who practice whole-person health for self, individuals and the community using nursing knowledge combined with spiritual care. They function in paid and unpaid positions as members of the pastoral team in a variety of religious faiths, cultures, and countries." (Westberg Institute, Definition of Faith Community Nursing n.d.)

While they seek to address all aspects of whole-person health care, assisting people to maintain and/or regain wholeness in physical, mental, emotional, social, spiritual and environmental aspects of life, the focus of their work is the intentional care of the spirit. They offer care to people of all faiths and none, working largely through local Christian churches of various denominations, but they may also be found working with other

H. A. Wordsworth (✉)
Parish Nursing Ministries, Westberg Institute for Faith Community Nursing, Peterborough, UK
e-mail: wordsworthh@churchhealth.org

A. Büssing (ed.), *Spiritual Needs in Research and Practice*,
https://doi.org/10.1007/978-3-030-70139-0_30

faith groups and faith-based organizations of different kinds. They receive specific training for this role through accessing a course based on the curriculum developed by the Westberg Institute for Faith Community Nursing, which is also available in an international version (Westberg Institute, Education for Faith Community Nursing n.d.).

History

The contemporary expression of Faith Community nursing began as "parish nursing" in Chicago in the 1980s through the initiative of Revd. Dr. Granger Westberg, a Lutheran hospital chaplain. He saw the potential for health promotion and support that could be offered through congregations, together with the spiritual care that could be provided alongside. But faith community nursing also had an older pedigree; well before the advent of modern health services, there were nurses employed by faith communities to reach out to the poor and the sick with both health-promoting activity and spiritual care. Religious orders offered care for the sick, and faith communities initiated hospitals as far back as 1123 in London, England (Barts Health NHS Trust, History of St Bartholomew's Hospital n.d.). Boulton (2007) records parish nurses as being present in London as early as the seventeenth century. Florence Nightingale and Mary Seacole were both inspired by their faith to engage in care for wounded soldiers (Coakley 1990; Catholic faith of Mary Seacole) and in the nineteenth century, churches employed deaconesses who had to do nurse training before they were sent out into local communities (Wordsworth 2015).

During the twentieth century, responsibility for health care was taken on by state-sponsored health systems and the role of faith communities became somewhat limited to health care chaplaincy and hospice care. In contrast, Westberg's experiment with six nurses in Chicago in 1986 led to an education program for qualified nurses, further growth among churches of different denominations, and international developments. The majority of these are based in the United States, but they may also be found in at least 29 other countries, including Finland, Canada, Australia, New Zealand, Nigeria, several Southern Africa countries, the Philippines, Taiwan, the United Kingdom, Germany, the Ukraine, Pakistan and Brazil (Westberg Insititute, International Faith Community Nursing n.d.).

Range of Practice

Faith Community Nurses work largely in a community context, and with the service user's permission, may liaise with other health providers as appropriate. They offer their service to people of all faiths and none, and from birth to old age. This gives them the opportunity to engage with service users and their families on a regular and long-term basis. Where a person requests to be referred to another faith group, or to another professional who is not working from a faith-based organization, they will action that request. Their practice covers health education and early detection of disease, through support for short- and long-term medical conditions, to end-of-life concerns.

Statistical data of 25 UK parish nurses over the three months from January to March 2020 indicated that:

- There were 5,570 service users, of which 1,987 were not regular worshippers with any faith community.
- The total number of interventions was 7,941.
- Of these, 1,662 interventions could be defined as spiritual care, involving issues related to meaning of life, the search for peace, connection with others, and transcendence. Of these 989 were with people who had long-term medical conditions. (Source, unpublished statistical returns to Parish Nursing Ministries UK, used by permission.)

Clearly, these nurses were making a significant impact in the field of spiritual care. In the following three months, during the COVID-19 outbreak and lockdown in the United Kingdom, the number of spiritual care interventions by parish nurses increased threefold.

Training

There is an international curriculum of 36.5 h for qualified nurses that can be offered by any approved institution with appropriately qualified faculty as an online or in-person course. Certification and faculty training is provided through the Westberg Institute for Faith Community Nursing, currently based in Memphis, Tennessee. The course can be contextualized for different cultures and consists of modules in spiritual care and prayer, professional practice, ethics, communication and collaboration, world faiths, leadership, volunteer coordination and management, among others.

In some countries, nurses who have a faith background face opposition in addressing the spiritual health needs of their patients. Faith Community nursing and its associated curriculum are founded on Judaeo-Christian values but both the practice and the course are accessible to all, and respect is offered to those from other faith or non-faith backgrounds. Nurses should not engage in discussion on politics or religion in inappropriate ways (NMC Nursing & Midwifery Council, Code of practice n.d.). But there appears to be considerable fear (some of which has occasionally been justified), of an overenthusiastic state-funded nurse persuading vulnerable patients to change their faith position. However, such caution should not result in the abandonment of spiritual care as part of nursing practice, and ways must be found to help all nurses rediscover the value of presence, active listening, spiritual assessment, intervention, and sometimes prayer, in the process of healing. As with other nursing interventions, choice should always be offered and respected, documentation completed and evaluation considered.

Faith Community nurses have an intentional focus on spiritual care, but even they sometimes find it difficult to know how to begin a conversation in this domain, given their secular training and experience in state-funded institutions. A professional assessment tool can therefore be the key to unlock discussion around this sensitive topic.

In the United Kingdom, several forms of assessment have been utilized, in the attempt to cover all aspects of whole-person care, including spiritual care. But for service users who have longer-term medical conditions, the need for a more in-depth spiritual care assessment has been recognized; hence the search for an effective, validated tool.

Exploring the Available Options

Faith Community nurses in the United States were using the HOPE (Anandarajah and Hight 2001) or FICA (Puchalski and Romer 2000) models of assessment. These gave a structure to the verbatim assessment but were not prescriptive of the wording to be used.

Hope stands for:

H—Sources of hope
O—Organized religion

P—Personal Spirituality
E—Effect on treatment

FICA stands for:

F—Faith and belief: What is their faith if they have one?
I—Importance: How important is it to them?
C—Community: What links, if any, do they have with a faith community?
A—Address in care: How may their religious needs be addressed in their care?

Neither of these worked well in a UK community context, largely because they concentrated on a person's religious needs and how those should be respected in a health care institution. UK parish nurses recognized that spiritual care with service users in their homes was more comprehensive and long-term in nature. Alternative sources were examined. Some focused on cancer patients only, others on specific age groups. Some were too long and complicated, and some omitted reference to anything of a transcendental nature.

The Spiritual Needs Questionnaire (SpNQ) (Büssing et al. 2010, 2018) was of interest because it was relatively short, covered all four domains of spiritual care, and had been validated with people suffering chronic pain conditions and cancer, which was similar to the largest category of service users benefitting from the attention of a Faith Community nurse. It also included questions about transcendent aspects of spirituality, and given that most Parish nurses work from a faith community, this was important.

One small problem was that the direct translation from the German required minor modification in order for the meaning to be understood by both the nurses and the service users. This was done using two fluent German speakers in order to be sure that the wording was as near to the original sense as possible.

Using the SpNQ to Form a Care Plan

Nursing assessments are only of use if the results are incorporated, either formally or informally, into the plan of care. Not all needs can be addressed in this way, and not all needs can be "fixed." But Parish nurses normally work with their service users to develop a personalized plan of care, involving achievable goals, ways of implementation and evaluation. It was therefore necessary to devise a way to use this questionnaire to feed into a typical nursing care action plan such as that in Table 30.1.

The suggested way to do this was to take those questions that had identified the strongest needs, and add them to the column on the left. For each line, an achievable goal would be agreed, ways of reaching that goal would be discussed, and action would be implemented. The spiritual care interventions would therefore be verbalized and evaluated. This would result in outcome data that could prove to be very useful in demonstrating the value of parish nursing to individuals, to faith groups and to funders. An example is offered to demonstrate this process in Table 30.1.

Pilot Testing with 25 Parish Nurses

The questionnaire and its accompanying action plan proforma, along with the example shown in Table 30.1, were then made available, with an hour of introduction and explanation, to a small pilot group.

Parish nurses used the questionnaire with service users needing long-term support. Twenty-five Parish nurses participated in the pilot study with 28 service users in all. Two nurses returned the SpNQ without an attached care plan, but had used it to inform their care planning for those service users.

Several parish nurses felt that the original meaning of the main question had been lost in translation. So "In the last time did you have had the needs?" became "In the past week have you felt that the following needs were unmet?" This small change clarified the question for the UK context.

The SpNQ responses yielded a variety of unmet needs. The average number of strong needs was 6 per patient/client (ranging from 0 to 9). The nurses had used these "very strong" ticks as a starting point for their care plans, and had recorded some very creative ways to address those needs. They had implemented the interventions and documented the outcomes. In most cases, the outcome had shown some progress toward a shared goal, and enabled discussion with the service user about next steps. A real benefit was that their spiritual care outcomes could now be demonstrated to their employers and potential funders of parish nursing, along with the outcomes already documented in the domains of physical health and mental health.

Table 30.1 Nursing action plan based on the Spiritual Needs Questionnaire

Client:	*Age: 69; Gender: female; Initials: YB; Condition if known: Chemotherapy*					
	Assessment		*Planning*	*Implementation*	*Evaluation*	
Date	Need (no.) as identified very strong by service user	Achievable aim	Planned interventions	Action taken and date	Outcome	Next steps
Sept 2018	For example, N28, N25 housebound lady needs to have more contact with family and grandchildren in particular	Learns to use "WhatsApp" or Facebook and communicates at least once a week	Purchase of mobile device, internet access and DBS checked volunteer to teach use	October 2018 Funds accessed from local rotary club for equipment and volunteer recruited	November 2018 Volunteer has visited, device set up and contact made with grandchildren	Motivate grandchildren! Volunteer to revisit weekly over four weeks PN to check outcome in January 2019
Sept 2018	For example, N20 wishes to pray themselves	Uses written prayers in own space and time	PN ascertains prayer concerns and writes/finds appropriate prayers. Holding cross or similar image may be helpful	October 2018 PN takes written prayers and reads them to her	November 2018 Service user requests more prayers	PN takes further prayer resources

Wordsworth (unpublished work)

Value to the Practice of Faith Community Nursing

Parish nurses tended to use the questionnaire with service users needing long-term support, but only felt comfortable in doing that once they had begun to establish a good working relationship with them. Some nurses found the questionnaire too long to be completed in one visit. In these cases, the 8-item SpNQ Screener could be used. Others said that the concentration levels of their service users were not sufficient, so they used the questionnaire as a guide, and asked only those questions that seemed most appropriate. There were several informal comments about the time it took to work through the questionnaire, but also that it seemed to be a worthwhile investment of time given the outcomes. Two written comments were received along with the responses:

> *I really enjoyed using them and they certainly highlighted needs that I wouldn't have realised were there. Definitely a useful tool to discover and action upon less obvious needs.* (LB)
>
> *I found the questionnaire most helpful and enlightening, showing that unmet spiritual needs can affect all areas of a service-user's life. The care plan helped to show that sometimes actual steer helped to move someone on when they were thinking that there was nothing that could be done.* (DW)

Value to the Organization and Parish Nurses

Parish Nursing Ministries UK already had output data from the nurses about their activities, including those in the area of spiritual care. Use of the SpNQ and associated care plan helped the nurses to understand their role in spiritual care more clearly and to measure the outcomes as well as the outputs. It enhanced the teaching of spiritual care to new parish nurses, and has provided the organization with a tool to explore in more depth the detail of spiritual care interventions and outcomes.

The nurses were used to documenting their work, since that is required of them by the Nursing and Midwifery Council. They were also familiar with the use of assessments and care plans. However, many of them had previously worked in a very secular health service facility, where spiritual care had been minimized by lack of time. In some cases, Christian nurses working in those institutions had been afraid to begin "spiritual" conversations for fear of being accused of proselytization. They consequently found that introducing the topic of spiritual need into a nursing context very difficult. The SpNQ gave them a way in to those essential conversations.

Conclusion

Faith Community nurses pay special attention to care of the spirit. They do this by means of presence, observation, active listening and codeveloped planning of responsive interventions. Use of the SpNQ assessment tool has been found to be helpful in beginning spiritual care conversations, prompting appropriate questions, identifying the most pressing needs, and then going on to develop a jointly owned care plan with the service user. The associated care plan proforma has enabled the formulation of step-by-step interventions, the outcomes of which can then be recorded, evaluated and made available to stakeholders. Furthermore, the SpNQ has become useful in teaching the practical delivery of spiritual care to new Faith Community nurses.

References

Anandarajah G, Hight E (2001) Spirituality and medical practice: using the HOPE questions as a practical tool for spiritual assessment. Am Fam Physician 63:81–89

Barts Health NHS Trust History of St Bartholomew's Hospital (n.d.). https://www.bartshealth.nhs.uk/st-bartholomews-our-history/ Accessed 27 July 2020

Boulton J (2007) Welfare systems and the parish nurse in early modern London, 1650–1725. Family and Community History 10(2):127–151

Büssing A, Balzat HJ, Heusser P (2010) Spiritual needs of patients with chronic pain diseases and cancer—validation of the Spiritual Needs Questionnaire. Eur J Med Res 15:266–273

Büssing A, Recchia DR, Koenig H, Baumann K, Frick E (2018) Factor structure of the Spiritual Needs Questionnaire (SpNQ) in persons with chronic diseases, elderly and healthy individuals. Religions 9:13. https://doi.org/10.3390/rel9010013

Coakley ML (1990) Faith of Florence Nightingale. Christianity Today 25. https://www.christianitytoday.com/history/issues/issue-25/ Accessed 10 August 2020

NMC Nursing & Midwifery Council (n.d.) Code of practice. https://www.nmc.org.uk/standards/code/read-the-code-online/ Accessed 10 August 2020

Puchalski C, Romer AL (2000) Taking a spiritual history allows clinicians to understand patients more fully. J Palliat Med 3:129–137

Werstberg Institute, International Faith Community Nursing (n.d.). https://westberginstitute.org/international-faith-community-nursing/ Accessed 27 July 2020

Westberg Institute, Definition of Faith Community Nursing (n.d.). https://westberginstitute.org/faith-community-nursing/ Accessed 24 June 2020
Westberg Institute, Education for Faith Community Nursing (n.d.). https://westberginstitute.org/ Accessed 10 August 2020
Wordsworth H (2015) Rediscovering a Ministry of Health: Parish nursing as a mission of the local church. Wipf and Stock, Oregon

CHAPTER 31

Physician's Perspectives on Addressing Patients' Spiritual Needs

Lubna Hammoudeh and Tracy Balboni

The Physician's Professional Role in Addressing Spiritual Needs

As first-line caregivers, physicians have an important role in caring for patients at times of serious illness. Physicians are highly trained to provide care to uphold patients' physical well-being, but they are also called upon to address the other domains of health, including emotional, social, and spiritual (Sulmasy 2002; Ramondetta et al. 2013), particularly to screen for needs and refer to specialty providers. Notable to a physician's responsibility in spiritual care, most seriously ill patients want their physicians to address the spiritual aspects of illness, including their spiritual needs (Maugans and Wadland 1991; King and Bushwick 1994; Balboni et al. 2013). Furthermore, spiritual care of patients with serious illness has been demonstrated to be associated with important outcomes (Wall et al. 2007;

L. Hammoudeh • T. Balboni (✉)
Supportive and Palliative Radiation Oncology Program, Brigham and Women's Hospital/Dana-Farber Cancer Institute, Harvard Medical School, Boston, MA, USA
e-mail: Lubna_Hammoudeh@dfci.harvard.edu; tbalboni@bwh.harvard.edu

A. Büssing (ed.), *Spiritual Needs in Research and Practice*,
https://doi.org/10.1007/978-3-030-70139-0_31

Astrow et al. 2007; Balboni et al. 2007, 2011; Williams et al. 2011) including better patient quality of life, greater transitions to hospice care, less aggressive end-of-life care, and greater satisfaction with medical care. However, physicians are not trained to be professional providers of spiritual care—that is a role for chaplains and other spiritual care professionals. This raises the question of what is the physician's professional role?

The National Consensus Project for Quality (2019) provides the most comprehensive guideline for the provision of spiritual care, domain five of eight palliative care domains, outlined in Table 31.1. Across each component of spiritual care, physicians have a clear, though circumscribed spiritual care role (Table 31.1). That role is, as a member of a larger interdisciplinary team that includes a spiritual care professional (e.g., chaplain), the physician participating in SC through spiritual history-taking and screenings (or supporting others on the interdisciplinary team to do this standardly, e.g., nurses doing spiritual histories and screenings at patient intakes); recognizing patient spirituality and attendant values and needs within illness; and supporting the spiritual care plan for patients and their families.

As an example, a physician upon meeting a newly diagnosed advanced cancer patient in consultation learns through a spiritual history that he is Muslim and that his faith plays a central role in his life and in his coping with illness. When that patient becomes an inpatient a few months later, the physician—informed by her prior spiritual history—screens for spiritual needs, including asking the patient if he would like to see a spiritual care professional, for example, his Imam or the Muslim chaplain. He indicates this would be helpful, and that he has already contacted his Imam. The physician indicates to the patient's nurse that the patient's Muslim faith is important to him, and she asks the nurse to call the Muslim chaplain. The patient's Imam, with whom he has a long relationship, visits him in the hospital to provide support to him and his family. The patient is provided a prayer rug by the chaplain, and the location of Mecca is indicated on the wall. Months later, the patient's illness has rapidly progressed and during a clinic visit, the physician discusses with him and his wife transitioning to hospice care. He is unsure about this decision, and the physician invites the patient to discuss this with his wife and his three adult children. She also suggests he discuss this with his Imam, indicating that if the patient wishes, she is happy to discuss this medical decision with his Imam as well. The patient declines this, but indicates he will discuss this decision with his family and with his Imam and will follow-up in the

Table 31.1 National Consensus Project for Quality Palliative Care spiritual, religious, and existential aspects of care components and the corresponding role of physicians

Spiritual care component	*Summary of spiritual care component*	*Physician spiritual care role*
Global aspects of spiritual care	Patient and family spirituality and related practices are recognized and respected. All members are trained in and recognize spiritual care as an important aspect of care. Chaplains are integrated into care as specialty providers of spiritual care.	Physicians recognize patient and family spirituality, including knowing when to refer to specialty palliative care providers.
Spiritual screening and assessment	Spiritual history and subsequent screenings are included as part of clinical assessments. A spiritual assessment, which includes exploration of spiritual needs, is prompted by spiritual history/screenings, and is performed by a trained spiritual care practitioner.	Physicians are trained in, and perform, spiritual histories as part of initial assessments, and spiritual screenings.
Spiritual care plan	Spiritual care plan is based on patient's/family's needs and goals. Spiritual care is documented in the chart. Patients/families are supported and accommodated in bringing their spiritual/cultural symbols into the health care setting (e.g., hospital room).	Physicians, as a member of the interdisciplinary team, supports the spiritual care plan for patients and families, and ensures they are aware of the spiritual care plan.
Ongoing spiritual care	Ongoing spiritual care is provided, with ongoing spiritual screenings and adjustments in the plan of care with changes in patient/family spiritual needs.	Physician, as a member of the interdisciplinary team, supports ongoing spiritual care provision by participating in ongoing screenings. and being aware of changes to the spiritual care plan.

future. The patient returns two weeks later and indicates he wishes to start hospice care at home.

This anecdote provides an example of the circumscribed but important role physicians have in providing SC, most notably in spiritual history-taking, screenings, and involving spiritual care specialists into care. One can readily see in this example how even if the physician has a very different spiritual background from the patient and family, such care can be provided in a patient-centered, respectful, and professional manner. Furthermore, this example demonstrates how SC acknowledges and respects a patient's spirituality, honoring it as an important aspect of the advanced illness experience.

Physician's Perceptions, Practices, and Barriers to Addressing Spirituality and Spiritual Needs within Care

A majority of physicians have a positive perception of spiritual care, viewing it as an important component of care within serious illness (Balboni et al. 2013, 2014). For example, in a study of 339 oncology and palliative care clinicians (Balboni et al. 2013), 80% of physicians and 87% of nurses thought that SC should be at least occasionally provided to cancer patients. However, only 24% of physicians and 31% of nurses had ever provided spiritual care to their last three patients seen in clinic. Notably, 68 advanced cancer patients were randomly sampled (response rate 73%) from the same institutions where the clinicians were surveyed (Balboni et al. 2013). Most of these patients believed spiritual care from doctors (86%) and nurses (87%) to be an important part of cancer care. However, they reported infrequent receipt of SC—6% of patients had ever received SC from physicians, and 13% had ever received spiritual care from nurses.

The wide disparity between perceptions of the importance of spiritual care and the actual practices of spiritual care raises the question of what barriers prevent physicians from providing spiritual care. As part of the survey of 339 physicians and nurses, barriers to provision of SC were evaluated (Balboni et al. 2014).

Physician perceptions of spiritual care barriers are summarized in Table 31.2. The most common barriers cited included lack of time, training, and believing spiritual care is best performed by others, endorsed by majorities of physicians. Sizeable minorities endorsed feeling uncomfortable providing SC, feeling personally uncomfortable discussing spirituality, and feeling that SC is outside the bounds of a physician's professional role. Similar minority proportions of physicians had concerns that SC could negatively impact the patient/physician relationship, including

Table 31.2 Top ten spiritual care barriers perceived by physicians and adjusted odds ratios estimating barriers' associations with actual spiritual care provision

Spiritual care barriers	*Proportion viewing barrier as a "moderate" or "very significant" impediment to SC provision (%)*	*MVA assessing barrier's associations with actual SC provision by physicians [AOR, 95% CI]*
Lack of time	73	NS
Lack of spiritual care training	62	0.49 (0.25–0.98)
Spiritual care better provided by others	62	NS
Feeling uncomfortable providing spiritual care	48	0.51 (0.26–1.00)
Feeling personally uncomfortable discussing spiritual issues	47	0.27 (0.14–0.54)
I do not believe it is my professional role to engage patient spirituality	45	0.37 (0.18–0.75)
I am worried that patients will feel uncomfortable	44	0.35 (0.18–0.70)
I am worried that the power inequity between patient and doctor makes spiritual care inappropriate	43	0.39 (0.20–0.76)
Lack of private space to perform spiritual care	39	NS
Spirituality/religion are not important to me personally	28	NS

Abbreviations: SC—spiritual care; AOR—adjusted odds ratio; CI—confidence interval; NS—not significant

causing patients to feel uncomfortable, and/or that SC might be inappropriate given the power dynamic between patients and physicians.

Interestingly, the barriers endorsed by physicians were not necessarily predictive of physician-reported spiritual care provision to their last three patients seen in clinic. Most notably, lack of time, endorsed by the most physicians, was not significantly related to SC provision. One possible explanation for this finding is that those who feel the barrier of time on their provision of SC may also be the clinicians most likely to be providing SC; in contrast those who don't provide SC may be less likely to experience the lack the time to provide it. Furthermore, viewing SC as best performed by others—also endorsed by a majority—was not predictive of SC provision. However, barriers related to training, discomfort with SC, and concerns about its impact on their professional role and on the patient–physician relationship were significantly related to SC provision.

Barriers that remained significant predictors of SC provision in multivariable analysis can be understood as interrelated. Given that most of these physicians (86%) had not received spiritual care training, concerns related to professional boundaries in spiritual care as well as the patient-centered nature of spiritual care may be due to the lack of an understanding of their circumscribed role in spiritual care. If physicians understood that their role is limited in scope primarily to patient-centered history-taking and screenings and working with spiritual care practitioners, for example, chaplains; and if they were trained in doing spiritual histories, screening, and SC referrals, then these perceived barriers would likely be mitigated. This highlights the importance of training clinicians in SC provision. It is also important to note that physician concerns regarding professionalism and potential harm to the patient–physician relationship are an apt concern. Spiritual care that is not patient-centered and lacks respect for professional boundaries indeed has the potential to harm vulnerable patients and their families. In contrast, the lack of spiritual care provision to patients leaves this aspect of care entirely unaddressed, arguably also a non-patient-centered approach to care as this central aspect of the illness experience is ignored. Spiritual care training should address this tension directly, outlining the need for patient-centered spiritual care, while also setting clear boundaries for clinicians regarding their role in professionally appropriate, patient-centered spiritual care provision.

Spiritual Care Training for Physicians

The 2009 Spiritual Care Consensus Conference identified key competencies for providers of spiritual care in the palliative care setting relevant to the training of physicians (Puchalski et al. 2009). These include that all members of the palliative care team should:

- have the fundamental knowledge of spiritual screening and history-taking;
- be aware of spiritual resources available to patients in the hospital;

- be trained in the variable spiritual cultures;
- be enrolled in the varying spiritual care duties of different health care providers and when to consult each;
- have training in spiritual care with their scope of practice;
- have essential training in how spiritual beliefs can impact the patient's family medical decisions;
- have training in active listening.

Spiritual care of patients is highly predicted by clinician training in SC. Previous reports indicate that medical professionals who have been trained in SC had 11-fold greater odds of providing SC to their patients with advanced disease stage due to better understanding of the clinician's proper role in SC provision, which highlights its importance within initial and continuing education for physicians (Balboni et al. 2013).

Major gaps identified in SC education (Puchalski et al. 2009) include a shortage of evidence-based curricula to train physicians in the spiritual care competency areas, as well as the lack of standardized schemes for assessing those competencies. Research is needed to determine and further refine each of the spiritual care components identified by the National Consensus Project and the Spiritual Care Consensus Conference (Balboni et al. 2017; Koenig et al. 2010; Rasinski et al. 2011). Furthermore, spiritual care interdisciplinary roles of physicians, nurses, social workers, and chaplains need to be specified to guide training for each member of the interdisciplinary care team. Finally, data are needed to establish the impact of SC training for physicians and other providers on outcomes, such as patient/family quality of life, medical decisions, and bereavement outcomes (Puchalski et al. 2009).

Conclusion

Physicians have an important role in caring for the whole person in the setting of serious illness, including patient spirituality (Balboni et al. 2013). Physicians largely recognize that patient spirituality and addressing their spiritual needs is an important aspect of medical care. However, they also experience many barriers to spiritual care provision, resulting in spiritual care being absent from the care of most seriously ill patients. Physicians not fulfilling their circumscribed role in spiritual care provision—spiritual history-taking, screening, and referrals—has important implications for patient spiritual well-being since physicians act as central providers of their care. Key to ensuring their participation in basic spiritual care is addressing the many barriers to SC experienced by physicians. In particular, training and concerns about harm to the patient–physician relationship due to crossing professional boundaries are paramount. These concerns are critical to framing patient-centered spiritual care that is always circumscribed to physicians' professional role. Training will require the establishment of evidence-based medical curricula addressing the SC roles of physicians, alongside professional providers of spiritual care and other members of the clinical care team (Puchalski et al. 2009; Balboni et al. 2017; Koenig et al. 2010; Rasinski et al. 2011).

Acknowledgments Tracy Balboni is supported by a John Templeton Foundation Grant (Principle investigator Tyler VanderWeele, PhD).

References

Astrow AB, Wexler A, Texeira K, He MK, Sulmasy DP (2007) Is failure to meet spiritual needs associated with cancer patients'perceptions of quality of care and their satisfaction with care? J Clin Oncol 25(36):5753–5757

Balboni TA, Vanderwerker LC, Block SC, Paulk MD, Lathan CS, Peteet JR, Prigerson HG (2007) Religiousness and spiritual support among advanced cancer patients and associations with end-of-life treatment preferences and quality of life. J Clin Oncol 25:555–560

Balboni T, Balboni M, Paulk ME, Phelps A, Wright A, Peteet J, Block S, Lathan C, Vanderweele T, Prigerson H (2011) Support of cancer patients' spiritual needs and associations with medical care costs at the end of life. Cancer 117(23):5383–5391

Balboni MJ, Sullivan A, Amobi A, Phelps AC, Gorman DP, Zollfrank A, Peteet JR, Prigerson HG, Vanderweele TJ, Balboni TA (2013) Why is spiritual care infrequent at the end of life? Spiritual care perceptions among patients, nurses, and physicians and the role of training. J Clin Oncol 31(4):461–467

Balboni MJ, Sullivan A, Enzinger AC, Epstein-Peterson ZD, Tseng YD, Mitchell C, Niska J, Zollfrank A, VanderWeele TJ, Balboni TA (2014) Nurse and physician barriers to spiritual care provision at the end of life. J Pain Symptom Manag 48(3):400–410

Balboni TA, Fitchett G, Handzo GF, Johnson KJ, Koenig HG, Pargament KI, Puchalski CP, Sinclair S, Taylor EJ, Steinhauser KE (2017) State of the science of spirituality and palliative care research part II: screening, assessment, and interventions. J Pain Symptom Manag 54(3):441–453

King DE, Bushwick B (1994) Beliefs and attitudes of hospital inpatients about faith healing, and prayer. J Fam Pract 39:349–352

Koenig HG, Hooten EG, Lindsay-Calkins E, Meador KG (2010) Spirituality in medical school curricula: findings from a national survey. Int J Psychiatry Med 40:391–398

Maugans TA, Wadland WC (1991) Religion and family medicine: a survey of physicians and patients. J Fam Pract 32:210–213

National Consensus Project for Quality Palliative Care (2019) Clinical practice guidelines for quality palliative care 4th edition. https://www.nationalcoalitionhpc.org/ncp/. Accessed 7 Aug 2020

Puchalski C, Ferrell B, Virani R, Otis-Green S, Baird P, Bull J, Chochinov H, Handzo G, Nelson-Becker H, Prince-Paul M, Pugliese K, Sulmasy D (2009) Improving the quality of spiritual care as a dimension of palliative care: the report of the consensus conference. J Palliat Med 12:885–904

Ramondetta LM, Sun C, Surbone A, Olver I, Ripamonti C, Konishi T, Baider L, Johnson J (2013) Surprising results regarding MASCC members' beliefs about spiritual care. Support Care Cancer 21:2991–2998

Rasinski KA, Kalad YG, Yoon JD, Curlin FA (2011) An assessment of US physicians' training in religion, spirituality, and medicine. Med Teach 33:944–945

Sulmasy DP (2002) A biopsychosocial-spiritual model for the care of patients at the end of life. The Gerontologist 42:24–33

Wall RJ, Engelberg RA, Gries CJ, Glavan B, Curtis JR (2007) Spiritual care of families in the intensive care unit. Crit Care Med 35(4):1084–1090

Williams JA, Meltzer D, Arora V, Chung G, Curlin FA (2011) Attention to inpatients' religious and spiritual concerns: predictors and association with patient satisfaction. J Gen Intern Med 26:1265–1271

CHAPTER 32

Relevance of Addressing Spiritual Needs for Clinical Support in Palliative Medicine

Stephan M. Probst

The Significance of Spiritual Care within Palliative Care

As a holistic practice, palliative care defines itself as "an approach that improves quality of life of patients with life-threatening illness and their families, through the prevention and relief of suffering by means of early identification, assessment and treatment of pain and other problems, physical, psychosocial and spiritual. Palliative care:

- provides relief from pain and other distressing symptoms;
- affirms life and regards dying as a normal process;
- intends neither to hasten or postpone death;
- integrates the psychological and spiritual aspects of patient care;

S. M. Probst (✉)
Palliative Care Unit, Klinik für Hämatologie, Onkologie und Palliativmedizin, Klinikum Bielefeld Mitte, Universitätsklinikum OWL Campus Klinikum Bielefeld, Bielefeld, Germany
e-mail: stephan.probst@klinikumbielefeld.de

A. Büssing (ed.), *Spiritual Needs in Research and Practice*,
https://doi.org/10.1007/978-3-030-70139-0_32

- offers a support system to help the family cope during the patient's illness and in their own bereavement;
- uses a team approach to address the needs of patients and their families, including bereavement counseling, if indicated;
- will enhance quality of life, and may also positively influence the course of illness;
- is applicable early in the course of illness, in conjunction with other therapies that are intended to prolong life, such as chemotherapy or radiation therapy, and includes those investigations needed to better understand and manage distressing clinical complications." (WHO 2007)

The existential and spiritual questions of patients and their families thus inevitably play a central role in palliative medicine. As the vagaries of life come to a head at end-of-life, the following existential opposing pairs reveal themselves ever more clearly and with concrete challenges:

- health versus sickness
- support versus helplessness
- life versus death
- freedom versus destiny
- autonomy versus dependence
- fulfillment versus meaninglessness

Patients wrestle with questions about their life's purpose and meaning amidst suffering. In anticipation of their death, spiritual considerations and the question of transcendence take on special meaning. Spirituality is experienced in palliative care as a person's search for existential meaning and purpose in life within a given life experience, which may or may not be related to traditional religious systems (Byrne 2002; Tanyi 2002). The therapeutic goal of enabling the ill person to live an active life as long as possible and remain true to what is most important to him or her often requires coming to terms with one's mortality. In the *Seven Advanced Lessons in the theory of Grief*, Irvin D. Yalom writes: "I understand that though the *fact* (the physicality) of death destroys us, the *idea* of death may save us" (Yalom 2000, p. 115). It may sound like a paradox, but the confrontation with one's one finite nature and recognition of the fragility of life may enrich the remaining time a terminally ill person has to live, thereby improving quality of life and dignity until the end. Coping with mortality touches the spiritual dimension of being human, and spiritual care can help lead to a positive conclusion. Edwards et al. identified the main themes of spiritual care as life review and reminiscence, involvement and control, a positive outlook, and death and dying (Edwards et al. 2010). Elizabeth Johnston Taylor posits that, "if left unaddressed [existential and] spiritual distress may [not only] stifle the opportunity for growth at the end of life [but also] lead to poorly controlled symptoms, and result in an '*unquiet death*'" (Taylor 2001, p. 395).

Palliative medicine is known for its strength in being solutions-focused and proactive in its actions while remaining an indispensable part of acute medicine. A basic tenet of palliative care is that it must make an allowance for the fact that there is not always a solution for every problem, and that immutable existential factors characterize our lives. There is no "solution" to death. The essential challenges to the foundation of palliative medicine as successfully practiced by palliative care professionals who support the dying and their families are as follows: Acceptance of the inevitability of death without illusion or defensiveness, plus the ability to care for the terminally ill by encountering helplessness together while remaining radically true and oriented to that person's values and needs. This basic tenet is the core of what they give the dying and their families as spiritual care in interpersonal relationships. Even the way in which the helpers meet the patients and their families can bring the dimension of spirituality to life.

The Meaning of Quality of Life and Spiritual Care from the Patient's Perspective

What is special about palliative care and what differentiates it from acute medicine is that practitioners are able to shift perspectives such as to meet patients in their subjectivity. Terminally ill patients do not always wish to gain as much time to live as possible or exhaust all of the possibilities that modern medicine has to offer, but rather they hope for quality of life worth living. Patients want to remain true to their own conceptualization of living life while maintaining dignity. Should they need to decide if it is worth it to lengthen their lives by weeks or months at all costs (even at the price of reductions to quality of life), or if the goal of therapy is a shorter life (with better quality of life and content), most people are willing to accept less quantity of life while hoping for more quality of life. Thus, the very definition of palliative care focuses intentionally on quality of life. The most important task of palliative care is to enhance quality of life via successful symptom management. Subjective and individually experienced quality of life of ill people is only determined in part by health-related quality of life. Especially when it comes to chronic and terminal illnesses, nonphysical determinants such as values, dignity and spirituality play an ever-increasing role as the disease progresses. According to Grant et al. (2004), spiritual determinants of main concern to terminally ill patients include:

- searching for meaning and identity within the illness experience.
- searching for peace of mind, and freedom from a pervasive fear of dying.
- searching for a guide to help the patient make sense of what is happening as death draws near.

The notion that "spirituality is known and experienced in relationship" (Burkhardt and Jacobson 2000, p. 95) underscores the importance of relationship in the spiritual well-being and the salience of spiritual care interventions that promote communion and connectedness. Studies show that patients with existentially threatening illnesses not only have a high level of spiritual needs, but also that they wish for doctors and caregivers to recognize these needs and consider them during treatment (Ehman et al. 1999; Fegg et al. 2005; Büssing et al. 2005; Balboni et al. 2007). Reliable data confirm that such spiritual accompaniment significantly improves the life quality of patients (Balboni et al. 2010; Bai and Lazenby 2015; Winkelman et al. 2011). In the interim, the spiritual needs of patients with life-limiting and terminal illnesses have been well-studied and a variety of models for spiritual assessment have been published (Maugans 1996; Puchalski and Romer 2000; Frick et al. 2006).

The Spiritual Needs Questionnaire (SpNQ) that this book is dedicated to proves to be a reliable instrument available that assesses needs by helping to measure spiritual, existential and psychosocial needs and to analyze the self-ascribed importance of the respective dimensions (Büssing et al. 2010, 2013). Spiritual needs must be recognized along with their meaning in the context of subjective individual quality of life. This makes it possible to correctly assess the patient's individual situation and classify concrete conflicts and challenges in order to work with the patient to determine the best route of accompaniment. Addressing these needs and facing unsolvable problems is of paramount importance for health care.

A working group at the Ludwig-Maximillians-University Munich was able to confirm that patients who faced ALS (Amyotrophic Lateral Sclerosis) and received palliative care administered via individual assessment scales (SEIQOL-DW in the form of a semi-structured interview) facilitated communication between physician and patient by pinpointing specific issues for discussions. The palliative care team used the results of individual QOL instruments as a guideline for planning and focusing interventions. Formulating their own priorities particularly regarding the nonphysical determinations of quality of life helped patients with terminal illness to develop appropriate strategies and ultimately to achieve meaning in the final stage of their lives. A successful palliative care accompaniment, which by definition is also spiritual care, could be of enormous help in leading to the improvement of a patient's individual subjective quality of life—even in the face of diminishing physical condition and impending death (Neudert et al. 2004).

A working group led by Borneman confirmed for FICA the feasibility and usefulness as a tool used for short spiritual assessment (Borneman et al. 2010). Frick and colleagues published in 2006 a study of the practicability and utility of a short, 15–30 min clinical interview for the assessment of cancer patients' spiritual needs and preferences. Physicians assessed the spirituality of their patients using the semi-structured interview SPIR (which is the German version of the FICA). It showed that neither doctors nor patients found the interview or questions about spirituality to be a burden or inappropriate, and that a short clinical assessment of spiritual needs and preferences may provide important data about coping, social support and patients' search for meaning, and may ultimately strengthen patient–physician relationship (Frick et al. 2006). Spiritual anamnesis based on SPIR is widespread in German-speaking countries and can be a pragmatic option for spiritual screening and a start to spiritual care for everyday use.

In any case, screening for spiritual needs (rather than for their fulfillment), can be seen as a task of the entire palliative care team and especially that of the physician, as patients tend to prefer to discuss these topics with their doctor and thus feel understood as a whole person and not just a patient (Ehman et al. 1999; Frick et al. 2006; Puchalski 2007).

Practical Issues

Assessment and diagnostic instruments may also be effective in creating space for spiritual topics and signal to the patient that he or she will be accompanied throughout the remainder of their disease process with awareness for and attention to spiritual needs. Information from the spiritual assessment is frequently used to help make decisions as well as formulate therapeutic goals for an individualized plan of care. Health care professionals learn via spiritual assessment about not only the needs, concerns and support required by the patients, but also sense and recognize the inner strengths and other resources the patient may use to process their illness while ideally maintaining quality of life. Whether or not the patient has specific religious needs that need to be considered during treatment comes quite often to light during a spiritual assessment. Let it be noted that it may not be assumed in all cases that people experiencing existential crises will automatically be aware of their spiritual resources and have them available for use. Thus, professionals must implement communication with the persons that are ill and their families about their convictions, as well as make clear the easy-to-access and continuous offer of support. Should the afflicted accept the offer, both sides tend to open to a multiplicity of positive and fulfilling experiences—including that of a fulfilled life being lived in the face of a terminal illness.

To this end, targeted interventions such as Dignity Therapy are available—patients who are especially experiencing feelings of loss of worthiness and meaning at end-of-life stand to benefit most (Chochinov 2012). The value of developing relationships in themselves is also stressed as being potentially therapeutic (Tanyi 2002; Anderson 2007). Even just the singular acts of "being there" and "caring presence" carry significant developmental, spiritual and existential meaning for patients as they face end-of-life issues. The process of being present unites the listener and the speaker in a spirit of compassion (Mowat and Swinton 2005).

Hinderances/Obstacles

It should be expected that assessment and diagnostic tools for many health care professionals offer a more simplified entry into spiritual care than perhaps an intuitive path via symbolic communication. The latter touches upon the indirectly addressed "secret" of the patient, his or her identity and experience of spirituality, bringing it to the fore and transcending the moment (Weiher 2014, p. 89 et seq.). Despite and even though palliative care explicitly defines itself by way of its attention to spiritual needs and thus plans for assessment thereof, many palliative care patients still feel lacking in an appropriate spiritual accompaniment or are loathe to burden their busy doctors and nurses with the topic.

On the other hand, professionals consider their own uncertainty (coupled with the resistance of the patient and hindering factors in the clinical arena) to be a barrier when it comes to carrying out spiritual care (Murray et al. 2004; Mayr et al. 2016). Clearly, the following factors also play a role:

- lack of sufficient training in spiritual assessment and end-of-life communication skills.
- lack of support environment in which to discuss issues of loss and death.
- extensive demands on time and busy clinical schedules.
- high (staff) turnover rates.
- pressure to be strictly evidence-based and time-effective with patients.
- lack of providers' attention to their own spiritual needs such as to be able to address this aspect with their patients.
- the marginalization and devaluing of psychosocial and spiritual care during medical training.

What is required of palliative care in order to implement spiritual care in alignment with its core tenets is a letting go of the need to control and an ability to be comfortable with mystery and the unknown (Chibnall et al. 2004; Oldnall 1996; Puchalski et al. 2004). There is always the danger that the inability to address spiritual needs may lead to an exaggerated pharmacological or solely bodily functional response to the despair and suffering of the patient, leading to a "medicalization" of death. However, an overemphasis on assessment using standardized scales for its own sake and without clinical consequences also poses the threat of "de-spiritualization" and "medicalization" of spiritual care itself. In all likelihood, every form of medicalization and "de-spiritualization" of death and dying is not only a catastrophe for the dying person, but rather also a possible risk factor for the generation of complicated grief on the part of the remaining relatives, and of burnout by the professionals. Even if reliable data on the subject does not yet exist, it must be possible to assume that attentive spiritual care following in the tradition of palliative care will help prevent complicated grief from arising for the dying person and their family members. Such care can likely help the grieving survivors hold lifelong thoughts and memories of the deceased—marked by beautiful, intensive, fulfilled and meaningful moments.

Acknowledgments I thank Ari Kloke, LCSW, very much for her great support in translating this chapter into English.

References

Anderson JH (2007) The impact of using nursing presence in a community heart failure program. J Cardiovasc Nurs 22:89–94

Bai M, Lazenby M (2015) A systematic review of associations between spiritual well-being and quality of life at the scale and factor levels in studies among patients with Cancer. J Palliat Med 10:286–298

Balboni TA, Vanderwerker LC, Block SD, Paulk ME, Lathan CS, Peteet JR, Prigerson HG (2007) Religiousness and spiritual support among advanced Cancer patients and associations with end-of-life treatment preferences and quality of life. J Clin Oncol 25:555–560

Balboni TA, Paulk ME, Balboni MJ, Phelps AC, Loggers ET, Wright AA, Block SD, Lewis EF, Peteet JR, Prigerson HG (2010) Provision of spiritual care to patients with advanced Cancer: associations with medical care and quality of life near death. J Clin Oncol 28:445–452

Borneman T, Ferrell B, Puchalski CM (2010) Evaluation of the FICA tool for spiritual assessment. J Pain Symptom Manage 40:163–173

Burkhardt M, Jacobson M (2000) Spirituality and health. In: Dossey B, Keegan L, Guzetaa G (eds) Holistic nursing: a handbook for practice, 3rd edn. Gaithersburg, Aspen

Büssing A, Ostermann TM, Matthiessen PF (2005) Spirituelle Bedürfnisse krebskranker Menschen: Einstellung und Praxis. Dtsch Z Onkol 37:13–22

Büssing A, Balzat HJ, Heusser P (2010) Spiritual needs of patients with chronic pain diseases and Cancer—validation of the spiritual needs questionnaire. Eur J Med Res 15:266–273

Büssing A, Janko A, Baumann K, Hvidt NC, Kopf A (2013) Spiritual needs among patients with chronic pain diseases and Cancer living in a secular society. Pain Med 14:1362–1373

Byrne M (2002) Spirituality in palliative care: what language do we need? Int J Palliat Nurs 8:67–74

Chibnall J, Bennet M, Videen S, Duckro O, Miller D (2004) Identifying barriers to psychosocial spiritual care at the end of life: a physician group study. Am J Hosp Palliat Care 21:419–426

Chochinov HM (2012) Dignity therapy: final words for final days. Oxford University Press, Oxford and New York

Edwards A, Pang N, Shiu V, Chan C (2010) The understanding of spirituality and the potential role of spiritual care in end-of-life and palliative care: a meta-study of qualitative research. Palliat Med 24:753–770

Ehman JW, Ott BB, Short TH, Ciamoa RC, Hansen-Flaschen J (1999) Do patients want physicians to inquire about their spiritual or religious beliefs if they become gravely ill? Arch Intern Med 159:1803–1806

Fegg M, Wasner M, Neudert C, Borasio GD (2005) Personal values and individual quality of life in palliative care patients. J Pain Symptom Manage 30:154–159

Frick E, Riedner C, Fegg M, Hauf S, Borasio GD (2006) A clinical interview assessing cancer patients' spiritual needs and preferences. Eur J Cancer Care 15:238–243

Grant E, Murray S, Kendall M, Boyd K, Tilley S, Ryan D (2004) Spiritual issues and needs: perspectives from patients with advanced cancer and nonmalignat disease. A qualitative study. Palliat Support Care 2:371–378

Maugans T (1996) The SPIRITual history. Arch Fam Med 3:129–137

Mayr B, Elhardt E, Riedner C, Roser T, Frick E, Paal P (2016) Die Kluft zwischen eingeschätzten und tatsächlichen Fähigkeiten bei der Erhebung der spirituellen Anamnese. Spiritual Care 5:9–16

Mowat H, Swinton J (2005) What do chaplain do? A report on a two year investigation into the nature of chaplaincy in the NHS in Scotland. Scottish Executive, Edinburgh

Murray S, Kendall M, Boyd K, Worth A, Benton T (2004) Exploring the spiritual needs of people dying of lung cancer or heart failure: a prospective qualitative interview study of patients and their carers. Palliat Med 18:39–45

Neudert C, Wasner M, Borasio GD (2004) Individual qualitiy of life is not correlated with health-related quality of life or physical function in patients with amyotrophic lateral sclerosis. J Palliat Med 7:551–557

Oldnall A (1996) A critical analysis of nursing: meeting spiritual needs of patients. J Adv Nurs 23:138–144

Puchalski CM (2007) Spirituality and the care of patients at the end-of-life: an essential component of care. Omega (Westport) 56:33–46

Puchalski CM, Dorff E, Hendi I (2004) Spirituality, religion, and healing in palliative care. Clin Geriatr Med 20:689–714

Puchalski CM, Romer A (2000) Taking a spiritual history allows clinicians to understand patients more fully. J Palliat Med 3:129–137

Tanyi RA (2002) Towards clarification of the meaning of spirituality. J Adv Nurs 39:500–509

Taylor EJ (2001) Spiritual assessment. In: Ferrell B, Coyle N (eds) Textbook of palliative nursing. Oxford University Press, Oxford and New York, pp 379–406

Weiher E (2014) Das Geheimnis des Lebens berühren – Spiritualität bei Krankheit, Sterben, Tod, 4th edn. Kohlhammer, Stuttgart

Winkelman WD, Lauderdale K, Balboni MJ, Phelps AC, Peteet JR, Block SD, Kachnic LA, VanderWeele TJ, Balboni TA (2011) The relationship of spiritual concerns to the quality of life of advanced Cancer patients: preliminary findings. J Palliat Med 14:1022–1028

World Health Organization (2007) WHO definition of palliative care 2007. Available via http://www.who.int/cancer/palliative/definition/en. Accessed 21 Jan 2020

Yalom ID (2000) Momma and the meaning of life. Harper Perennial, New York

CHAPTER 33

Addressing Spiritual Needs and Spiritual Care from a Volunteers' Perspective

Torsten Ernst

Background

Whenever things get difficult, when one's own life gets into borderline situations, many people open up to the transcendent. To put it in a saying: "Need teaches you to pray." Now we are living in a time when an increasing erosion of the religious can be observed in several European societies. More and more people have not learned to find access to their own spirituality. If you have not learned to pray, you will not know how to access this resource, particularly in difficult situations.

This opening of the human being to "something more" in life is a process that urges accompaniment, has always urged accompaniment. The question arises, *how* should this accompaniment be? As a natural aspect of human coexistence, this accompaniment is part of our everyday togetherness, where people listen to one another and are there for one another, in the circle of friends, in the family, in the group of colleagues, in the sports

T. Ernst (✉)
Anhalt Hospice and Palliative Care Society, Deaconess Foundation Dessau, Dessau, Germany
e-mail: ternst@ada-dessau.de

A. Büssing (ed.), *Spiritual Needs in Research and Practice*,
https://doi.org/10.1007/978-3-030-70139-0_33

club, in the parish, and so on. Or does this accompaniment require special skills, does it need the classic mediator, the priest, the consecrated person, the expert for borderline questions in life?

As in many other fields of life too, the pendulum moves back and forth between the two poles, because both are necessary: (1) a general awareness that there is more than what is in front of our eyes in our everyday concerns and a corresponding sensitivity toward it; and (2) at the same time, however, it also requires the 'professionals' who take on this aspect of life, awaken sensitivity and accompany on a meta-level. However, everything that happens in this professional setting will only be complete when it finds a resonance space in which it can unfold.

In the following, I will try to shed some light on the importance of volunteering in the context of spiritual needs and spiritual care. First of all, it is important to clarify what volunteering actually means—and this especially in a time of multiple professionalization, in which increasingly only what is (financially) rewarded has value. This is the reason why there are discussions about honorary pay and honorary flat rates to value this kind of commitment. At the same time, one can observe how, especially in more complex contexts, volunteer work is viewed with some kind of professional reservation, which in many cases expresses an arrogance that can perhaps be formulated as follows: "I am the professional and have training and knowledge—you are that Unaware and require my instructions for your actions."

Volunteering in Hospice Work and Palliative Care

In the last few decades, hospice and palliative care work in particular (but not only this) has brought about a significant development in the understanding of cross-professional cooperation and has underlined the terms therapeutic or multiprofessional team. In such a team, the different professional groups come together to find the best approach for the people entrusted to them together with their respective competencies. In hospice work, the profession of volunteering has been of particular importance from the very beginning, since this field of work has developed from a strongly civic/voluntary movement in the twentieth century. To this day, the work of all forms of hospice care has been shaped by this voluntary commitment in the outpatient hospice services, which are a constitutive part of hospice and palliative care.

At the beginning of modern hospice work, volunteering was essential because there was no general funding for this form of human care at the end of life. Over the years, a special profession has developed under this honorary position, which is expressed in the development of different training programs for this voluntary service in terminal care (e.g., the so-called *Celler Model* in its different stages of development from the church). Key words that describe this profession can be found in the structure of the new edition of the original *Celler Model*: "The Art of Dying Care" (Vol. 1) and "Dying Care—Cordially and Carefully" (Vol. 2) (Godzik 2013, n.d.).

Three things can be determined so far: (1) Hospice and palliative work is incomprehensible without the involvement of volunteers. (2) In addition to the people in the therapeutic/multiprofessional teams who are responsible for the medical, nursing and psychosocial care of persons in need, there are those who try to listen to and care for the affected persons—beyond the traditional professions. (3) Spiritual encounter takes place on all levels of relationship in such an event.

Despite the above-average staffing levels in the remunerated areas (i.e., nursing, medical service, social work, psychological support, housekeeping) in hospice and palliative work, I am convinced that volunteers in particular are predestined in favor of the spiritual encounter, as they are driven by an empathetic human impulse of mercy,[1] without a classic care mandate when they face the affected persons and their relatives. In this combination lies the chance for the freedom of spiritual experience.

At the core of their tasks, there are very different aspects, all of which can be easily assigned to the ambiguous term spirituality (Streib and Keller 2015). If spirituality in the sense of Peter Zimmerling is understood as "faith that takes on external form and which encompasses the three aspects of justifying faith, the practice of piety and the way of life" (Zimmerling 2017), then the essentials of what is understood by spiritual concern are described here. Or, in other words, without the theological connotation inherent in the concept of faith: wherever a basic conviction of life takes shape in practical action, there is spiritual concern, because here there is room for the man's inherent knowledge of the greater part of his existence. Oskar Föller understands spirituality similarly as a synonym for

[1] Mercy as an active aspect of spirituality—Mercy is understood here as listening to the "barmen" (Middle High German term for "lament") of one's own heart and the actions derived from it. Here affection (heart) and subsequent reaction (hand) come together.

spiritual life or piety. For him, spirituality is "'*praxis pietatis*', ... practiced faith(s) in devotion to God and the world" (Föller 2002).

In this respect, hospice and palliative work with its extensive opportunities for voluntary engagement has created spaces in which people can discover and develop their own spirituality and thus come into a situation in which faith in the broadest sense can be trained. This is also expressed by Traugott Roser when he sees spirituality as an anthropological category that describes in particular existential human life in life-threatening situations. In doing so, "the attribution of spirituality determines people as an open being (process-oriented and open in a temporal perspective), relational (based on physical, social, spatial and transcendent relationships) and fragmentary (vulnerable and finite)" (Roser 2017).

The model of spiritual needs by Arndt Büssing and Harold Koenig also takes up the aspects of developing faith and affection/sociality when spiritual needs are differentiated into the four categories of social, emotional, existential and religious, and assigned to the human core dimensions of Connectedness, Peace, Meaning and Transcendence (Büssing and Koenig 2010).

Conclusions

It can thus be stated that with regard to volunteer workers in hospice and palliative work, there are no formal differences from other professions with regard to their spiritual needs or their possibilities for spiritual care. However, there is a clear distinction: Without a direct professional group assignment as volunteer employees (please do not label them as "helpers"), the volunteer hospice workers can turn to persons in need in a completely different way and explore their life concerns with them. In doing so, they are driven by their own beliefs and convictions, which are expressed in their devotion to other people and the will to give the world a better face even in the greatest need.

In this way, these employees become "drivers" in dealing with those affected and become role models, although as a rule they do not claim to be. In this way, volunteers make a decisive contribution to a spiritual culture in their respective institution. It is important that the actions of these employees are consistently given the appropriate importance; there should not be a gap between those employees who earn money with their actions and those who work voluntarily without payment. And it is further necessary to organize structures in such a way that volunteers can also experience good self-efficacy.

If we bring all this together and place it in the borderline situations of life described at the beginning, we will find that the "unprofessional" profession of volunteering can make a decisive contribution in dealing with spiritual needs and shaping spiritual care.

References

Büssing A, Koenig HG (2010) Spiritual Needs of Patients with Chronic Diseases. 0Religions 1: 18–27

Föller O (2002) Geistliches Leben und Evangelisation. Faktoren missionarischer Motivation und Müdigkeit in Deutschland. In: Klement HH (ed) Evangelisation im Gegenwind. Zur Theologie und Praxis der Glaubensverkündigung in der säkularen Gesellschaft. Brunnen, Gießen

Godzik P (ed) (2013) Die Kunst der Sterbebegleitung. Handbuch zur Begleitung Schwerkranker und Sterbender. Rosengarten, Hamburg

Godzik P (n.d.) Sterbebegleitung – herzlich und zugewandt. http://www.pkgodzik.de/fileadmin/user_upload/Hospiz_und_Sterbebegleitung/Das_alte_Celler_Modell_neu_zugaenglich.pdf. Accessed 25 Sep 2020

Roser T (2017) Spiritual care. Der Beitrag von Seelsorge zum Gesundheitswesen, 2nd edn. Kohlhammer, Stuttgart

Streib H, Keller B (2015) Was bedeutet Spiritualität? Befunde, Analysen und Fallstudien aus Deutschland. Vandenhoeck & Ruprecht, Göttingen

Zimmerling P (2017) Handbuch Evangelische Spiritualität. Idee und Vorgeschichte. In: Zimmerling P (ed) Handbuch Evangelische Spiritualität 1: Geschichte. Vandenhoeck & Ruprecht, Göttingen

CHAPTER 34

Concluding Suggestions

Arndt Büssing and Harold G. Koenig

What have We Learned from International Studies?

Spiritual needs are expressed with varying intensity in different groups of patients with chronic diseases and are often specific to the individual patient. They are also expressed by patients' relatives, especially their caregivers. Spiritual needs are also present among healthy young persons stressed by their external life situations (e.g., soldiers, refugees or mothers of sick children or of children with special needs), also by elderly living in retirements homes, and by persons with special needs (e.g., those with

A. Büssing (✉)
Professorship Quality of Life, Spirituality and Coping, Faculty of Health, Witten/Herdecke University, Herdecke, Germany

IUNCTUS—Competence Center for Christian Spirituality, Philosophical-Theological University of Münster, Münster, Germany
e-mail: Arndt.buessing@uni-wh.de

H. G. Koenig
Center for Spirituality, Theology and Health, Duke University Medical Center, Durham, NC, USA

Department of Medicine, King Abdulaziz University, Jeddah, Saudi Arabia
e-mail: harold.koenig@duke.edu

A. Büssing (ed.), *Spiritual Needs in Research and Practice*,
https://doi.org/10.1007/978-3-030-70139-0_34

autism, dementia or Down's syndrome). Perhaps all persons at some level have unmet spiritual needs, depending on their circumstances, personality traits, cultural and religious background, and available resources to cope with the various stressors in life.

Health professions need to identify unmet spiritual needs in patients and their families. Doing so is not optional, given their impact on health outcomes. These are not 'secondary' as Maslow's (outdated) hierarchy of needs would suggest. Addressing these needs indicates that the healthcare professionals value and respect the person with their specific life situation, biographical background, current sense of purpose and meaning in life, hope, changing priorities, moral values, religious and nonreligious convictions, and spiritual rituals important to them, depending on the resources available to them. However, this requires time, interest, and competence, which can vary across healthcare professionals. Thus, it may be important to differentiate more general from specific spiritual care competences and responsibilities. The role and availability of professional pastoral care providers will depend on the importance that societies place on religion and spiritual matters. As noted, even nonreligious persons have spiritual needs, whether acknowledged or not, which require support. Currently an increasing number of healthcare professional and volunteers are trained to enable them to provide spiritual care, which is not identically with pastoral care as some critics assume.

Having unmet spiritual needs is not simply the opposite of spiritual well-being. Both constructs might be interrelated in that research indicates they may be negatively related, positively related, or both, or not at all—depending on the situation in which a person may find themselves, and depending on their religious background. The construct of 'spiritual well-being' is related to psychological well-being in dealing with issues related to meaning and purpose in life, while having unmet 'spiritual needs' is a broader concept that indicates a general longing to fill unmet psychological, social, and personal needs related to the transcendent or the immanent. These needs might be triggered by a reduction in well-being (e.g., states of depression, loneliness, existential fear); although addressing them may not necessarily result in greater psychological well-being as the underlying health condition may not have changed. When spiritual needs are the result of what is longed for in comparison to what is available, this may result in different scenarios. When something is lacking in life, people will strive to obtain this needed 'something' in order to improve their situation. When one is satisfied with the current situation, no significant spiritual needs may be evident. However, persons' expectations could also be higher than what they can realistically achieve, and when those spiritual needs are strong and remain unmet, this often results in dissatisfaction. When persons' life circumstances are poor and the perception is that they cannot be changed, then a sense of depression, frustration, and loss of hope can result, which the healthcare professional must address.

For some individuals, their meaning and purpose in life have slowly vanished and nothing is expected anymore. In that case, spiritual needs may no longer be perceived (due to a state of depression, hopelessness, and disinterest). In other cases, when physical, mental, social, or spiritual integrity is threatened, then spiritual needs may be reactively triggered, as the longing for a more complete and meaningful life increases. In either situation, it is important to appreciate the possible existence of spiritual needs, assess the person's level of distress and available resources, and then get them connected to someone from the spiritual care/healthcare team who can address those acknowledged or unacknowledged spiritual needs.

Support Plans

When spiritual needs of inpatients are identified, the spiritual care team (consisting of different health care professions, pastoral workers, social workers, volunteers, etc.) should discuss what might be done to address those unmet needs. A decision has to be made on who could communicate with the patient about these issues, what can be achieved, and what resources are available to meet unmet spiritual needs (the action or support plan). The entire process should be viewed from a team perspective, including the patient on the team as a key member. It is important to emphasize that not all needs can be met and not all problems in life can be solved by the spiritual care team. This is not their goal and therefore excessive demands on them should be avoided. Beginning to communicate about these issues is the first step in a process that will require 'inner work' by the patient and sensitive guidance by the healthcare professional (including clergy and pastoral care workers). The spiritual care team should seek to 'jump start' the process and help to clear the 'spiritual windows', while the patient will need to 'drive' the car (although with supporting passengers).

The situation is very different when inpatients are leaving the hospital or when it comes to very old people. In that case, the health professional or pastoral care person will need to identify what resources exist in the community to support their spiritual needs. There may not be persons and structures available in the community to address unmet spiritual needs. When available, it may be that family and friends are the best supporters depending on the specific spiritual needs. However, patients may be afraid of burdening others with their problems or feel ashamed to discuss their spiritual struggles with others, particularly family or friends. Thus, other, more neutral persons might be required who are trained to listen to these individuals and organize resources to support their spiritual needs.

Spiritual support teams in palliative care units and hospices are perhaps those who are most organized and prepared to address the spiritual needs of patients. There is a clear demand to identify spiritual needs, to identify spiritual struggles, and to provide resources to meet those needs, including specific spiritual rituals that have been helpful to patients in the past (e.g., prayer, receiving the Eucharist and other Sacraments, formal blessings, mindfulness meditation, music and singing, lighting a candle, and so forth). Talking about spiritual issues in such situations is clearly recognized as important and necessary. Nevertheless, as noted above, patients who are not dying and may not even be that physically ill may also have spiritual needs that require attention. In that case, social workers, pastoral care specialists, counselors, community clergy, and other trained professionals may be called upon to address these unmet spiritual needs. However, a clear assignment to care for these issues outside of the health care structure is often missing and structures rarely available.

However, with whom should people talk about their spiritual needs when trained individuals to meet those needs are not available to them? The pastor might not be the first person that a nonreligious person may ask; consultation of a psychologist or psychotherapist might be viewed by some as indicating that they are mentally 'ill'; community nurses have more 'concrete' tasks that they are responsible for. Apart from the systems in place developed for palliative care patients, there is also a need for those with and without chronic nonterminal illnesses to have their spiritual needs addressed, preferably in the early stages of disease or at difficult life situations. This remains an important task of future healthcare systems that wish to more comprehensively care for the healthcare needs of patients, and of religious communities to ensure that spiritual concerns of all persons, independent of their religious orientations, are met in and outside healthcare settings.

Appendix: Questionnaires

SpNQ for Adults (Extended Version)

The following statements were mentioned by several other persons, and they must not necessarily apply to yours. Please read these statements carefully and then indicate how true each is for you and your current situation by circling one number per line. When you do have a respective need ("Yes"), then indicate how strong it is. Otherwise, circle the "No" option. Please be as honest and true as possible: There is no 'right' or 'wrong' answer.

During the last time, did you have had the needs …		**Agreement**		**If YES, how strong is this need?**		
		No	**Yes**	**some-what**	**strong**	**very strong**
N2	To talk with others about your fears and worries?	❍	❍ →	1	2	3
N3[a]	That someone of your religious community (i.e. pastor) cares for you or comes to see you?	❍	❍ →	1	2	3
N4	To reflect back on your life?	❍	❍ →	1	2	3
N5	To dissolve/clarify open aspects of your life?	❍	❍ →	1	2	3
N6	To plunge into beauty of nature?	❍	❍ →	1	2	3
N7	To dwell at a place of quietness and peace?	❍	❍ →	1	2	3

(continued)

A. Büssing (ed.), *Spiritual Needs in Research and Practice*,
https://doi.org/10.1007/978-3-030-70139-0

(continued)

N8	To find inner peace?	❍	❍ →	1	2	3
N10	To find meaning in illness and/or suffering?	❍	❍ →	1	2	3
N11	To talk with someone about the question of meaning in life?	❍	❍ →	1	2	3
N12	To talk with someone about the possibility of life after death?	❍	❍ →	1	2	3
N13	To turn to someone in a loving attitude?	❍	❍ →	1	2	3
N14	To give away something from yourself?	❍	❍ →	1	2	3
N15	To give solace to someone?	❍	❍ →	1	2	3
N16	To forgive someone from a distinct period of your life?	❍	❍ →	1	2	3
N17	To be forgiven?	❍	❍ →	1	2	3
N18	To pray with someone?	❍	❍ →	1	2	3
N19	That someone prays for you?	❍	❍ →	1	2	3
N20	To pray for yourself?	❍	❍ →	1	2	3
N21	To participate at a religious ceremony (i.e., Sunday service)?	❍	❍ →	1	2	3
N22	To read religious/spiritual books?	❍	❍ →	1	2	3
N23	To turn to a higher presence (i.e., God, Allah, Angels, Saints)?	❍	❍ →	1	2	3
N25[a]	To feel connected with family?	❍	❍ →	1	2	3
N26	To pass own life experiences to others?	❍	❍ →	1	2	3
N27	To be assured that your life was meaningful and of value?	❍	❍ →	1	2	3
N28[a]	To be re-involved by your family in their life concerns?	❍	❍ →	1	2	3
N29[a]	To be invited by friends?	❍	❍ →	1	2	3
N30[a]	To receive more support from your family?	❍	❍ →	1	2	3
In case you have further specific needs you would like to let us know:						
X1			❍ →	1	2	3
X2			❍ →	1	2	3
X3			❍ →	1	2	3

[a]Optional items that may be used in elderly living in residential/nursing homes, etc.

SpNQ for Adolescents (Reduced Variant Version)

The following statements were mentioned by several other persons, and they must not necessarily apply to yours. Please read these statements carefully and then indicate how true each is for you and your current situation by circling one number per line. When you do have a respective need ("Yes"), then indicate how strong it is. Otherwise, circle the "No" option. Please be as honest and true as possible: There is no 'right' or 'wrong' answer.

During the last time, did you have had the needs …		**No**	**If YES, how strong is this need?**		
			some-what	**strong**	**very strong**
N2	To talk with others about your fears and worries?	0	1	2	3
N7	To dwell at a place of quietness and peace?	0	1	2	3
N6	To plunge into beauty of nature?	0	1	2	3
N8	To find inner peace?	0	1	2	3
N10	To find meaning in illness and/or suffering?	0	1	2	3
N11	To talk with someone about the question of meaning in life?	0	1	2	3
N27	To be assured that your life was meaningful and of value?	0	1	2	3
N13	To turn to someone in a loving attitude?	0	1	2	3
N18	To pray with someone?	0	1	2	3
N19	That someone prays for you?	0	1	2	3
N20	To pray for yourself?	0	1	2	3
N23	To turn to a higher presence (i.e., God, Allah)?	0	1	2	3
N38	That there is someone there for you who is always at your side?	0	1	2	3
N43	That your situation is improving for the better?	0	1	2	3
N44	To have someone to assure you how to proceed (in a positive way).	0	1	2	3

SpNQ Screener (Reduced Version)

The following statements were mentioned by several other persons, and they must not necessarily apply to yours. Please read these statements carefully and then indicate how true each is for you and your current situation by circling one number per line. When you do have a respective need ("Yes"), then indicate how strong it is. Otherwise, circle the "No" option. Please be as honest and true as possible: There is no 'right' or 'wrong' answer.

During the last time, did you have had the needs ...		**No**	**If YES, how strong is this need?**		
			some-what	**strong**	**very strong**
N2	To talk with others about your fears and worries?	0	1	2	3
N7	To dwell at a place of quietness and peace?	0	1	2	3
N8	To find inner peace?	0	1	2	3
N11	To talk with someone about the question of meaning in life?	0	1	2	3
N17	To be forgiven?	0	1	2	3
N20	To pray for yourself?	0	1	2	3
N21	To participate at a religious ceremony (i.e. Sunday service)?	0	1	2	3
N23	To turn to a higher presence (i.e., God)?	0	1	2	3

Index[1]

A

Accompaniment, 29, 38, 54, 460, 461, 463, 467, 468

Acquired Immunodeficiency Syndrome (AIDS), 193, 196, 197, 201, 430

Adolescents, 3, 88, 103–109, 155, 184, 185, 266, 297–308, 430

Anxiety, 27, 30, 34, 39–41, 97, 98, 139, 142, 143, 174, 194, 210, 215, 222, 233, 252, 258, 298, 300, 303, 353, 398, 402, 414, 427

Application, 3, 79–85, 128, 186, 194, 202, 217, 328

Areligious persons, 80

Assessment, ix, 3, 27–43, 47, 54, 61–63, 67–69, 72–74, 79, 80, 83, 85, 96, 104, 112, 113, 126, 143, 147, 156, 163–166, 168, 208, 209, 216, 217, 240, 244, 253, 254, 257, 259, 260, 271, 275, 328, 352, 385–386, 427, 431, 440, 441, 444, 445, 457, 460–463

Attention, 18, 51, 53, 59, 95, 104, 105, 108, 128, 154, 162, 167, 188, 190, 208, 213, 217, 221, 231, 234, 243, 252, 254, 257, 282, 290, 304, 314, 319, 370, 386, 390, 413, 415, 416, 424, 441, 445, 463, 476

Attentiveness, 50–55, 398

Autism, 88, 265, 268–270, 274, 357, 474

Autism spectrum disorder (ASD), 265–275

Autonomy, 47, 48, 287, 288, 290, 325, 372, 458

B

Breast cancer, 173–180

[1] Note: Page numbers followed by 'n' refer to notes.

A. Büssing (ed.), *Spiritual Needs in Research and Practice*, https://doi.org/10.1007/978-3-030-70139-0

C
Cancer, 20, 22, 30, 32, 67, 72, 92–94, 96, 98, 117–119, 124–127, 138, 139, 147–156, 159–168, 173–180, 189, 195, 208, 240–244, 252, 257–259, 318, 319, 371, 441, 448, 450
Chaplains, vii, viii, 33, 35, 37, 41, 54, 66, 68, 229–231, 402, 409–417, 438, 448, 452, 453
Chemotherapy, 173–180, 458
Children, 4, 39, 88, 97, 98, 104, 155, 160, 184, 245, 265–269, 274, 283, 286, 297–300, 308, 315, 330, 351–364, 352n1, 376, 388, 404, 448, 473
Chronic diseases, 3, 87–100, 103–109, 113, 117, 119–122, 126, 128, 138–140, 154, 160, 161, 166–168, 189, 194, 195, 202, 210, 211, 213, 215, 216, 257, 259, 297–308, 319, 351, 363, 374, 379, 473
Chronic pain, 31, 34, 90, 92–94, 96, 119, 127, 135–144, 164, 189, 259, 441
Cognitive decline, 122, 208, 215
Comfort, 104, 208, 209, 213, 216, 243, 335
Community nurse, 476
Competence, 53, 54, 148, 155, 217, 232, 243, 260, 291, 325, 416, 428, 429, 474
Coping, 2, 10, 19–21, 31, 32, 37, 59, 73, 99, 104, 124, 136–139, 142, 143, 153, 184, 193, 201, 234, 252, 258, 259, 268, 298–302, 307, 308, 314, 319, 327, 328, 336, 337, 351, 352, 362, 371, 373, 402, 427, 448, 459, 461
Cultural differences, 124, 128, 153, 202
Culture, 3, 11, 12, 14, 17, 31, 51, 70, 117, 121, 148, 159, 160, 163, 166, 324, 325, 327–329, 335, 338, 370, 387, 415, 422, 426, 437, 439, 453, 470
Cystic fibrosis (CF), 183–190, 300

D
Dementia, 88, 113, 122, 207–217, 373, 474
Depression, 30, 34, 40, 98, 126, 143, 163, 194, 210, 222, 228, 230, 233, 283, 298–300, 303, 336, 357, 364, 371, 372, 427, 474, 475
Dignity, 3, 4, 16, 29, 33, 208, 213, 216, 217, 370–372, 425, 426, 459, 460
Down syndrome (DS), 88, 281–291, 352, 356–359, 363, 364, 404

E
Education, 28, 42, 50, 51, 54, 149, 154, 159, 197, 216, 227, 228, 232, 243, 270, 274, 291, 315, 324, 337, 352, 360, 361, 416, 420, 422, 424–426, 428, 429, 438, 439, 453
Elderly, 3, 67, 68, 87–100, 113, 141, 160, 163, 257, 307, 327, 369–391, 404, 473
Emergency room, 68, 251–260, 397–400, 402–404
Escape from illness, 97, 98, 142, 178–179
Ethics of care, 47–55

F
Factorial structure, 88–91, 100, 123, 128

Faith, viii, 2, 3, 14, 17, 18, 20, 30, 36, 39, 41, 95–97, 100, 135, 141, 148, 153, 154, 160, 162, 167, 184, 186, 194, 196, 201, 229, 231, 239, 241, 259, 268–270, 272, 274, 283, 285, 289, 290, 305, 314, 326, 328, 337, 352, 353, 355, 372, 377–379, 387–389, 414, 421–423, 437–445, 448, 469, 470
Faith development, 35, 470
Fear, 3, 34, 38, 54, 82, 84, 88, 91, 92, 95, 105, 118–120, 122, 127, 135, 141–143, 149, 152, 166, 167, 174, 178, 189, 194, 196, 227, 242, 243, 284–287, 289, 302–304, 308, 317, 319, 320, 323, 324, 353, 354, 356, 361, 376, 379, 386–389, 403, 415, 440, 444, 460, 474

G
Generalist spiritual care, 410, 415, 416
Guardian angel, 268, 285, 286, 288, 290

H
Happiness, 13, 15, 79, 149, 153, 155, 156, 288, 326, 362, 389
Health, vii–ix, 2–4, 9–22, 28–30, 32, 35–37, 40–42, 47, 48, 51, 52, 54, 60n1, 67, 68, 72, 80, 83, 97–99, 104, 112, 113, 120, 121, 123, 125, 126, 141–143, 147–149, 152–154, 156, 159, 161, 163, 167, 168, 174, 175, 179, 180, 184–186, 194, 195, 200, 202, 208–210, 214–217, 225, 231, 232, 234, 239–243, 252–254, 260, 266, 281, 282, 299, 300, 306–308, 320, 324–326, 329, 337, 351–355, 359–363, 370, 371, 382, 384, 387, 390, 409–411, 413–417, 421, 423, 424, 438–442, 444, 447, 453, 458, 461, 462, 474–476
HIV infection, 193
Holistic, 43, 69, 148, 155, 156, 168, 195, 213, 217, 246, 314, 320, 352, 370, 420, 422, 425, 426, 428, 431
Hope, 1–3, 32, 35, 38, 80, 84, 88, 99, 104, 108, 120, 124, 125, 136, 138, 139, 144, 160, 161, 167, 168, 174, 178, 184, 189, 194, 209, 239, 282, 288–290, 319, 321, 326, 335, 337, 353, 356, 362, 372, 373, 381, 388, 389, 399, 404, 409–417, 421, 423, 428, 459, 474, 475
Hospice work, 468–470

I
Implementation, 71, 72, 79–85, 156, 441
Inclusion, 32, 61, 62, 72, 128, 283, 288–291, 326, 391
Interpretation of illness, 99, 138

L
Languages, 51, 70, 72, 73, 111, 113, 117, 118, 121–123, 128, 195, 208, 326, 414, 415
Life expectancy, 184, 185, 282
Life satisfaction, 97–99, 108, 109, 120, 138–139, 149, 154–156, 167, 174–180, 186, 188, 228, 230, 241, 242, 257, 270, 282, 284–290, 300, 304–307, 323–338, 352, 354, 355, 358–363, 374–376, 379–383, 385

Loneliness, 153, 289, 371, 380–382, 390, 474
Longitudinal, 174, 428, 429
Love of God, 16
Love of neighbor, 21, 22
Lung transplantation, 184–186, 189

M

Meaning, 2, 10, 11, 18–21, 30, 32, 34, 36, 38–41, 47, 61, 81, 84, 87, 88, 91, 96, 97, 99, 104, 105, 108, 112, 117–122, 124, 125, 127, 135, 136, 139, 141–143, 149, 161, 164, 167, 184, 193–195, 201, 202, 209, 216, 223, 227, 228, 234, 239, 241, 258, 271, 272, 274, 283–285, 291, 303, 305–307, 314, 316, 324, 325, 331, 335, 336, 352, 353, 355, 359–361, 370, 372, 373, 376, 377, 379, 386, 388, 389, 398–400, 409, 411, 412, 414, 416, 417, 421, 423, 424, 428, 439, 441, 442, 458–461, 470, 474, 475
Mood states, 98–100, 307, 355, 356, 358, 359, 372, 376, 385, 390
Mothers, 49, 88, 96–98, 160, 274, 352–364, 404, 473

N

Nurses, vii, viii, 27, 31, 54, 62, 68, 70, 155, 180, 223, 225, 226, 229, 231, 244–246, 352, 385, 386, 416, 419, 420, 422–431, 437–442, 444, 445, 448, 450, 453, 463

O

Old persons, 378, 389

P

Pain diseases, 92–94, 96, 119, 127, 135–144, 164, 189
Palliative care, 4, 9, 30, 33, 51, 67, 68, 73, 83, 88, 97, 104, 155, 180, 194, 209, 215, 239–246, 320, 386, 413, 414, 421, 422, 427, 448–450, 452, 457–461, 463, 468–470, 476
Parents, 41, 185, 268, 284–286, 298, 299, 351–364, 400, 402, 412
Parish nurse, 386, 438, 439, 441, 442
Participation, 30, 137, 142, 195, 223, 283, 288–290, 315, 352, 377, 391, 454
Patients, vii–ix, 4, 9, 27, 47, 59–74, 80, 87–100, 113, 135–144, 147–156, 159–168, 173–180, 184, 194, 208, 239–246, 251–260, 265, 301, 313–321, 352, 371, 397–404, 409, 422, 440, 457, 473
Phases of treatment, 179
Praying, viii, 15, 70, 84, 88, 95, 99, 105, 108, 126, 136, 137, 139, 141, 154, 162, 167, 184, 185, 188, 189, 283, 285–288, 305–308, 319, 336, 355, 356, 361, 373, 374, 378, 381, 382, 400, 402, 403, 410
Psychotherapy, 221–235, 242, 267, 270, 272, 275, 314, 320, 371

Q

Quality of life, 10, 20, 21, 29, 30, 59, 87–100, 108, 124, 142, 160, 163, 174, 176–177, 184, 194, 201, 202, 213, 215, 216, 266, 267, 270, 271, 273–275, 282, 288, 289, 291, 307, 326, 352, 357, 362, 364, 372, 373, 381, 414, 421, 427, 448, 453, 457–461

Questionnaires, 3, 47–55, 59–74, 80, 123, 125, 126, 164, 195, 202, 210, 211, 225, 234, 244, 253, 254, 268, 270, 271, 284, 286, 315, 329, 330, 359, 386, 410, 413, 442, 444

R

Relatives, 4, 9, 32, 68, 88, 153, 161, 190, 267–269, 397–404, 463, 469, 473
Religion, vii, ix, 2, 13–17, 19–21, 28, 30, 39, 70, 112, 120, 126, 148, 149, 153, 155, 156, 162, 166–168, 184, 188, 196, 197, 201, 202, 209–211, 214, 226, 232, 253, 257–259, 274, 282, 283, 305, 323, 325–330, 337, 338, 352, 370, 372, 373, 402, 414, 416, 420, 421, 440, 474
Religious freedom, 18
Resources, 1, 22, 30, 32, 33, 35, 37, 42, 43, 52, 59, 79, 80, 88, 95–97, 137, 141–143, 160, 167, 184, 194, 196, 216, 222, 228, 233, 234, 239, 243, 254, 259, 267, 268, 270, 272, 274, 275, 282, 290, 291, 298, 299, 301–303, 307, 314, 324, 325, 327, 328, 337, 353–355, 357, 362, 370, 372, 379, 381, 383, 385, 388, 399, 409–417, 419, 420, 430, 431, 452, 467, 474–476
Responsibility, 21, 49, 51–53, 55, 83, 225, 226, 240, 242, 289, 421, 428, 438, 447, 474
Responsiveness, 17, 54, 55, 289
Retirement home, 88, 90, 93, 96, 98, 371, 373, 374, 379, 381

S

Satisfaction with life, 149, 272, 326, 359
Self-efficacy expectation, 174, 186–188, 300, 304–307
Sensory interventions, 213
Sick children, 353, 359, 361, 473
Social care, 9–22, 47, 48, 51, 52
Specialist spiritual care, 410, 413, 414, 416
Special needs, 3, 283, 289–291, 357, 363, 473
Spiritual care, 3, 20, 21, 27–43, 47, 53, 54, 59–62, 67–70, 73, 74, 79–85, 100, 104, 124, 143, 148, 155, 156, 160, 189, 190, 240, 242–246, 257, 260, 300, 320, 379, 385, 388–390, 409–416, 420–423, 427–430, 437–442, 444, 445, 447, 448, 450–454, 457–463, 467–471, 474, 475
Spirituality, 1, 2, 4, 12, 16, 19, 20, 22, 28–33, 36–39, 41, 42, 47, 59–62, 60n1, 67–70, 72, 73, 95–96, 103, 104, 112, 113, 117, 120, 121, 124, 125, 137, 148, 156, 159–162, 164, 167, 168, 184, 185, 190, 194, 196, 201, 202, 208–210, 213, 215–217, 221, 225, 228–232, 239, 240, 253, 257–259, 267–270, 274, 275, 282–286, 290, 291, 299, 300, 325–329, 335–338, 351, 352, 357, 362, 370, 372, 373, 377–379, 385, 387–389, 399, 411, 412, 414–417, 420–424, 426–429, 441, 448, 450–451, 453, 458–462, 469, 469n1, 470
Spiritual wellbeing, 33, 63–68, 72, 73, 96–97, 100, 137, 215, 216, 241, 355, 359, 361, 362, 391, 427, 428, 453, 460, 474

Stress, 27, 38, 88, 98, 126, 167, 258, 298, 299, 318, 324, 327, 328, 330, 353, 355–358, 415
Support plan, 83, 84, 385, 475–476
Support satisfaction, 242

T

Tumor patients, 138, 179, 239–246

V

Validation, 66, 88, 113, 117, 118, 120, 121, 123, 127, 128, 166, 330
Validity, 66, 125, 234
Volunteering, 468–471
Volunteers, vii, 4, 440, 467–471, 474, 475

W

Wellbeing, 2, 18, 21, 29, 32, 48, 50, 96, 97, 100, 108, 147, 148, 155, 190, 213, 216, 241, 242, 268, 269, 282, 285, 290, 308, 324–328, 336–338, 357, 370–372, 380–382, 388, 390, 410, 424, 427, 431, 447, 474

The manufacturer's authorised representative in the EU is Springer Nature Customer Service Centre GmbH, Europaplatz 3, 69115 Heidelberg, Germany. If you have any concerns regarding our products, please contact ProductSafety@springernature.com

Printed and bound by CPI Group (UK) Ltd, Croydon, CR0 4YY
30/09/2026
02225700-0020